One Hundred
ORTHOPEDIC CONDITIONS
Every Doctor
Should Understand

One Hundred
ORTHOPEDIC CONDITIONS
Every Doctor
Should Understand

SECOND EDITION

EDITED BY

Roy A. Meals, MD

Clinical Professor of Orthopedic Surgery,
David Geffen School of Medicine,
University of California at Los Angeles,
Los Angeles, California

Scott A. Mitchell, MD

Resident in Orthopedic Surgery,
David Geffen School of Medicine,
University of California at Los Angeles,
Los Angeles, California

Quality Medical Publishing, Inc.

SAINT LOUIS, MISSOURI
2006

PUBLISHER   Karen Berger
PROJECT MANAGER   Donna Rothenberg
EDITORS   Keith Roberts, Michelle Berger
PRODUCTION   Carolyn Garrison Reich
BOOK DESIGN   Susan Trail
COVER DESIGN   David Berger
ILLUSTRATOR   William M. Winn

Quality Medical Publishing, Inc.
2248 Welsch Industrial Court
St. Louis, Missouri 63146
Telephone: 800-348-7808, 314-878-7808
Website: *http://www.qmp.com*

LIBRARY OF CONGRESS CATALOGING-IN-PUBLICATION DATA

One hundred orthopedic conditions every doctor should understand /
    edited by Roy A. Meals, Scott A. Mitchell. — 2nd ed.
        p.   ;   cm.
    Includes bibliographical references and index.
    ISBN 1-57626-235-9 (pbk.)
    1. Orthopedics—Miscellanea. I. Meals, Roy A. II. Mitchell, Scott A.
1975-   .
    [DNLM: 1. Musculoskeletal System—injuries. 2. Musculoskeletal
Diseases. 3. Orthopedic Procedures.   WE 140 O58 2006]
RD732.M39 2006
616.7—dc22

2006001231

QM/VG/VG
5   4   3   2   1

Contributors

Keith J. Cannon, MD
Graduate, David Geffen School of Medicine, University of California at Los Angeles, Los Angeles, California

†Robert Eric Carlson, MD
Graduate, David Geffen School of Medicine, University of California at Los Angeles, Los Angeles, California

Raymond J. Chang, MD
Graduate, Cedars-Sinai Medical Center, Los Angeles, California

Karl Christoffersen, MD
Graduate, St. Louis University School of Medicine, St. Louis, Missouri; currently Orthopedic Surgeon, Santa Cruz, California

Eugene DellaMaggiore, MD
Graduate, David Geffen School of Medicine, University of California at Los Angeles, Los Angeles, California; currently Orthopedic Surgeon, San Jose, California

Thomas L. Gautsch, MD
Graduate, David Geffen School of Medicine, University of California at Los Angeles, Los Angeles, California; currently Orthopedic Surgeon, Southern Sports Medicine Institute, Gallatin, Tennessee

Robert Gutierrez, MD
Graduate, David Geffen School of Medicine, University of California at Los Angeles, Los Angeles, California; currently Orthopedic Surgeon, Hand and Upper Extremity Surgery, Las Vegas, Nevada

†Deceased.

David J. Hak, MD
Orthopedic Residency, David Geffen School of Medicine, University of California at Los Angeles, Los Angeles, California; currently Associate Professor Orthopedic Surgery—Trauma, University of California Davis, Sacramento, California

Michiyuki Kono, MD
Graduate, David Geffen School of Medicine, University of California at Los Angeles, Los Angeles, California; currently Orthopedic Surgeon, Kaiser-Permanente, Orange County, California

Viet K.P. Le, MD
Former Resident, Harbor UCLA Medical Center, Los Angeles, California

James E. Li, MD
Graduate, David Geffen School of Medicine, University of California at Los Angeles, Los Angeles, California

Gregory J. Loren, MD
Graduate, David Geffen School of Medicine, University of California at Los Angeles, Los Angeles, California; currently Clinical Instructor, Department of Orthopedic Surgery, University of California at San Diego, San Diego, California

James H. Lubowitz, MD
Orthopedic Residency, David Geffen School of Medicine, University of California at Los Angeles, Los Angeles, California; currently Assistant Clinical Professor, Department of Orthopedic Surgery and Rehabilitation, University of New Mexico School of Medicine, Albuquerque; Director, Taos Orthopedic Institute, Taos, New Mexico

Roy A. Meals, MD
Clinical Professor of Orthopedic Surgery,
David Geffen School of Medicine, University
of California at Los Angeles, Los Angeles,
California

Russell Meldrum, MD
Graduate, University of Utah School of
Medicine, Salt Lake City, Utah; currently
Assistant Professor of Orthopedic Surgery,
Indiana University School of Medicine,
Indianapolis, Indiana

Kevin Mikaelian, MD
Graduate, David Geffen School of Medicine,
University of California at Los Angeles,
Los Angeles, California; currently Orthopedic
Surgeon, Stockton, California

Scott A. Mitchell, MD
Resident in Orthopedic Surgery, David Geffen
School of Medicine, University of California
at Los Angeles, Los Angeles, California

Edward H. Parks, MD
Orthopedic Residency, David Geffen School
of Medicine, University of California at Los
Angeles, Los Angeles, California; currently
Orthopedic Surgeon, Western Orthopedics,
Denver, Colorado

Ronald K. Robinson, MD
Graduate, David Geffen School of Medicine,
University of California at Los Angeles,
Los Angeles, California; currently Orthopedic
Surgeon, Stockton, California

Nicholas E. Rose, MD
Graduate, David Geffen School of Medicine,
University of California at Los Angeles,
Los Angeles, California; currently Orthopedic
Surgeon, California Orthopedic Specialists,
Newport Beach, California

Kevin G. Shea, MD
Graduate, David Geffen School of Medicine,
University of California at Los Angeles,
Los Angeles, California; currently Associate
Clinical Professor, Department of Ortho-
pedics, University of Utah School of
Medicine, Salt Lake City, Utah

Lawrence Shin, MD
Orthopedic Residency, David Geffen School
of Medicine, University of California at Los
Angeles, Los Angeles, California; currently
Orthopedic Surgeon, Baltimore, Maryland

J. Scott Smith, MD
Graduate, David Geffen School of Medicine,
University of California at Los Angeles,
Los Angeles, California; currently Orthopedic
Surgeon, Southwest Orthopedics, Midland,
Texas

Michael C. Stephen, MD
Graduate, David Geffen School of Medicine,
University of California at Los Angeles,
Los Angeles, California

Yong Sung, MD
Graduate, University of Western Ontario,
Ontario, Canada

Gary L. Zohman, MD
Graduate, David Geffen School of Medicine,
University of California at Los Angeles,
Los Angeles, California; currently Director of
Orthopedic Trauma, Department of Surgery,
Kern Medical Center, Bakersfield, California

Ira Zunin, MD
Graduate, David Geffen School of Medicine,
University of California at Los Angeles,
Los Angeles, California; currently Director,
Manakai O. Malama, Integrative Health Care
Group and Rehabilitation Center, Honolulu,
Hawaii

To

the effective teachers in our lives—

on your methods rode
indelible messages

Preface

The first edition of _One Hundred Orthopedic Conditions Every Doctor Should Understand_ was enthusiastically received by medical students, residents, and even practitioners. Various readers praised the case-study format and the lighthearted tone for catalyzing retention of practical information regarding our bones and joints. A reviewer for JAMA even described the book as a combination of Dr. Seuss and O. Henry on musculoskeletal conditions. Mission accomplished.

In the ensuing 14 years, however, much has changed. We are beginning to understand the molecular foundations of bone formation and repair. Growth factors and tissue engineering strategies have moved from the laboratory into clinical use. Osteoporosis is a four-letter word and is aggressively treated. Diagnostic imaging continues to expand its role in patient care, and MRI in particular has become ubiquitous. Surgical instrumentation seems to improve constantly, and minimally invasive approaches ranging from arthroscopy to even total joint replacement continue to refine our techniques.

What has not changed is the way people learn. Perhaps a dry dissertation of facts can be memorized, but the information is unlikely to be retained. Doctors learn best when presented with real-life situations or at least simulations, so in this new edition the case-study formats remain. Facts, theories, and novel treatment principles have been updated where appropriate. Controversies that have developed in the field are mentioned, although their exploration is left to the curious through the advanced reading references. We have also enhanced the number and quality of images both to reflect their clinical prevalence and importance and to reinforce findings introduced by each case.

We are pleased that nearly all of the original authors agreed to participate in shaping the second edition. Their diligence and creativity was and is paramount to the book's success. We also congratulate all of the professionals at Quality Medical Publishing for doing exactly what the company's name describes. From the efforts of all involved, we hope that you will share our enthusiasm and awe for the ever-expanding realm of orthopedics.

Roy A. Meals, MD
Scott A. Mitchell, MD

CHAPTER TOPICS BY CATEGORY

If you choose to focus your reading on a specific disease type, a specific anatomic region, or both, use this table to locate pertinent chapters.

SITE

ETIOLOGY	General	Spine	Shoulder & Arm	Elbow & Forearm	Wrist & Hand	Hip & Thigh	Knee & Leg	Ankle & Foot
Congenital/ Developmental	5, 14, 55, 58	21, 48			29, 44, 56	3, 52, 53	3, 34	3, 17, 39, 50
Trauma	28, 32, 33, 35, 59, 60	20, 31, 48	7, 26	11, 24, 41, 46	2, 13, 19, 29, 38, 43, 49	16, 27, 34	8, 15, 18, 34, 53, 54, 62	22, 25, 30, 45, 47, 53
Infections	9, 12, 28, 60, 62				2, 19	9	62	
Metabolic/ Autoimmune	4, 12	37			12, 29	1		
Tumors	4, 5		61		6, 36, 40	36, 51, 61	36, 51	
Degenerative		10, 31	42		19	1, 53	23, 54	50, 57
Vascular	23, 33	10		11	49	1, 52	23, 60, 62	

Contents

1

Quentin B. Tull, Crime Fighter

March 3

Dear Inspector,

Here's my full report on our recent "houseguest." As you saw yesterday, we live in a secluded area, which probably contributed to his choice of temporary residence. I say "his" because my new *Field and Stream* and *Maxim* magazines were all tattered, while my wife's *Glamour* and *Cosmo* weren't touched. There was a Red Cross brochure for autologous blood transfusion among the magazines and junk mail, and he had underlined different portions with pen and pencil. Judging by the music he chose from our extensive collection of compact discs, he is at least 60 years old or else a very nerdy teenager.

By the dates on the newspapers, he lived here nearly a week, and although he made himself at home on the main level, nothing was disturbed in the bedrooms upstairs or in the basement. The scoundrel obviously slept on the couch in the living room, and by the arrangement of the pillows, he preferred several behind his knees. Despite his concern for comfort while sleeping, he did all his sitting on a bar stool and even lifted down the TV from the high cabinet so he could see it better from the bar area. From that vantage point, he used the old manual can opener to open nearly every can of food we had and ate the contents directly. My extensive supply of booze, however, went untouched.

Then there was the curious rearrangement of the bathroom. He backed up a dining room chair on each side of the commode to make a narrow stall, like he needed to use his arms to get up from a low sitting position. He also opened a new bottle of aspirin and, calculating from the number remaining, he took at least nine tablets daily. He muddied four pairs of my shoes going back and forth to the garage—all but one pair were the slip-on type. He took the shoestrings out of the only tie-up pair. His footprints showed an intriguing gait pattern, which I have sketched.

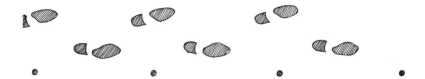

Judging by the odometer and the gas gauge, the culprit made one 60-mile round trip in my Jeep, presumably before he found the keys to the other cars. I say that because when he left for good, he took my beloved '66 Caddy instead of the Jeep or my son's Corvette.

All this may seem like so much gibberish to you, Inspector, but to a Baker Street Irregular like myself, the evidence is irrefutably conclusive. The man has, or I should say had, osteoarthritis of his left hip. The pain led him to the aspirin. The painful, limited motion precluded use of the stairs and made it awkward to sit down or rise from a low position; hence the bar stool and the chairs in the bathroom. For these same reasons, he chose the biggest car with the easiest entry. Attaining enough hip flexion to tie shoes was also difficult, and a hip contracted in a partially flexed position makes sleeping in a knee-flexed posture a necessity; thus the intriguing arrangement of pillows on the couch.

Of course, any novice could get this far with the evidence, and I'm sure your team would have done so eventually, but time is of the essence. Briefly, his left side is arthritic because the footprints show a typical external rotation deformity on that side and use of a cane on the right. Anybody with a bad hip learns that using a cane on the *opposite* side relieves weight-bearing forces without the need to shift the center of gravity from side to side with each step. Interestingly, during normal gait, the forces directed across the hip joint are significantly greater than just one's body weight, as might be expected. This happens because as weight is applied to a single limb and the contralateral limb is unweighted, the hip abductors on the weighted side must fire to prevent the pelvis from falling toward the unweighted limb. Because the abductors are positioned obliquely relative to the hip joint, some of this force is used to stabilize the pelvis, whereas a large proportion is transmitted to the articular surfaces, increasing contact forces across the joint. In someone with an arthritic hip, this causes a worsening of the pain. Thus by using a cane on the contralateral side, the patient is able to balance the pelvis when weighting the affected hip, relieving some of the work of the hip abductors. This results in a decrease in contact forces across the joint and thus reduces pain.

PRINCIPLE:	One of the most sensitive indicators of intraarticular hip pathology is pain with internal rotation. Thus patients typically assume a position of external rotation with ambulation.

Although osteoarthritis is the most common cause of arthritis in the hip, there are a number of other possible causes that often must be differentiated. If this person had rheumatoid arthritis, I doubt he or she would have been strong enough to lift down the large TV set, to open the childproof aspirin bottle, or to repeatedly use the manual can opener. Rheumatoid arthritis seldom affects the hip joint in isolation, and often patients are also disabled because of multiple painful joints, most commonly those in the hands and wrist. The other common explanation for hip arthritis is avascular necrosis of the femoral head with collapse and secondary destructive changes. Alcoholism is probably the most common cause of avascular necrosis, and although the subject certainly made himself at home, he didn't touch the hooch.

At some point he must have decided on surgical correction. With the uncertainty about blood transfusions these days, he made a preliminary trip to the hospital to donate some of his own blood so he could get it back at the time of surgery. We have several hospitals in the area, but the closest one equipped for total hip replacement is 28 miles away. I say he had a total hip replacement because artificial joints work so well for the hip these days that there is little call for arthrodesis or realignment osteotomy of this commonly arthritic joint.

PRINCIPLE:	For elective surgery in which a blood transfusion may be required, return of autologous banked blood is the safest.

A check of my calendar indicated that 3 weeks ago nearly all of the orthopedists were out of town attending a meeting of their academy, which coincided with his stay in my home. On the assumption that he checked into the hospital for his hip replacement when he left here, I realized that he might still be there, especially if he encountered one of the more common complications: early infection (related to the massive amount of foreign material implanted), thromboembolism (related to venous sludging in the lower limbs), or nerve palsy (related to intraoperative stretching). That's why your boys found me in the hospital's x-ray file room looking over films of older men with osteoarthritis who had recently undergone left total hip replacement. All this was too much to explain at the time, so I diverted their attention (by pulling down the shelf on them) and escaped to the visitor parking lot to look for my Caddy. I didn't find it there, but at home I discovered that our friend had returned just long enough to exchange the Cadillac for the Corvette, pick up my skis, and drop off a case of canned food and a new bottle of aspirin. From the muddy footprints he left on my carpet, it looks like he's discarded the cane and regained a normal gait pattern. Perhaps he has had one of the new minimally invasive techniques of total hip replacement to account for this rapid return to activity. I'm off to search the local ski areas. Please post men at the airport in case he prefers Utah or Colorado.

Yours in crime fighting,

Quentin

Quentin B. Tull

✦   ✦   ✦

March 8

Dear Inspector,

To help your investigation while I'm staking out the ski resorts, I have enclosed x-rays showing common forms of hip arthritis. I'm certain our adversary has either primary or secondary osteoarthritis.

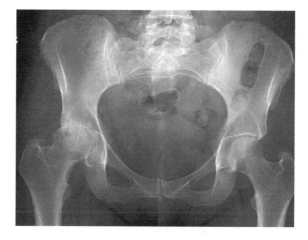

Primary osteoarthritis of the right hip. Subchondral sclerosis of bone, osteophyte formation, loss of cartilage space, and cyst formation, seen here in the femoral head, are characteristic.

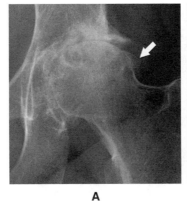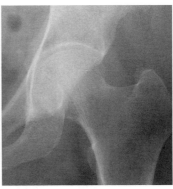

A

B

A, Note the loss of joint space and large subchondral cysts in the femoral head. Arrow is pointing toward an osteophyte.
B, Normal-appearing hip for comparison.

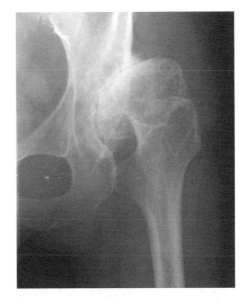

Right hip osteoarthritis secondary to developmental hip dysplasia. The acetabulum is dysplastic (shallow, incompletely formed) and does not completely cover the weight-bearing portion of the femoral head. Degenerative changes characteristic of osteoarthritis have developed secondary to the increased stresses across the narrowed contact area between the acetabulum and the femoral head.

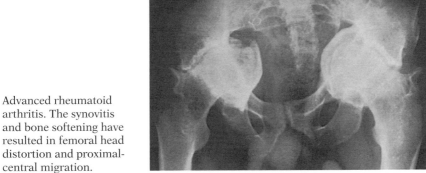

Advanced rheumatoid arthritis. The synovitis and bone softening have resulted in femoral head distortion and proximal-central migration.

Avascular necrosis. A large wedge of the right femoral head is sclerotic *(black arrow),* indicating loss of its blood supply. Cystic lesions *(white arrow)* are also characteristic of this stage of avascular necrosis. What do you notice about the left femoral head? Remember that avascular necrosis is bilateral in at least 50% of cases.

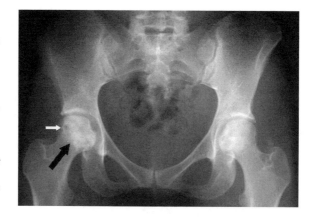

T1-weighted MRI showing bilateral avascular necrosis. Nearly the entire left femoral head is involved, but only a small portion of the right femoral head is affected *(arrows).*

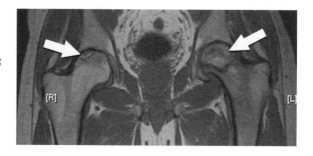

A, In avascular necrosis, loss of mechanical integrity of the femoral head results in collapse of the articular surface *(between the arrows).* If untreated, the deformed femoral head will cause secondary arthritic changes in the acetabulum. **B,** Late-stage avascular necrosis of the left hip demonstrating severe collapse of the femoral head, ultimately leading to joint space narrowing and degenerative changes in the acetabulum.

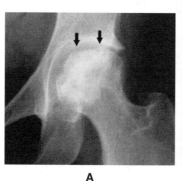 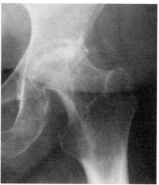

A   B

Yours in crime fighting,

Quentin B. Tull

✦ ✦ ✦

March 10

Dear Inspector,

It's been a year since my last report. I was unable to find our visitor at the ski slopes, although I looked for him every day through April. Since then, I have maintained a regular watch at the hospital because even though hip arthroplasty is quite successful in relieving pain and improving function, there are a number of complications that can occur. Loosening of the components, referred to as aseptic loosening, remains the most common late complication with total hip replacements, especially in younger, active people who put the hip to strenuous use. The risk of infection, while relatively low, is lifelong, particularly if the immune system is suppressed by diabetes or a large number of possible comorbid conditions. These patients are susceptible to infection caused by bacteremia from simple dental or genitourinary procedures, and as such, prophylactic antibiotics must often be considered.

Instability of the hip, either subluxation or frank dislocation, is also a risk. Although highest in the first few months after surgery, this risk is also lifelong. Patients must learn to adapt the positioning and movements of their hips to avoid instability. Finally, the presence of a strong metal prosthesis shields the normal bone around the acetabulum and proximal femur from the stresses it would otherwise encounter, causing localized loss of bone density (known as stress shielding). Another cause of bone loss is referred to as osteolysis, which is essentially an inflammatory reaction around the implant caused by wear debris. Both osteolysis and stress shielding weaken the surrounding bone, which can lead to fractures at the tip of the prosthesis as well as loss of bone stock, which would make revision surgery much more difficult. Ten-year follow-up studies of total hip replacements show rates of revision up to 10%.

I'm waiting for him; he owes me for gas, and I want my Corvette and my skis back. I'm tired of checking eBay to see when he's going to post them for sale. Since you still don't agree with my analysis of the clues, I recommend you do some additional reading, perhaps beginning with the works listed below.

Yours in crime fighting,

Quentin

Quentin B. Tull

ADVANCED READING

Beaule PE, Matta JM, Mast JW. Hip arthrodesis: Current indications and techniques. J Am Acad Orthop Surg 10:249-258, 2002.

Berry DJ. Venous thromboembolism after a total hip arthroplasty: Prevention and treatment. Instr Course Lect 52:275-280, 2003.

Bomalaski JS, Schumacher HR Jr. Arthritis and allied conditions. In Steinberg ME, ed. The Hip and Its Disorders. Philadelphia: WB Saunders, 1991.

Bozic KJ, Rubash HE. The painful total hip replacement. Clin Orthop Relat Res 420:18-25, 2004.

Buckwalter JA, Saltzman C, Brown T, et al. The impact of osteoarthritis: Implications for research. Clin Orthop Relat Res 427:S6-S15, 2004.

Hanssen AD, Spangehl MJ. Treatment of the infected hip replacement. Clin Orthop Relat Res 420:63-71, 2004.

Lieberman JR, Berry DJ, Mont MA, et al. Osteonecrosis of the hip: Management in the 21st century [review]. Instr Course Lect 52:337-355, 2003.

Padgett DE, Warashina H. The unstable total hip replacement. Clin Orthop Relat Res 420:72-79, 2004.

Schurman DJ, Smith RL. Osteoarthritis: Current treatment and future prospects for surgical, medical, and biologic intervention. Clin Orthop Relat Res 427:S183-S189, 2004.

2

The Roustabouts

One Monday morning, four young oil field workers drive into town to see you. Each complains of pain in the right-hand resulting from a brawl in a roadside tavern 2 nights previously. Although there seem to be some gaps in their recollections of the events, they are able to provide you with some of the highlights.

Mr. Brawley recalls striking his clenched fist against the wall when his adversary ducked. His speech is a bit difficult to understand because of a massively swollen upper lip. Examination of the hand shows swelling with tenderness centered at the metacarpophalangeal (MP) joint of the small finger. The range of motion of the interphalangeal joints is normal but hesitant secondary to pain, and MP joint motion is restricted. The skin is locally contused but intact. You examine his x-rays.

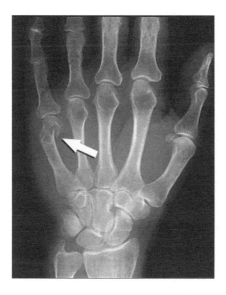

Palmarly angulated and impacted fracture of the fifth metacarpal neck.

Mr. Katz was bitten by the barkeeper's cat when he crawled over its tail while trying to escape the scene unnoticed. Examination shows multiple skin puncture wounds over the right thenar eminence with local acute inflammation. There is no evidence of abscess, but a faint red streak extends up the anterior surface of his forearm to his elbow. Epitrochlear and axillary nodes are not tender.

Mr. Ruff was bitten by his own dog who was apparently aiming for the cat. Examination shows several jagged, open, 1 cm skin lacerations palmarly and dorsally along the ulnar border of his right hand. They came close to, but did not disturb, a quite explicit tattoo. Mild tenderness and local bruising are present. Active range of motion is somewhat hesitant but full.

Mr. Mann states that he doesn't remember what happened to him, but in private he later grudgingly admits that he may have actually struck Mr. Brawley in the mouth. To his relief, you promise to keep this information confidential. Examination shows active finger flexion restricted by swelling on the dorsum of the hand. You note a 5 mm skin break over the metacarpal head of the middle finger. Any motion at the MP joint of the middle finger causes exquisite pain.

The x-rays on Katz, Ruff, and Mann are normal. A couple of phone calls verify that the pets are fully immunized against rabies. Being complete gentlemen, the four men insist that you treat the most seriously injured first. Which one is that? Katz, Ruff, and Mann have each taken several ampicillin tablets since the melee. Does that change your plan?

Mr. Brawley has a closed fracture, and that can wait. Katz, Ruff, and Mann have open injuries inoculated by cat, dog, and human saliva, respectively. Mr. Mann not only shows evidence suggestive of a joint infection, but he was also inoculated with human saliva, the vilest saliva of the bunch. The wound over the metacarpal head needs to be opened widely in the operating room and cultured, and the MP joint must be thoroughly irrigated and debrided of any small fragments of bone, cartilage, or tooth. Intravenous antibiotics should be continued until the local cellulitis has subsided and the wound is granulating cleanly. This common human "bite" injury initially may be discounted by patient and physician alike because of the deceivingly innocuous skin laceration and a lack of awareness of the impending disaster.

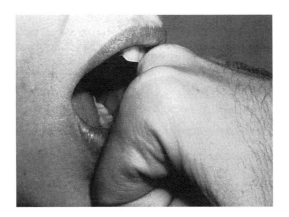

Mechanism of human bite injuries: Incisor tooth inoculates MP joint with mouth flora.

Human saliva is teaming with aerobic and anaerobic bacteria, and when these bacteria are introduced into a joint, their proliferation is poorly checked by white cell and macrophage migration. Their proteolytic enzymes wreak havoc on the cartilage. To delay treatment almost guarantees total destruction of the joint.

In general, cat and dog saliva is much cleaner. In the absence of evidence of joint penetration, significant joint inflammation, or abscess formation, these bites usually can be treated with local cleansing and oral antibiotics. Compared to dog bites, cat bites tend to puncture the skin without tearing it; therefore these wounds are often deceptively deep, but bleed less and place the patient at higher risk of infection. Overall, about 30% of animal bites to the hand become infected. But wait. Mr. Katz also has ascending lymphangitis, as evidenced by the red streak on his forearm. If left unchecked, this can lead to sepsis and its dire consequences. So while Mr. Mann is en route to the operating room, Mr. Katz needs to be admitted for limb elevation and immobilization, and for systemic antibiotics.

Of course, all three patients with the open injuries need to have their tetanus immunizations reviewed and updated if necessary. Infections stemming from cat, dog, and human bites are typically polymicrobial, but there are some particular organisms in each that should be considered when selecting empiric antibiotics. For both cat and dog bites, *Pasteurella multocida* is a gram-negative organism that can be resistant to both synthetic penicillins and first-generation cephalosporins. Most infections can be managed with either amoxicillin/clavulanate or a third-generation cephalosporin. Quinolone derivatives are also acceptable for adult patients. Guidelines for human bite infections remain somewhat controversial, but in most circumstances a similar antibiotic regimen is appropriate. Staphylococcus species are the most common offending agents and should be covered, but *Eikenella corrodens,* a nasty anaerobe in human saliva, has a relatively unusual resistance profile that must also be considered. It does not respond well to many semisynthetic penicillin derivatives, although it remains quite sensitive to penicillin, amoxicillin, and cephalosporins.

PRINCIPLE: All open joint injuries require operative debridement. Unchecked joint space infections have disastrous consequences.

Finally, it's time for Mr. Brawley. He has an angulated fracture of the fifth metacarpal neck with the apex directed dorsally, a result of the wall forcing his metacarpal head into his palm. This commonly occurring "boxer's fracture" may also affect the fourth metacarpal, particularly in patients who have had previous fractures through the fifth metacarpal neck. The resulting shortening exposes the fourth metacarpal to the greatest deforming force during a roundhouse blow with a clenched fist.

With local anesthesia, it is easy to reduce boxer's fractures by flexing the MP joint and pushing on the digit to correct the angular deformity. It is more difficult, however, to hold this reduction with plaster for the 3 to 4 weeks required for healing. Fortunately, angular malunions in the fourth and fifth metacarpal necks of 30 degrees or even more are not associated with functional or cosmetic deformities since the adjacent MP joint and the nearby carpometacarpal joint are quite supple. However, as with all long-bone fractures, rotational malalignment of the fragments will not be apparent on the x-rays and must be sought carefully on examination. The digits may appear normal in extension, except for a nail lying in a different plane from the others, but in flexion the rotated digit will cross over the adjacent one, creating a deficient grasping pattern.

PRINCIPLE: Examine for rotational malalignment in all long-bone fractures. Even with children in whom deformities in the flexion-extension and abduction/adduction planes may correct spontaneously with further growth, axial rotational deformities are permanent and therefore best prevented.

Whenever the MP joint is immobilized, it should be placed into flexion because in this position the collateral ligaments are stretched over the cam-shaped metacarpal head. Subsequent recovery of joint extension is easy. Conversely, if the joint is immobilized in extension and the lax collateral ligaments are allowed to contract, recovery of joint flexion will be difficult.

Follow-up Note: About a month later, all four men stop by in their work clothes to express their gratitude for your treatment. They insist on taking you and your parrot out for drinks.

ADVANCED READING

Arons M, Femando L, Polayes IM. Pasteurella multocida—The major cause of hand infections following domestic animal bites. J Hand Surg 7:47-52, 1982.

Brook I. Microbiology and management of human and animal bite wound infections. Prim Care 30:25-39, 2003.

Burkhalter WE. Hand fractures. Instr Course Lect 39:249-253, 1990.

Faciszewski T, Coleman DA. Human bite wounds. Hand Clin 5:561-569, 1989.

Hausman MR, Lisser SP. Hand infections. Orthop Clin North Am 23:171-185, 1992.

Hunter J, Cowan N. Fifth metacarpal fractures in a compensation clinic population. A report on one hundred thirty cases. J Bone Joint Surg Am 52:1159-1165, 1970.

Lee SG, Jupiter JB. Phalangeal and metacarpal fractures of the hand. Hand Clin 16:323-332, 2000.

Murray PM. Septic arthritis of the hand and wrist. Hand Clin 14:579-587, 1998.

3

Overheard in the Garage

"Where've you been?"

"I've started a course on front-end alignment at Community College, so I'll be out on Thursdays for a while. And whadda yuh mean, where've I been? You weren't here yesterday afternoon. Toss me that spark plug, will yuh?"

"I took my kids to the doctor; my husband couldn't get off."

"Oh dear, your kids are sick, Harriet?"

"I thought so, but Dr. Eldridge says not. Yesterday morning I got my two boys in shorts for the first time this year. I had a good look at their knees. They've got some alignment problems of their own."

"I know all about alignment. Bent tie rods? Worn ball joints? Improperly adjusted wheel bearings?"

"No, silly. The young one's got bowlegs, and the older one's got knock-knees. Dr. Eldridge called them 'genu varum' and 'genu valgum.'"

"What's that mean? Sounds insulting. It's not contagious, is it?"

"Latin, she said. Genu means knee, and varum means that from the front, the legs bend *in* from the knees—you know, bowlegs. Valgum means the opposite; the legs slant *out*—knock-knees."

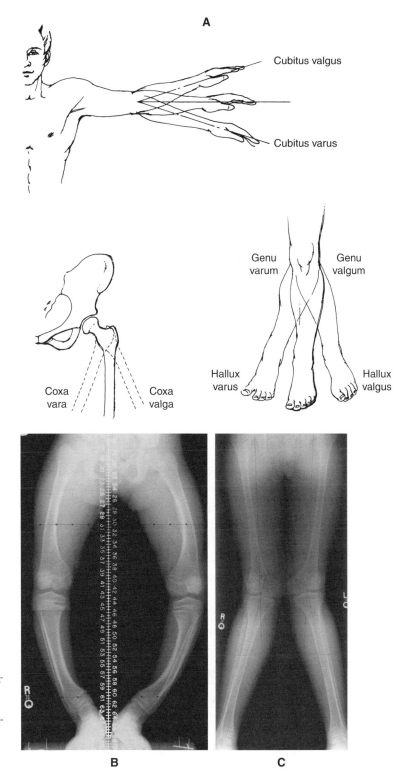

A, For joints in varus alignment, the limb segment distal to the joint deviates medially from the midaxial line. For joints in valgus alignment, the distal segment deviates laterally. **B,** Radiographs of a child with genu varum secondary to rickets. **C,** Lower extremity radiographs of an adult patient demonstrating bilateral genu valgum.

"Just like the camber on a wheel. You can tell a lot about front-end alignment just by looking at tire wear. I wonder if it works with kids? Have a look at their shoes."

"Well, if this class is making you so smart, why isn't Dr. Eldridge worried about my boys? And what did she say to calm me down?"

"I've only been to one class, but I know that on cars some variation is allowed; it's called tolerance."

"Same's pretty much true for kids, too. Dr. Eldridge told me that when kids first begin to walk, they're all a little bit bowlegged and some get more so, but this corrects naturally by about the age of 3, so Ricky should straighten out in about a year."

"What about David?"

"A little genu valgum is normal in adults. Sometimes when kids grow out of their bowlegs, they swing a little too much the other way and get accentuated knock-knees. But they usually correct themselves too after a year or two of growth."

NOTE: *Normal lower extremity alignment progresses from 10 to 15 degrees of varus at birth to a maximal valgus of 10 to 15 degrees at 3 years of age. This progressively decreases to adult values (3 to 6 degrees of valgus) by 6 to 9 years. Patients with physiologic genu varum typically present at around 12 to 14 months of age as they begin to walk and their bowlegged stance is first noticed. Patients with physiologic valgus typically present at around 3 years of age.*

"What about that lecherous old goat with bowlegs and a cane who comes in here now and then? He must not have outgrown his."

"Well, the way I understand it, most bowlegs and knock-knees are just part of growing up, and the kids will simply outgrow them. But the doctor has gotta check for fracture malalignment, uneven growth, arthritis on one side of the knee, and bone-softening disorders."

"I learned that one of the more common causes of bowlegs, er sorry, genu varum, is named after a guy named Blount. Dr. Eldridge said that while in almost all cases normal bowing like Ricky has will resolve with age, kids who have Blount's disease may not, and might even need surgery."

"I guess nothing is simple in medicine, huh?"

"You got that right. Dr. Eldridge said that in some cases it can be a little tricky to tell the two apart, and that's why she will sometimes take x-rays and make measurements or see the kids back in a couple of months to make sure things aren't getting worse."

NOTE: *Blount's disease results from a disturbance in the growth of the medial aspect of the proximal tibial physis. Depression and even fragmentation of the physis are seen radiographically, and a prominent metaphyseal beak is typically present beneath the disturbed physis. Occasionally a bony bar will form across the physis linking the metaphysis to the epiphysis, resulting in severe progression of the deformity with growth.*

"You know, I just had a funny thought. What if cars could out-grow a bent tie rod? It'd put us right out of business."

"Then maybe we could get jobs helping Dr. Eldridge. She said I was the third parent yesterday with lower limb alignment problems in their kids—very common, she said. She spent a lot of time looking my boys over to make sure they didn't have some other disease and then spent more time explaining it all to me. She was quite reassuring."

"Did she take x-rays?"

"Said it wasn't necessary right now because everything checked out. She used some sort of plastic angle measurer to record the angle at their knees; then she stood them both up and measured the distance between Ricky's knees and the distance between David's ankles. She wants to see them back in 6 months."

"So what if they don't get better? I've seen some adults with pretty gnarly knees."

"I asked her about that. She said that before children finish growing, it's possible to slow the growth down on the convex side of the knee to let growth on the other side catch up and correct the deformity. Even later, after they've quit growing, either the bone just above the knee or just below the knee can be cut and re-aligned."

"Sounds good. I've got to make a run to the parts store. I'll see you Monday."

Tuesday

"Good morning, Harriet."

"Hey, must've been some weekend. The rest of us worked yesterday, you know."

"I know, I know. After what you said about Ricky and David, I went home and had a good look at the way Sheri walks. I couldn't believe it. Even while I'm becoming a front-end alignment expert, my own daughter is walking around pigeon-toed, and I hadn't even noticed it! So I took her to Dr. Eldridge yesterday and really gave her a surprise when I told her I thought my daughter had genu varum."

"What'd she say?"

"Not so. Her knees looked fine. 'Intoeing' is what she called it. Same as what we use in alignment class. And the neat thing is that

Dr. Eldridge went about diagnosing the cause systematically, just like I do with a wheel that's out of alignment. Started with Sheri's hips, looking for 'femoral anteversion.' You see, the neck of the femur can point more directly ahead than normal, so then the only comfortable way the kid can keep the hip joint in the socket without stretching the front capsule (which is painful) is to rotate the femur in, but then the knees and toes will point in, too. When Sheri is standing, I can see that her kneecaps seem to be kissing rather than facing straight ahead."

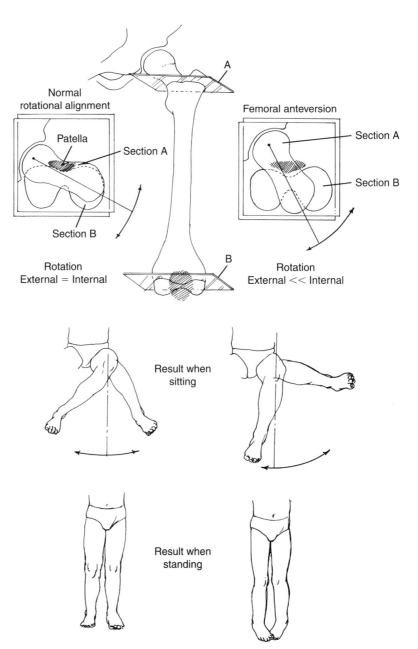

Femoral anteversion.

"You're *right*. I remember her checking my boys like that. Did she roll Sheri's hips around on the examining table?"

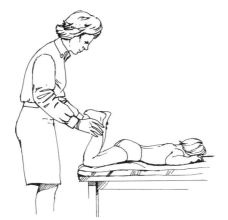

In this position, femoral anteversion, internal tibial torsion, and metatarsus adductus can be easily identified.

"Yep. Face down, knees flexed. Dr. Eldridge said that internal and external rotation motions of the hips should be roughly equal, but with femoral anteversion, internal rotation is increased and external rotation is diminished."

"What'd she do next?"

"Checked the alignment of Sheri's tibias. Just like there can be a rotational deformity of the femur in femoral anteversion, Dr. Eldridge explained that the natural internal rotation of the tibia that is seen in newborn babies can persist—'internal tibial torsion,' she called it. While Sheri was still face down and still had her knees flexed, Dr. Eldridge checked the alignment of her feet with her thighs. Normally, feet point out a bit. If the tibias are internally rotated, the kneecaps still point straight ahead since the femurs are fine, but the feet point in."

A, Internal tibial torsion. The knee points forward and the whole foot points in. **B,** With the knees flexed 90 degrees in the prone position, the axis of the foot normally is slightly externally rotated compared to the thigh (the so-called thigh-foot angle), shown on the left. With internal tibial torsion, shown on the right, the axis of the foot is internally rotated relative to the thigh.

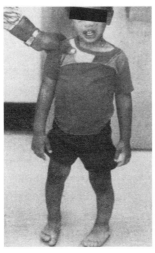

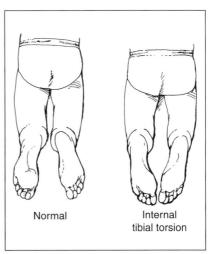

Normal   Internal tibial torsion

A   **B**

"Seems logical. Just like in a car. Start with the steering wheel and work your way right out to the tires. Was that all?"

"No, Dr. Eldridge also checked her feet. 'Metatarsus adductus,' she called it, or forefoot varus. I accused her of tossing around strange words, but she said at least she explained them, not like some mechanics she knows who use terms like 'rack and pinion' and 'McPherson strut' as if they're second-grade concepts."

"I guess we all have our jargon. We probably need to give simpler explanations to our customers, too. But what about Sheri's feet?"

"They're fine. In this metatarsus adductus, the hindfoot lines up normally with the leg, but the forefoot bends in."

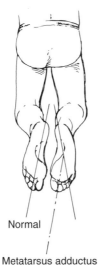

Metatarsus adductus, also known as forefoot varus. Compare the affected right foot with the normal-appearing left foot.

Modified from Alexander IJ. The Foot: Examination and Diagnosis. New York: Churchill Livingstone, 1990, p 153.

Normal

Metatarsus adductus

"Dr. Eldridge says she can see this easily when the child is face down with knees bent. Like with internal tibial torsion, metatarsus adductus usually is what Dr. Eldridge called a 'persistent adaptation to fetal positioning,' with hips and knees flexed up and feet turned in."

"So what's wrong with Sheri?"

"Femoral anteversion."

"What's to be done about it? It can't be very efficient or graceful to bang your knees together or hit your toes against your opposite ankle with every step."

"She prescribed patience, just like for your boys. I wonder if that's why they call us patients? Anyway, spontaneous derotation occurs until kids are at least 8 years old, so Sheri's got a couple of years to go. Dr. Eldridge also said that doctors used to think that persistent femoral anteversion was a cause of osteoarthritis. Not so, but if it continues and it is severe, it can *look* bad, and it's possible to fix it by 'cutting the femur transversely and derotating it,' according to Dr. Eldridge."

"What did she say about tibial torsion and metatarsus adductus?"

"Tibial torsion is normal in babies and gradually disappears with growth and weight bearing. Like femoral anteversion, if it's persistent and severe, corrective surgery can help. Metatarsus adductus is the most common foot deformity in children and is seen at birth. She mentioned that metatarsus adductus is one component of clubfoot, whatever that is. At any rate, a mild case of forefoot varus can be corrected by the parents just by stretching the baby's foot during the first few weeks of life; the more rigid, complex forms of metatarsus adductus are usually corrected by a series of casts over several weeks or months but sometimes require surgery."

"Pretty cushy job Dr. Eldridge has. All she says is, 'Your kids have bowlegs, knock-knees, femoral anteversion, and tibial torsion, Ma'am. We'll just watch 'em, and for your little ones with metatarsus adductus, just give those pudgy forefeet a push every time you change their diapers.'"

"Right. Just imagine somebody bringing their car in complaining that the car veers to the side or the front end shimmies. I'd like to tell 'em, 'Oh, don't you worry. Just be patient. With time, it'll probably go away.' They'd go bananas."

"I guess that's why Dr. Eldridge is good. She really explained things and put my mind to rest. Sometimes it's really hard just to wait and let nature fix it. Let's get some lunch."

"Thanks, but I'm going to study."

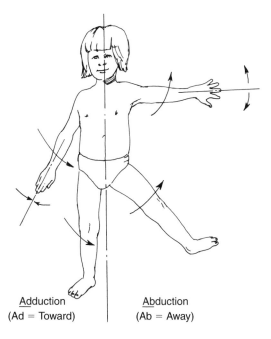

Joint motion in the frontal plane: Adduction and abduction.

Adduction
(Ad = Toward)

Abduction
(Ab = Away)

ADVANCED READING

Cozen L. Knock-knee deformity in children. Clin Orthop Relat Res 258:191-203, 1990.

Greene WB. Genu varum and valgum in children. Instr Course Lect 43:151-159, 1994.

Hoppenfeld S. Physical Examination of the Spine and Extremities. New York: Appleton-Century-Crofts, 1976.

Kling TF. Angular deformities of the lower limbs in children. Orthop Clin North Am 18:513-527, 1987.

Lincoln TL, Suen PW. Common rotational variations in children. J Am Acad Orthop Surg 11:312-320, 2003.

Martin PR. Auto Mechanics for the Complete Dummy. Long Beach, CA: Motormatics Publications, 1982.

Spero C. Orthopedic disorders. In Rajkumar S, Toback C, eds. Principles and Practice of Ambulatory Pediatrics. New York: Plenum Press, 1988.

Staheli LT. The lower limb. In Morrissy RF, ed. Lovell and Winter's Pediatric Orthopaedics, 5th ed. Philadelphia: JB Lippincott, 2000.

◆ *If a patient who is accurately described as having windswept knees is facing south and a "wind" is blowing from the east, which knee has the valgus deformity? Did Charlie Chaplin have femoral anteversion?*

4

Ruby and Rose

I don't know whether I have ever mentioned them before, but Ruby Malinewski and Rose Rose were the two elfin spinsters who lived next door while I was growing up. Eccentric to say the least but nonetheless charming, they tolerated the neighborhood children's pranks in good humor and even offered a few of their own. Ruby liked to smoke cigarettes she had rolled herself, and she also liked to read *National Geographic* to Rose in her heavy Baltic accent. When Ruby ventured outside, even on the hottest days, she kept every inch of skin covered with varying combinations of scarves and floppy hats in addition to her ever-present housecoat. Rose, on the other hand, enjoyed being outdoors. Her father had been a noted plant breeder, and Rose carried forth his love of horticulture. She was exceedingly generous with her garden bounty, and I remember several dinners staring down such offerings as tomato leaf and violet petal salad. Together Rose and Ruby shared a love of cats and cards, usually caring for at least six of the former, and seemingly forever sitting in the window at night playing gin rummy.

Because they had always seemed ancient to me, I instantly recognized Ruby in my waiting room, although I hadn't seen her in probably 10 years. When she stood up, she seemed shorter than I remembered, but then I had more than doubled my height since first meeting her. That day she reiterated her distrust of doctors and berated me for choosing such a career. She complained of pain in the middle of her back that had started with a coughing episode several weeks previously. Ruby said she was having difficulty lying flat in bed and felt better propped up on a large pillow. The same pillow boosted her up enough so that she could see the discard pile when she was playing gin rummy. She would let me do only a quite limited examination. A prominent thoracic kyphosis was present, and there was tenderness over the spinous processes at about T8. She denied having any radiating pain, numbness, or weakness.

I persuaded her to have x-rays taken of her spine. As I expected, the cortical bone and the medullary trabeculae were thinned. Multiple vertebral body compression fractures were present with the characteristic codfish-shaped vertebral bodies resulting from disc protrusion into the soft bone.

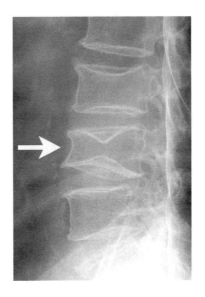

Marked osteoporosis of the thoracic and lumbar spine with collapse of multiple vertebral bodies. Note the characteristic "codfish" vertebra at L4.

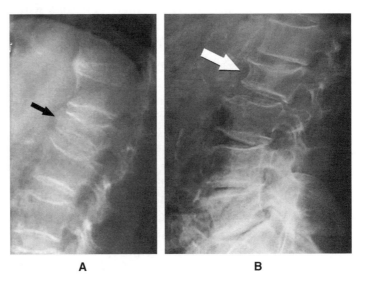

Thoracic **(A)** and upper lumbar **(B)** anterior compression fractures characteristic of osteoporotic vertebrae.

A   **B**

She hadn't breast-fed any of her babies or touched any alcohol, but she had most of the other risk factors predisposing women to osteoporosis: postmenopausal age, weight below normal, northern European ancestry, cigarette smoking, and limited sun exposure. She also reminded me of her lifelong aversion to milk, so her calcium intake was almost certainly deficient.

I told her about my working diagnosis of osteoporosis, an incompletely understood uncoupling of bone production and bone resorption. I didn't mention that her osteoblasts weren't producing the necessary bone matrix to keep up with her osteoclasts because of a loss of hormonal stimulus. This is typical of postmenopausal women. Rather, I explained that the bone she had was fine, but there just wasn't enough left to withstand much stress. She had been losing cortical bone by at least 3% per decade since age 30 and up to 10% per decade from menopause to age 60. (I didn't have the nerve to ask her age.) Her vertebrae were collapsing, which accounted for her complaints. I pointed out that this thinning of the bone also predisposed her to fractures of the proximal femur, distal radius, and proximal humerus, and by that I convinced her to at least start taking calcium and vitamin D supplements. I didn't expect the treatment to rebuild bone, but I hoped it would help slow further loss. Given her obstinacy, however, I knew that I should consider this a victory and decided to wait and discuss additional pharmacologic options during her next checkup.

Several days of bed rest is appropriate for new compression fractures. However, because further disuse would accentuate the bone loss to as much as 1% per week, I emphasized the importance of limiting this period of inactivity as much as possible. Bracing can be quite helpful in this setting to facilitate mobilization while stabilizing the fracture and helping to minimize pain. I also demonstrated the thoracic spine extension exercises designed to minimize the kyphotic deformity (Ruby called it her dowager's hump) due to the presence of multiple osteoporotic compression fractures. As Ruby was quite pleased to hear, nonsurgical management is typically the rule. However, in patients with chronic pain from poorly healing fractures or with progressive vertebral collapse and kyphotic deformity, percutaneous vertebral cementation techniques may be indicated.

After we had completed the exercises together and she seemed more relaxed, I brought up the need for laboratory tests. She wouldn't agree until I discussed in detail the other diagnostic possibilities, including osteomalacia, hyperparathyroidism, hyperthyroidism, bone marrow dyscrasias, and malignancies. These could be mostly excluded if her serum calcium, phosphorus, alkaline phosphatase, and urea nitrogen values were normal along with her creatinine clearance and urinary hydroxyproline excretion. The best assessment of bone density and predictor of fracture risk can be made using dual-energy x-ray absorptiometry (DEXA). But Ruby would have nothing to do with more x-rays.

PRINCIPLE: Plain radiographs are often of little use in evaluating osteoporosis because they appear relatively normal until at least 30% bone loss has occurred.

Why she called Mother 3 days later to get her laboratory results she never said. Maybe it was to verify that Milo Oldenbuchs (that's me) had, in fact, gone to medical school. The test results were normal, characteristic of osteoporosis, and essentially excluded most other diagnoses. Even so, I asked her to have a complete general medical evaluation to rule out underlying causes such as thyrotoxicosis, acromegaly, Cushing's syndrome, hematologic disorders, liver disease, and chronic steroid use. She refused.

As expected, her back pain subsided over several more weeks as the most recent vertebral compression fracture healed. She bought some mauve jogging shoes and began walking regularly to maintain her bone mass. She also agreed to begin taking an oral bisphosphonate after I explained to her how the medication inhibits the osteoclasts from resorbing bone. Bisphosphates have been shown to retard bone loss and prevent fractures in critical areas such as the proximal femur and vertebral bodies. Estrogen therapy continues to remain somewhat controversial, so I decided not to bring it up with Ruby. Although it does seem to prevent the dramatic increase in bone loss typically experienced in the early postmenopausal years, it does not seem to be as useful when initiated well past menopause. Additionally, it has been suggested that hormone replacement may increase a woman's risk of heart disease and breast cancer. Certain classes of selective estrogen receptor modulators, such as raloxifine, also appear to help maintain bone density but without some of the risks of estrogen replacement. Unfortunately, however, current medications are all limited in their ability to restore bone mass in patients with significant preexisting osteoporosis. Parathyroid hormone preparations have become available clinically that appear to stimulate bone production. Thus regular exercise and adequate dietary calcium intake begun early in life (a woman reaches her peak bone mass near age 25), along with early pharmacologic intervention in high-risk groups, continue to be the best means of prevention.

NOTE: *Current "antiresorptive" medications for osteoporosis inhibit bone turnover, suppressing bone resorption more than bone formation. Recently introduced recombinant parathyroid hormone (given as daily injections) acts as an anabolic agent to stimulate bone formation, improving bone density and architecture to reduce fracture risk.*

One day Ruby came by with a magazine article on osteoporosis and asked me to clarify the terms "osteopenia," "osteoporosis," and "osteomalacia." Fortunately, I had just read up on these. I explained that osteopenia is a generic term meaning sparse bone from any cause. Osteomalacia, bad bone, means that the collagen matrix of bone isn't mineralized normally. Although there are a multitude of possible causes, the common problem is a lack of available calcium and phosphate required to mineralize newly formed collagen matrix, also known as osteoid. Rickets in children is the classic example (although the same process is referred to as osteomalacia in adults). In osteoporosis, on the other hand, the available collagen bone matrix is mineralized normally; there is simply not enough of it. I explained that osteoporosis is a problem of quantity, rather than quality, of bone.

Almost as an afterthought Ruby told me she had been sharing her calcium and vitamin pills with Rose because she too had developed a hump. Ruby asked me for a pain prescription for Rose since her back pain had still not subsided after 2 months. I explained I couldn't do that without first seeing her, so Ruby agreed to have Rose make an appointment. After she left, I wondered whether Rose really had osteoporosis since pain from that type of compression fracture usually subsides relatively quickly. Also, Rose was as rotund as Ruby was thin, and obesity seems to protect against osteoporosis because of the increased peripheral conversion of androgens to estrogen. Only 2 days later, Rose was in the emergency room with a new pathologic fracture.

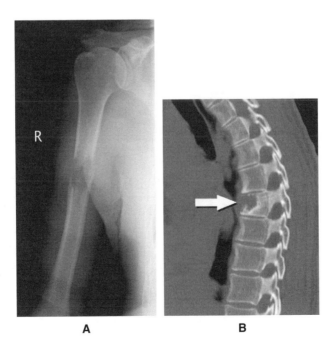

A, Pathologic fracture of the humerus. Note the lytic lesion in the humeral diaphysis through which the fracture line passes. **B,** CT scan of a vertebral body lytic lesion.

A **B**

I heard the wailing and saw the distress on the nurses' faces the instant I walked in. I wouldn't have recognized Rose if Ruby hadn't been with her, although it was Ruby who was bawling. Rose was no longer obese, just hunched over, frightened, and sick. The emergency room doctor shouted in my ear that she had snapped her humerus while opening a window that morning. He already had the x-rays; they showed a transverse fracture through a lytic area approximately 2 cm in diameter.

Nearly a box of Kleenex later, along with much hand-holding and reassurance, Rose said her back and right arm had been hurting for several months and thought it was the same "ah-stereo-poor-sis" that Ruby had. More tears. We obtained an admission chest x-ray in the emergency room. It showed an osteoporotic spine with several collapsed vertebral bodies and several punched-out lytic rib lesions. This wasn't something nice, and Rose, Ruby, and I were all filled with dread. They didn't want to talk about it. I applied a long-arm splint and ordered laboratory tests for the morning. Ruby crept home to feed their cats

In adults, the most common malignancy in bone is metastatic cancer. Breast, lung, thyroid, kidney, and prostate carcinomas account for the vast majority of bone metastasis. (Mnemonic: BLT with a kosher pickle.) But with multiple lytic lesions, multiple myeloma is also likely.

✧ *Which metastatic carcinomas produce blastic rather than lytic lesions?*

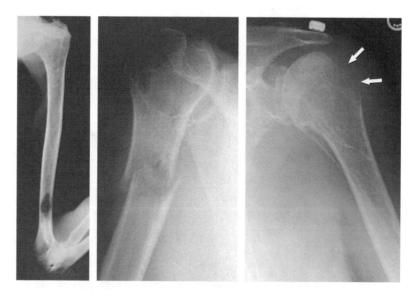

Examples of metastatic lytic lesions of the humerus.

As I suspected, the blood smear showed an abundance of plasma cells, and serum protein electrophoresis showed a prominent monoclonal spike. The light-chain metabolite of the immunoglobulin, the so-called Bence-Jones protein, was also detected by protein electrophoresis of a 24-hour urine concentrate. Radionucleotide bone scans are of minimal value in multiple myeloma because the tumor suppresses osteoblast activity, making the scans most often negative. Rose's complete skeletal x-ray survey showed an additional lesion in the neck of the right femur. The skull, which is frequently involved along with the ribs and spine, was unaffected. Bleeding can be a major problem in multiple myeloma because of thrombocytopenia and altered coagulation factors, but Rose's tests showed satisfactory hemostatic capacity. Rose and Ruby, now in better spirits after some sleep, easily understood the need to fix the humerus fracture, but they looked at me like I was selling snake oil when I added that her hip also needed to be fixed before it broke. An explanation of the relative ease of fixing it prophylactically versus the difficulties of fixing a shattered eggshell sufficed, along with a discussion of further osteoporosis related to disuse if prolonged bed rest was required. Rose, bless her soul, wanted to know whether methylmethacrylate bone cement, which is used to help stabilize the metallic hardware in the weakened bone, was harmful to the environment.

At surgery, I curetted the humeral and hip lesions, and our pathologist confirmed the diagnosis of multiple myeloma. I packed both cavities with methylmethacrylate. While the cement was still soft, I placed an intramedullary rod across the humerus fracture. For the femur, I also used a long intramedullary rod with two screws placed through the rod up into the femoral neck. This type of reconstruction protects the entire femur should further lesions develop along its length.

The next day the nurse pointed out that on the operated side Rose was numb over the dorsal radial aspect of her hand and couldn't extend her wrist or fingers. I practically sank through the floor. A radial nerve paralysis and I'd missed it! In the turmoil of the emergency room and of psychologically preparing Rose and Ruby for the surgery, as well as dealing with my own feelings about Rose's delayed diagnosis, I had overlooked a fundamental point. I hadn't initially checked and recorded her peripheral neurovascular status. A lawyer could hang me out to dry since I couldn't say whether the nerve injury occurred at the time of fracture or at surgery—possibly from the dissection, manipulation of bony fragments, the surgical hardware, or the exothermic reaction of the methacrylate cement. It is hard to be methodical and thorough, especially in stressful situations, but it is ever so important.

After the skin healed and Rose was up and around on a walker, all of her identified lesions were irradiated. She refused to even consider chemotherapy. For different reasons, the visiting nurse and I were relieved when Rose's radial nerve palsy resolved sufficiently so she could again hold her own gin rummy cards. Unfortunately, however, Rose's renal tubules slowly failed from the protein overload inflicted by the myeloma, and about a year after her humerus fracture occurred, she died.

I still see Ruby occasionally, looking lonely and walking not so briskly or elflike up and down Windsor Avenue. I think of her often and wonder whether her life could have been a little brighter if, long ago, she had developed good habits to preserve her bone mass.

ADVANCED READING

Aaron AD. Treatment of metastatic adenocarcinoma of the pelvis and extremities [review]. J Bone Joint Surg Am 79:917-932, 1997.

Kim DH, Silber JS, Albert TJ. Osteoporotic vertebral compression fractures. Instr Course Lect 52:541-550, 2003.

Lin JT, Lane JM. Osteoporosis: A review. Clin Orthop Relat Res 425:126-134, 2004.

Mirra J. Lymphoma and lymphoma-like disorders. In Mirra J, Picci P, Gold R, eds. Bone Tumors: Clinical, Radiologic, and Pathologic Correlations. Philadelphia: Lea & Febiger, 1989.

Mirra J. Metastases. In Mirra J, Picci P, Gold R, eds. Bone Tumors: Clinical, Radiologic, and Pathologic Correlations. Philadelphia: Lea & Febiger, 1989.

Rougraff BT, Kneisl JS, Simon MA. Skeletal metastases of unknown origin. A prospective study of a diagnostic strategy. J Bone Joint Surg Am 75:1276-1281, 1993.

Walker MP, Yaszemski MJ, Kim CW, et al. Metastatic disease of the spine: Evaluation and treatment. Clin Orthop Relat Res 415:S165-S175, 2003.

Zizic TM. Pharmacologic prevention of osteoporotic fractures. Am Fam Physician 70:1293-1300, 2004.

◆ *How do you position your forearm for taking change? Using a keyboard? Washing your face? Would you rather have your forearm stiff in full pronation, neutral rotation, or full supination? Why?*

5

Sans Souci

Robert Eric Carlson ✦ *Scott A. Mitchell* ✦ *Roy A. Meals*

Mrs. Stevens sounded quite anxious when she phoned to make a same-day appointment with her pediatrician. Later in the office she explained: "Oh, Dr. Eldridge, thank you so much for seeing us today. Wilfred, show the doctor your knee. Look at that bump on his thigh, Doctor."

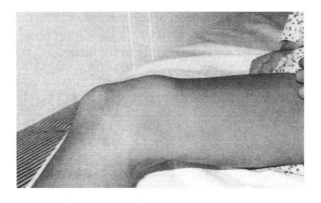

Bony mass on anterior distal thigh.

"He's only 11 years old. The weather is warming up, and he started wearing shorts today. That's when I noticed it. You know, I don't mean to worry, but several of our relatives have had cancer. Do you think its something bad?"

"Well, let's just see what we have here. Does it ever hurt, Wilfred?"

"No."

"How about when I push on it?"

"No."

"Did you ever notice it before today?"

"I guess."

"Has it been getting larger?"

"Nope."

"Do you have any other bumps?"

"I don't think so."

Wilfred had no complaints or symptoms, and his mother could not recall any relatives with bony growths similar to those in her son. Examination did not reveal any similar bumps elsewhere, and the remainder of Wilfred's neuromuscular examination, including strength, sensation, and circulation, was entirely normal.

"First, Mrs. Stevens, let me tell you that I don't think this is anything serious. You see, what we have here is a hard, painless mass, which is near a joint and appears to be growing from his bone—his femur, to be exact. My suspicion is that this bump is what we call an osteochondroma, also known as an exostosis. It's the most common bone tumor, but don't worry, in nearly all cases such as Wilfred's, it is entirely benign. These tumors are usually discovered between 10 and 20 years of age, as they tend to grow right along with the normal bones during this period. While they deserve attention, there is no need for alarm.

"But all you can see is this bump? How can you be certain it's not something rare and dangerous?"

"I hear you, and I do want to obtain an x-ray to confirm the diagnosis. An osteochondroma has a quite unique and easily identifiable appearance on x-ray that helps to exclude those rare dangerous things. But we also have the information that Wilfred so generously provided us—that there is no pain, tenderness, or evidence of rapid growth—all of which are encouraging. It would be quite unusual for a dangerous bone or soft tissue tumor to be entirely asymptomatic.

✧ *What "rare and dangerous" processes would you consider in the differential diagnosis of a symptomatic enlarging mass around the knee in an 11-year-old boy?*

"Nothing serious? You sure?"

"Let's get the x-ray, and then I'll explain it to you more fully."

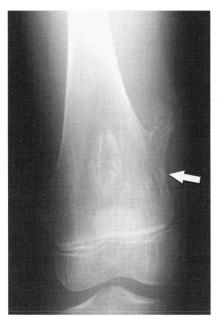

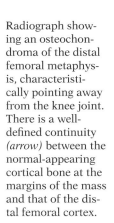

Radiograph showing an osteochondroma of the distal femoral metaphysis, characteristically pointing away from the knee joint. There is a well-defined continuity *(arrow)* between the normal-appearing cortical bone at the margins of the mass and that of the distal femoral cortex.

"What did you think of the x-ray machine, Wilfred?"

"OK, I guess."

"Here's the film. It's exactly as I suspected. This is the classic appearance of an osteochondroma. The continuity of the medullary canal from the normal bone into the base is characteristic. Sometimes CT scans are necessary to see it though."

"What exactly is an exostosis?"

"I'll draw you a picture. This area, near the end of the bone—the clear space on the x-ray—is the growth plate. The cartilage cells in this region are responsible for the longitudinal growth of children's bones. As these cells divide, they are pushed away from the growth plate. This newly formed cartilage is then gradually replaced by bone through a process called endochondral ossification. Sounds complicated but what it really means is that bone forms from cartilage. You with me so far?

PRINCIPLE: There are two primary mechanisms of bone formation: (1) Endochondral ossification is the formation of bone through a cartilaginous model. This method is responsible for the formation and growth of long bones and most of the axial skeleton. (2) Intramembranous ossification is the direct deposition of bone in condensations of mesenchymal tissue without a cartilage intermediate. This occurs in the flat bones such as the skull, mandible, and clavicle.

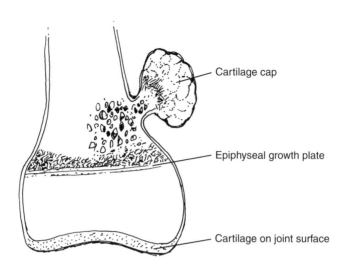

Cartilage cap

Epiphyseal growth plate

Cartilage on joint surface

Osteochondroma.

"I think, but I'm still worried."

"Occasionally a portion of the growth plate gets separated and begins to grow in the wrong direction, out to the side, away from the joint. Because the rest of the growth plate continues to grow normally and make the bone longer, the end of the bone grows away from the confused portion. Now that mixed-up portion still contains normal growth plate cartilage, admittedly pointing in the wrong direction, so as long as the child is growing, it continues to grow too. In the same way that the newly formed cartilage from the growth plate is replaced by bone, so too is the newly formed cartilage in this disoriented portion. So, as the exostosis grows, the stalk turns into bone while the cap remains cartilage. And since cartilage doesn't show up on an x-ray, the lump always feels bigger than it looks on the film. So the bottom line is this: Wilfred's bump is normal tissue growing in an abnormal direction."

"You said you didn't feel any others. How do you know where to look?"

"Osteochondromas can form on any bone that's derived from cartilage, and that's most of our bones; but they occur most commonly on the bones that grow the longest—in other words, femur, tibia, and humerus. Exostoses on the pelvis or scapula are hard to feel, but like osteochondromas elsewhere, they can draw attention to themselves if they impinge on an artery, nerve, tendon, or another bone."

PRINCIPLE: Epiphyseal growth plates with the most growth potential also have the greatest potential for developing pathologically.

"Is Wilfred going to get more of them? How about his brothers and sisters?"

"Most osteochondromas are solitary—just a fluke of nature. Boys and girls are equally affected. Occasionally, however, several members of the same family have large numbers of osteochondromas, sometimes even causing curved or otherwise misshapen bones. They are said to have hereditary multiple osteochondromas and this disorder is inherited in an autosomal dominant pattern. That means that if it did run in your family, I would expect you or your husband to have the tumors along with about half of your boys.

"Can these things turn into cancer?"

"Well, occasionally an osteochondroma can undergo malignant transformation, but this occurs most often in patients with the multiple, hereditary condition. Even then the risk is probably less than 10%. Rarely, in less than one in a hundred patients, a solitary one can turn bad, usually later in adult life.

"Oh dear. How can you know if it goes bad?"

"Well, we'd have a couple of clues. First of all, the cartilage cap of the osteochondroma, similar to the cartilage in the growth plates, ceases to grow after skeletal maturity. So if an exostosis in an adult begins to enlarge, then it probably deserves treatment, even if only to exclude malignancy. Malignant lesions are also likely to become painful, perhaps even before enlargement becomes apparent.

"Shouldn't Wilfred's tumor be removed?"

"No, not merely for the risk of malignant transformation— that's just too remote to justify the risks of surgery. Asymptomatic lesions such as Wilfred's typically require no treatment and are best just observed with routine clinical examination. If the lesion becomes painful or changes in size, then further investigation would be warranted. And just so I don't make you too nervous, I should tell you that even though pain can be a sign of malignancy, it is far more likely to be the result of simple mechanical irritation of the overlying soft tissues. The surrounding tendons, muscles, or nerves may become stretched or inflamed from rubbing over the exostosis. It is not uncommon for a bursa to form between the osteochondroma and these soft tissues, which also may become inflamed. Also, sometimes the stalk of the osteochondroma may fracture as a result of a relatively minor trauma. So if the exostosis causes impaired function or is unsightly, then I would consider removing it. But Wilfred's tumor just doesn't seem to be bothering him much now.

"Thanks, Dr. Eldridge. I feel better. Like I said, I get worried about lumps."

"People should at least be knowledgeable about their lumps and bumps, and watch carefully for any changes. For your peace of mind, I am going to refer you to a colleague of mine, Dr. Carlson. He's a fine orthopedic surgeon, and I respect his opinion highly. Also, he is easy to talk to, and he can describe the condition in more detail. He'll be willing to answer any other questions that you, your husband, or Wilfred may have. He will want to see Wilfred periodically and maybe take some other x-rays. Dr. Carlson could remove Wilfred's osteochondroma if it becomes symptomatic."

"Thank you so much, Dr. Eldridge. You don't know how much better I feel. Thanks for taking the time to explain this to me. I was so worried."

"It's been my pleasure. Bye, Wilfred."

"Bye."

A   B

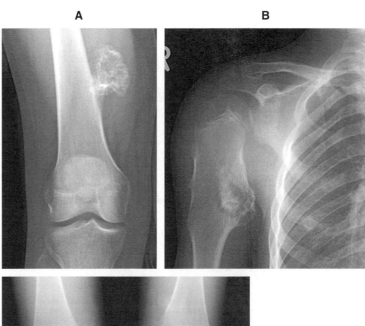

Examples of osteochondromas:
A, Pedunculated osteochondroma of the distal femur in a skeletally mature patient with a narrow stalk and a large ossified cap.
B, Osteochondroma with a large sessile base arising from the proximal humerus.
C, Multiple hereditary osteochondromatosis. Note multiple bilateral exostoses around the knee in this patient.

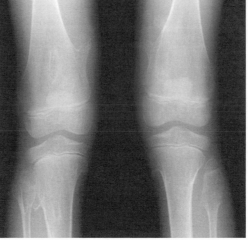

C

ADVANCED READING

Ballock RT, O'Keefe RJ. The biology of the growth plate. J Bone Joint Surg Am 85:715-726, 2003.

Biermann JS. Common benign lesions of bone in children and adolescents. J Pediatr Orthop 22:268-273, 2002.

Springfield DS. Bone and soft tissue tumors. In Morrissy RI, ed. Lowell and Winter's Pediatric Orthopaedics, 5th ed. Philadelphia: JB Lippincott, 2000.

Temple HT, Scully SP, Aboulafia AJ. Benign bone tumors. Instr Course Lect 51:429-439, 2002.

Zaleske DJ. Cartilage and bone development. Instr Course Lect 47:461-468, 1998.

◆ *Which bones fall outside the domain of orthopedics?*

6

Suddenly

Seth Rankin, a 25-year-old stockbroker and avid tennis player, noted the sudden appearance of a mass on the dorsum of his dominant right wrist. He claims that it appeared overnight. Now, 2 weeks later, it is somewhat smaller but still hurts when he does pushups and other forceful wrist extension activities. Other than a broken ankle in college, his general health has been excellent. His family history is positive for cancer.

Examination shows a firm, nontender spherical mass about 2 cm in diameter, on the dorsal radial aspect of his wrist.

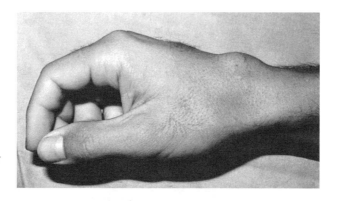

The common tumor shown here is not a neoplasm.

It is fixed to the deep tissues but not to the skin. Excursion of the adjacent extensor tendons is normal. Active and passive wrist extension/flexion is 70/70 degrees on the affected side as compared with 75/80 degrees on the left. If the room is darkened and a penlight is used, the mass transilluminates more than the surrounding tissues.

PRINCIPLE: Use a goniometer to measure joint angles and compare the results with the opposite side. Your eye will miss subtle abnormalities.

The patient is concerned about the possibility of the mass being cancer. Are you? What simple procedure could confirm your diagnosis?

Ganglion cysts are by far the most common tumors in the hand. Ganglion means knot, and this non-neural knot is actually a pseudocyst. Remember, a true cyst has an endothelial lining, whereas a pseudocyst does not. A ganglion arises from a joint capsule or tendon sheath and is filled with a clear, viscous fluid consisting of hyaluronic acid. The most common location is the dorsal radial aspect of the wrist; the next most common location is the anterior radial aspect of the wrist beneath the radial artery; and third is the flexor tendon sheath at the proximal digital flexion crease. The cause is uncertain, but most likely it is related to a small chronic tear and irritation of the underlying ligament or sheath, and in fact most ganglions are connected by a narrow stalk to this disrupted capsule or ligament. In the case of dorsal wrist ganglions, this most often involves the scapholunate interosseous ligament. At times the fluid can accumulate quickly, which accounts for the sudden appearance of ganglion cysts—they occur far more quickly than a solid neoplasm could enlarge. This feature, along with the ganglion's tendency to wax and wane in size and its capacity to transmit light, makes the diagnosis easy, particu1arly when the mass occurs in one of the three classic locations.

N O T E :   *Another classic location for ganglion cysts is over the dorsum of the distal interphalangeal joints, where it is referred to as a mucous cyst. At times the cyst can produce a longitudinal groove in the fingernail from chronic pressure on the germinal matrix of the nail bed. Mucous cysts are always associated with an underlying osteophyte (Heberden's node) that must also be removed to prevent recurrence.*

Aspiration of clear viscous fluid through a large-gauge needle confirms the diagnosis and may prove curative in about one-half of patients. Aspiration of an anterior wrist ganglion is risky because of the proximity of the radial artery. So for these ganglions and for those at other sites that have recurred after aspiration, surgical removal of the pseudocyst along with the underlying patch of responsible capsule or sheath is typically curative.

Follow-up Note: Aspiration confirmed the diagnosis of a ganglion cyst, but the mass reappeared within several months and interfered with Seth's tennis game. He underwent surgical excision of the ganglion and the offending portion of the underlying wrist joint capsule. While back at work with a postoperative bandage, he met Lucy Thompson, the woman of his dreams. Two weeks later, Seth gave her an engagement ring. She refused it, however, ostensibly because it wouldn't fit over a lump on her left ring finger. After much cajoling he convinced her to come to your office for aspiration of a presumed ganglion.

Lucy is uncertain about how long this painless mass has been present. Examination reveals a firm, somewhat spherical, but irregularly contoured, mass that is 1 cm in diameter on the anteroulnar border of the ring finger's proximal segment. It is slightly fixed to the flexor tendon sheath. The overlying skin moves easily. Digital motion is full, sensibility is intact, and a digital Allen test shows patency of both digital arteries. You darken the room. A penlight does not transilluminate the mass.

Is this a ganglion? Do you recommend aspiration?

This mass does not have the characteristics of a ganglion. It is not in a classic location, it has an irregularly contoured surface, and it does not transilluminate. Another reason not to attempt aspiration is the proximity of the digital neurovascular bundle.

Ganglion cysts are the most common tumors in the hand; but remember, tumor means swelling, and swelling is not synonymous with neoplasm. The most common true neoplasm in the hand is localized nodular tenosynovitis. If you use its alias, giant cell tumor of the tendon sheath, be careful that you do not confuse this condition with the entirely different giant cell tumor of bone. Localized nodular tenosynovitis is a benign growth of fibrous and fatty tissues with a generous sprinkling of multinucleated giant cells. Usually next to a tendon, the mass is firm, generally spherical, and multilobulated, giving the surface the feel, and sometimes even the transcutaneous appearance, of a tiny head of cauliflower. Other possible diagnoses include neurilemoma, lipoma, and epithelial inclusion cyst, but malignancy cannot be excluded without histologic examination. The patients are generally and justifiably concerned that the presence of a mass indicates cancer, and excisional biopsy is indicated.

N O T E :   *Nodular tenosynovitis is referred to as a giant cell tumor of the tendon sheath due to the abundance of giant cells on histologic examination. Just to confuse things, it bears a cursory resemblance to giant cell tumor of bone under the microscope (it too contains multinucleated giant cells). Despite this, the two tumors have nothing else in common. Giant cell tumor of bone is a locally aggressive, destructive lesion that is potentially limb-threatening.*

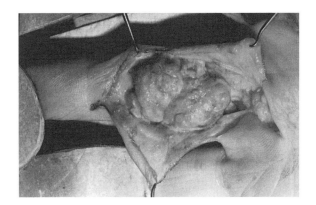

Multilobulated appearance of localized nodular tenosynovitis.

Follow-up Note: With the patient under local anesthesia, you excise the mass after you identify and protect the adjacent digital neurovascular bundle. On inspection, the mass has the typical appearance of localized nodular tenosynovitis, a lumpy-surfaced nodule with a mottled yellowish brown coloration—hence its other aliases, xanthofibroma and fibroxanthoma (*xantho-* means yellow). The pathologist confirms your clinical diagnosis and reminds you that although the mass is benign, localized nodular tenosynovitis can recur locally.

When you see Lucy in your office several weeks later, the surgically induced inflammation is subsiding nicely and she has recovered full digital motion. On inquiry about Seth, Lucy relates that they have had less to talk about since their surgeries and that Seth is moving to Singapore. She asks if you happen to know a medical student she has seen at her apartment complex with his left arm in a sling.

ADVANCED READING

Angelides A, Wallace P. The dorsal ganglion of the wrist: Its pathogenesis, gross and microscopic anatomy, and surgical treatment. J Hand Surg 1:228-235, 1976.

Glowacki KA, Weiss AP. Giant cell tumors of tendon sheath. Hand Clin 11:245-253, 1995.

Moore J, Weiland A, Curtis R. Localized nodular tenosynovitis: Experience with 115 cases. J Hand Surg Am 9:412-417, 1984.

Nahra ME, Bucchieri JS. Ganglion cysts and other tumor related conditions of the hand and wrist. Hand Clin 20:249-260, 2004.

Nelson CL, Sawmiller S, Phalen GS. Ganglions of the wrist and hand. J Bone Joint Surg Am 54:1459-1464, 1972.

Plate AM, Lee SJ, Steiner G, et al. Tumor-like lesions and benign tumors of the hand and wrist. J Am Acad Orthop Surg 11:129-141, 2003.

7

Not Covered by Tuition

Russell Meldrum ✦ *Scott A. Mitchell* ✦ *Roy A. Meals*

"Mom? Is that you? Wow, I can't believe I get reception up here."

"Yeah, hi to you too. I've got some good news. This afternoon I thought I was going to have to drop out of med school, but the doctor says I'm going to be OK. Hello? Mom? I can't hear you."

"Hi, Dad. Is Mom OK?"

"Where am I? I'm up on the ski slopes. Remember, I told you I was going snowboarding for several days at the beginning of Christmas vacation?"

"What happened? That's what I was trying to tell Mom. I kind of dislocated my shoulder on the terrain park."

"What? No, I wasn't doing something stupid. Dude, you should have seen it. I even had people cheering at me from the lift."

"No Dad, I didn't hit my head."

"OK, I'll slow down. So you know that big snowboard park that just opened? Well, I had just finished coming through the pipe, and right after it they have one of those huge hits. No, not that kind of hit; you know, a big jump. So anyway, I guess I had a little too much speed because I overflew the landing. That's what all the people were cheering about. It must have looked spectacular. If only I had that one on film. But then I came down a little too far on my backside edge and slam, it was all over from there. Flipped my way down another hundred yards or so, I think. Tried to recover, but every time I moved my left shoulder, wow, I've never had pain like that before."

"Did they what? Of course not. I didn't feel like making a big commotion of it all, so I just boarded right on down to the first aid station at the bottom. Its ski-in, ski-out, you know."

"Hi, Mom, you're on the line too? Didn't mean to scare you. More good news, Mom. They didn't have to cut off the sweater you knitted for me. The doctor was great. I told him I was a medical student interested in orthopedics, so he explained everything to me. He says that as I fell, I probably reached out instinctively and forced my shoulder into abduction and external rotation. He checked me over and compared the shape of one shoulder with the other. He knew right then what was wrong. It's a common injury for people my age, especially during ski season. He checked my pulse as well as the sensation and strength in my hand. And he also checked the sensation over the outside of my shoulder. Sometimes a nerve can get stretched from the dislocation, and the deltoid or other muscles can be paralyzed."

P R I N C I P L E :   Always compare the symptomatic limb with the normal one.

"No, Mother. I am not paralyzed."

"The x-rays were fine, Dad. Just a garden variety anterior dislocation."

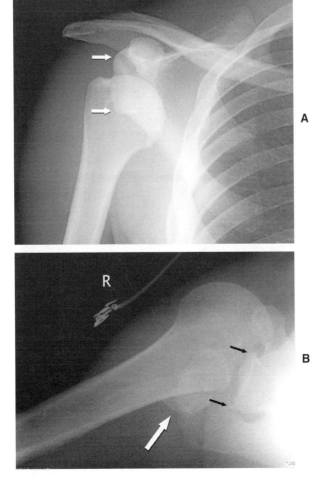

A, Anterior glenohumeral dislocation. The arrows delineate the superior and inferior margins of the glenoid cavity. The humeral head should be centered between the arrows. NOTE OF CAUTION: Not all dislocations are readily apparent on an anteroposterior film. Always obtain an axillary view. **B,** Axillary view of an anterior dislocation associated with a greater tuberosity fracture. The large white arrow points to the displaced tuberosity fragment. The humeral head should normally be centered on the glenoid cavity *(black arrows)*.

"Nope, no greater tuberosity or humeral neck fracture. Once he'd seen the x-rays, he gave me some Versed and reduced the dislocation by having me lie prone on the stretcher with my left arm dangling down over the side. Said that was the safest way. In a few minutes one of his associates pulled down on the arm while he put his thumbs in my armpit and pushed the head back in place. Clunk. I felt better right away."

"Uh huh. I'm in a sling. He told me not to abduct or externally rotate my shoulder for at least 4 weeks. He said in my age group, it's almost always the anterior labrum that gets torn off—called it a Bankart lesion. That's where the thickened capsular ligaments insert onto the glenoid rim; you know, the socket. With extreme abduction and external rotation, these structures can get pulled right off of the bone. Since I'm interested in orthopedics, he drew a sketch of this for me. He even showed me an MRI from a patient with this type of injury."

Glenohumeral joint stability.
A, A fibrous rim, the labrum, normally deepens the glenoid cavity.
B, Anterior dislocation with avulsion of the anterior glenoid labrum and impaction fracture of the posterior humeral head.
C, Reduction after anterior dislocation. **D,** Chronic instability in external rotation.

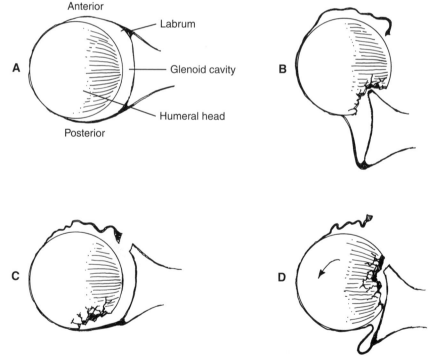

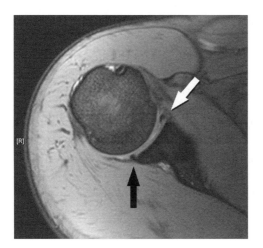

Axial MRI revealing disruption of the anterior labral capsuloligamentous insertion *(white arrow)* and intact posterior labrum *(black arrow)*.

"These types of ligament avulsions don't heal so well and sometimes need to be reattached to prevent recurrences. Also, the lip of the glenoid sometimes punches a crater in the humeral head during the dislocation. This makes recurrences more likely too, but my x-ray looked OK to him."

"He said recurrent dislocation is still the most common complication in my age group. The younger the patient at the time of initial dislocation, the greater the risk of redislocation. In people over the age of 30, this risk starts to decrease—then it's stiffness that becomes the biggest problem. For me, he said, I just need to let the tissues heal a bit by wearing this sling. If I were a little younger, maybe still in my teens, then he said we might actually consider early surgery to reattach the labrum. Especially in people who are active in contact sports, the risk of recurrent dislocation is high enough that some patients opt for surgery right away. For others, he keeps them in the sling for a few weeks and then starts physical therapy to strengthen the rotator cuff and periscapular muscles that help stabilize the joint. But if they continue to dislocate, they will probably need surgery."

"Apparently, in elderly people this same injury mechanism usually fractures the humeral neck rather than dislocating the joint because the osteoporotic bone becomes weaker than the ligaments. But if they do happen to dislocate, patients older than 40 tend to get rotator cuff tears rather than Bankart lesions."

"Are you still there? Good. Maybe just to scare me into always using my sling, he told me about the various surgical treatments for recurrent dislocation. If the labrum is torn off, it can be reattached. Otherwise, there are various ways to tighten up the joint capsule to reduce the laxity. This can even be performed arthroscopically. Unfortunately, surgery sometimes works a little too well and may limit an athlete's ability to throw because of decreased external rotation. Good thing I'm right-handed."

"What? No the Versed's not making me high—well maybe a little. Don't worry, there's somebody here to drive me back home. No, not her, that didn't work out. Uh, no, not her either. Different one this time. Oh, here she is. Can't talk now. Tell you about it later. Tell Dad I said bye."

Follow-up Note: I've taken care of many patients with shoulder dislocations and humeral neck fractures since then. Having had such an injury myself, I can easily empathize with patients regarding their pain and disability. I was lucky, I guess. I was doing my surgery clerkship at the time. I kept my arm in the sling for about 5 weeks except when I scrubbed. It was a little tricky getting into a surgical gown. Typical for someone in his twenties, I quickly got my motion back and fortunately I haven't had any recurrences. For at least 2 years, however, I would get a sharp pain with sudden, forceful shoulder elevation, like when blocking a spiked volleyball or diving into a pool. Even now, many years later, I still can't externally rotate my left shoulder quite as much as my right.

P R I N C I P L E :   Posttraumatic collagen remodeling continues around moving joints for many months.

In elderly people the bone becomes brittle, making the humeral neck the weak link during a fall; so a fracture occurs there with possible fragmentation of the humeral head. With simple fracture patterns, the humeral shaft usually is impacted into the head, and with the broad, well-vascularized surface of cancellous bone available, the neck fracture heals readily.

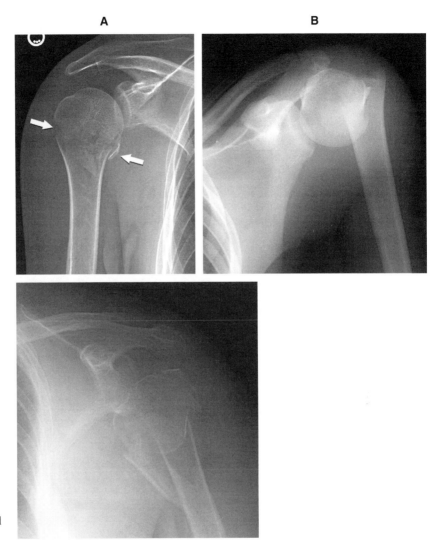

A, Simple impacted proximal humerus fracture in osteoporotic bone. This fracture will likely heal with nonoperative treatment. **B,** Displaced two-part fracture of the humeral neck with preserved bone stock, amenable to internal fixation. **C,** Complex proximal humerus fracture through osteoporotic bone with multiple fragments. This fracture will likely require prosthetic humeral head replacement.

However, in more complex fractures with multiple fragments, the blood supply to the humeral head can become disrupted, resulting in avascular necrosis. Depending on the degree of comminution (and thus the risk of avascular necrosis), open reduction and internal fixation may be required in younger patients, or even prosthetic replacement in the elderly. But regardless of the type of treatment, the importance of doing gentle pendulum-type exercise of the limb, even during the first week, to minimize capsular fibrosis and joint stiffness cannot be overemphasized. Even so, unfortunately, full motion rarely returns.

ADVANCED READING

Bigliani LU. Fractures of the proximal humerus. In Rockwood CA Jr, Matsen FA III, eds. The Shoulder, 2nd ed. Philadelphia: WB Saunders, 1998.

Cole BJ, Millett PJ, Romeo AA, et al. Arthroscopic treatment of anterior glenohumeral instability: Indications and techniques. Instr Course Lect 53:545-558, 2004.

Matsen FA III, Thomas SF, Rockwood CA Jr. Anterior glenohumeral instability. In Rockwood CA Jr, Matsen FA III, eds. The Shoulder, 2nd ed. Philadelphia: WB Saunders, 1998.

Neer CS. Displaced proximal humeral fractures. I. Classification and evaluation. J Bone Joint Surg Am 52:1077-1089, 1970.

Rose CR, Colville M. Fractures of the adult shoulder, the glenohumeral joint. In Rowe CR, ed. The Shoulder. New York: Churchill-Livingstone, 1988.

◆ *If you had to have your shoulder fused, which position would be best?*

8

The Ultimate Mystery

Gregory J. Loren ✦ *Roy A. Meals*

"How was work today, Dear?"

"I was a little tired from the weekend, but actually it was very interesting. Pass the salad, please."

"So what happened?"

"Thanks. When I got to the office, a young man was sitting on the front step. Gym shorts, a tattered rugby jersey, and a pair of those $200 athletic shoes."

"Don't tell me his feet hurt."

"That would have been fitting. But no, it was knee pain. I could see that his right knee was swollen, and when he walked into the office, he was limping to relieve pain on that side. He's an ultimate Frisbee competitor."

"What's that?"

"He told me it's kind of a cross between polo and football, but with a Frisbee. It involves sprinting and leaping, both finesse and endurance, and even some physical contact. This is why it's interesting; it turns out I took care of his younger brother several years ago; he also had knee pain. They play on the same team."

"So is this some sort of contagious ligament or cartilage tear?"

"Not really. Neither one could recall any specific injury. Just gradual onset of swelling and vague pain over several months that worsens with activity."

"Sounds like my old patellar problem. What did you call that?"

"Chondromalacia of the patella. Good guess, but that occurs mainly in young women, and the roughened cartilage causes pain and tenderness under the patella. This young man's patella is fine, but the medial femoral condyle is tender, and there's some quadriceps wasting."

"What does that mean?"

"If there's enough knee pain to make a person favor the other leg, the quadriceps muscles will atrophy. It takes just a couple of weeks. You may not be able to see the diminished muscle mass immediately, but it's evident when you measure the circumference of the thighs."

PRINCIPLE: Knee pain results quickly in quadriceps atrophy.

"Of course. Remember how scrawny my thigh was after my powder-puff football ligament injury. But you said the fellow today hadn't injured his knee. Salt, please."

"Right. That's why I was mystified at first, but one look at his x-rays and bingo."

"So what did his x-rays show?"

"Osteochondritis dissecans. In the classic location, too—medial femoral condyle."

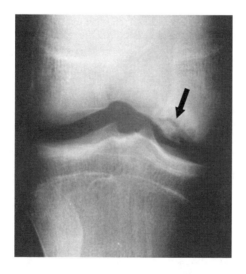

Osteochondritis dissecans of the medial femoral condyle.

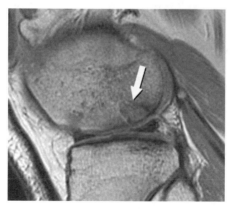

MRI images can often define the shape and extent of separation more clearly than x-rays. Pictured here is a lesion with evidence of partial separation.

"Translate that into English, please."

"Well, literally, I suppose it means something like dissecting inflammation of bone and cartilage, but there's actually no inflammation."

"Oh great, another example of lofty medicalese supplanting a simple and accurate description. Just think what patients would say if you called it the 'big hole' rather than 'foramen magnum.'"

"Come on, calm down. I didn't name it, and we're stuck with it. Remember, a rose by any other name would smell . . . "

"OK, OK, so tell me about osteoconfucius destitute, or whatever it is."

"Osteochondritis dissecans is the loss of blood supply to an area of bone that is next to a joint surface. The dead bone and the overlying cartilage gradually loosen and cause pain. If the osteochondral fragment breaks loose into the joint, locking can occur, and the resulting joint surface irregularity predisposes a person to degenerative arthritis. It is most commonly seen on the lateral aspect of the medial femoral condyle, but the same thing can happen in the distal humerus, proximal femur, dome of the talus, or metatarsal head. Notably, all are on convex surfaces."

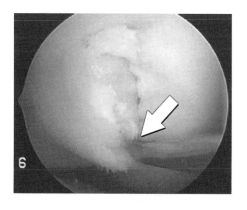

Arthroscopic view of a lesion of the medial femoral condyle. A probe has been placed beneath the detached border of the lesion. By contrast, a normal femoral condyle seen arthroscopically would have a smooth convex surface.

"So if there's no inflammation, what's the cause?"

"Most cases arise spontaneously, usually in active adolescent or young adult males. One cause may be a minute subchondral fracture, perhaps even from unrecognized trauma, which leaves the overlying cartilage undamaged. The cartilage continues to receive its nourishment from the synovial fluid, but the underlying bone undergoes avascular necrosis from the disruption of its blood supply. Another theory is that a thrombus or embolus in an end artery initiates the insult. Or finally, an accessory center of ossification may induce the lesion. Whatever the cause, there must be some hereditary predisposition, since several joints of the same patient or several members of the same family may be affected."

"Is this what his brother had? How about dessert?"

"Yes and no, thank you. Just some coffee. His brother had a similar defect in the same location. He was a bit younger at the time, though. That defect healed spontaneously after he spent several months on crutches, as is commonly the case in skeletally immature patients. Unfortunately, older individuals usually aren't so lucky."

"Why, what happens?"

"Joint motion and repeated impacts prevent the capillaries from growing into the necrotic bone fragment. The overlying cartilage eventually separates, allowing synovial fluid to interpose between the normal bone and avascular fragment. This further impairs healing, and ultimately the osteochondral fragment breaks loose into the joint causing sudden locking accompanied by sharp pain, instability, and effusion."

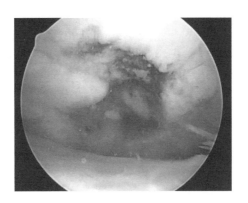

Arthroscopic view of a crater left in the femoral condyle after detachment of an osteochondral fragment. Also note the degenerative changes in the surrounding cartilage, which are likely due to the resulting joint surface irregularity.

"So how do you treat it?"

"I try to reattach the fragment to get it to heal."

"How do you do that without messing up the joint surface even more?"

"That's the problem. If the overlying cartilage is still relatively intact, we stabilize the osteochondral fragment with pins or headless screws countersunk into the cartilage, hoping to establish a new blood supply.

"If the fragments are loose but still in good shape, we scrape the cavity down to fresh bone, add cancellous bone graft as necessary, and secure the fragment in position. Fragments that are unsuitable for replacement are removed, and the cavity is drilled or abraded to stimulate fibrocartilage ingrowth."

"What's fibrocartilage?"

"Well, in this case, it's almost exactly what it sounds like—kind of a combination between fibrous tissue and hyaline cartilage. It's how the body tries to repair cartilage defects that are deep enough to penetrate subchondral bone. It has some of the load-absorbing properties of hyaline cartilage, but is unfortunately much less durable over time to compressive and shear forces. So procedures that stimulate ingrowth of fibrocartilage may alleviate symptoms for a time, but eventually joint degeneration will ensue.

"If such procedures fail or if the defect involves a large weight-bearing area, more extensive surgery may be required. One option is an osteochondral transplant. One or several osteochondral plugs may be taken from a nonarticular area of the knee and transferred to the defect. Alternatively, donated cadaver osteochondral grafts may be used. With advances in tissue engineering, treatment options continue to evolve, utilizing biologic scaffolds or autologous chondrocyte implantation techniques that attempt to regenerate articular cartilage."

"Will that get him back to ultimate Frisbee?"

"It'll give him a good shot, but any residual incongruity in the joint surface will predispose to osteoarthritis, which may not be evident for many years. So I spent a long time talking to him, sketching the problem and the surgery, and so forth. What did you do today?"

"I'll tell you while we're doing the dishes. We don't have much going on this weekend. How 'bout some ultimate Frisbee? Sounds interesting."

"You're kidding. My knee's not up to it, and I don't think yours is either."

"Of course not, Dear. Let's go watch."

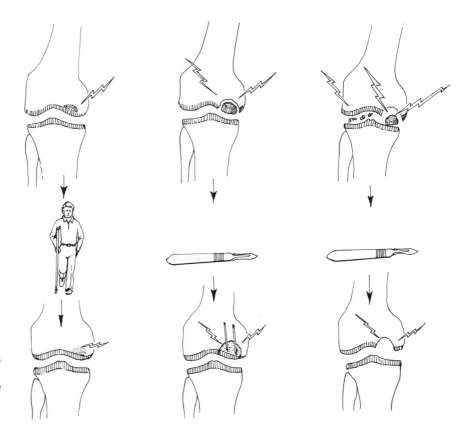

The symptoms, treatment, and outcome of osteochondritis dissecans depend on the fragment's degree of detachment. The lightning bolts represent pain.

ADVANCED READING

Crichton M. Medical obfuscation: Structure and function. N Engl J Med 293: 1257-1259, 1975.

Flynn JM, Kocher MS, Ganley TJ. Osteochondritis dissecans of the knee. J Pediatr Orthop 24:434-443, 2004.

Moti AW, Micheli LJ. Meniscal and articular cartilage injury in the skeletally immature knee. Instr Course Lect 52:683-690, 2003.

Schenick RC Jr, Goodnight JM. Osteochondritis dissecans. J Bone Joint Surg Am 78:439-456, 1996.

Wall E, Von Stein D. Juvenile osteochondritis dissecans. Orthop Clin North Am 34:341-353, 2003.

9

Zeke

The pediatrician down the hall, Dr. Eldridge, calls and asks you to see Ezekiel Walton, the first child born in your town's new hospital. Now 6 months old, he has recently been treated for otitis media, and Mrs. Walton notes that he has become irritable and unwilling to eat after several days of feeling well. She observes that her baby is particularly uncomfortable during diaper changes. On the phone Dr. Eldridge tells you that the child is afebrile and his middle ears are no longer inflamed. His white blood cell and differential count are normal.

Examination of this kid with extraordinarily blond and curly hair shows that he holds his right hip partially flexed, abducted, and externally rotated. He resists your efforts to move the hip. When you try to test the hip for dislocation, he cries intensely and urinates on your sleeve. The musculoskeletal examination is otherwise unremarkable. You study the x-ray.

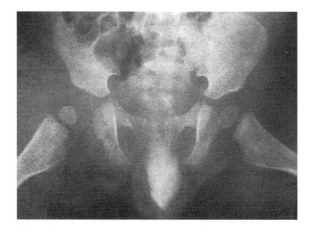

Lateral displacement of right femoral epiphysis. Purulent joint fluid in the right hip has pushed the femoral head away from the acetabulum.

What's wrong? Can you give his mom more antibiotic and see them again next week?

Despite the lack of systemic signs pointing to infection, this child has a septic hip joint and needs immediate surgical treatment. Acute suppurative arthritis can occur at any age and at any joint, but it is particularly common in infants and very young children. The larger joints are most commonly affected, and *Staphylococcus aureus* is the usual infectious organism in most age groups. In infants younger than 6 months, *Streptococcus pneumoniae* and to a lesser extent now *Haemophilus* species may also be seen. From the bloodstream the bacteria reach the joint either directly by seeding the synovium or indirectly by settling in the metaphyseal bone and breaking through into the joint. This second mechanism is common in infantile septic hip arthritis because the joint capsule extends to the base of the femoral neck and encompasses proportionately more of the proximal femoral metaphysis than in the older child. Bacterial proliferation in this poorly defended area is brisk, leading to a purulent joint fluid with a white blood cell count of more than 50,000/mm^3, a decreased glucose concentration, and an increased protein concentration. The bacteria compete with the chondrocytes for synovial fluid nourishment and degradative enzymes in the pus rapidly destroy the cartilage matrix.

Accumulating pus distends the capsule, causing the joint to be held in the characteristic position of midflexion, abduction, and external rotation to minimize pressure and pain. Movement of the joint from this position will be painful and limited. The increased intraarticular pressure also may result in subluxation or dislocation, which is seen on the x-ray as varying degrees of lateral displacement of the femur. The blood vessels supplying the femoral head run up the femoral neck inside the joint capsule, and increased pressure also can diminish blood flow to the vulnerable femoral head, resulting in bone necrosis with ensuing epiphyseal growth arrest and arthritis.

Particularly in young infants, the systemic response to this potentially devastating infection may be minimal. You should not be deceived by a normal temperature and white blood cell count. Also, in children older than about 1 year of age, lateral subluxation of the affected femoral head is not reliably present on x-rays. Capsular distention from the purulent effusion may at times only be apparent on **MRI** or ultrasound images. In unclear cases, these modalities are often quite useful for identifying an effusion, and ultrasound may be used to guide percutaneous aspiration. In any case, if the diagnosis is at all uncertain, joint aspiration and fluid analysis are mandatory to exclude infection. The presence of more than 50,000 white blood cells in the synovial fluid or a positive Gram stain warrants emergent surgical intervention. Drainage of the infected hip should be supplemented with appropriate intravenous antibiotics (typically a penicillinase-resistant cephalosporin). After the infection is controlled, gentle active and passive exercises are carried out to restore joint motion and improve cartilage nutrition. A delay of 5 days or more in diagnosis and treatment greatly increases the risk of permanent deformity, limb-length discrepancy, and early osteoarthritis.

P R I N C I P L E :   Cartilage lacks a blood supply, and the chondrocytes survive by synovial fluid diffusion. Joint motion pumps metabolites through the cartilage.

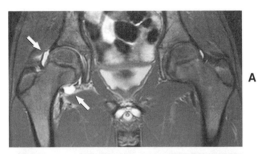
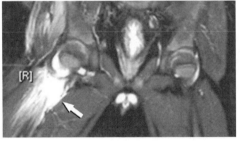

A, T2-weighted MRI of a left hip effusion, suspicious for infection. The accumulated fluid in the joint shows high signal intensity *(white arrows)*. **B,** T2-weighted MRI showing spread of infection into the right hip from a focus of osteomyelitis in the proximal femoral metaphysis *(white arrow)*.

Follow-up Note: Four weeks later, Mrs. Walton brings Zeke into your office for a checkup. She has been performing the range-of-motion exercises to both hips, and she states that he is much improved. Follow-up will be necessary for many years to ensure that the infection has not disturbed the growth of the femoral head. Should you take off his diaper to measure hip motion? Indubitably. Otherwise how do you know whether any restriction is caused by his diaper or by capsular fibrosis? Should you take your watch off first?

A common diagnostic dilemma that arises in young children is differentiating transient synovitis from septic arthritis of the hip. Transient synovitis is thought to represent a sterile reactive inflammatory process that typically follows a viral infection, and it is the most common cause of hip pain in children between 3 and 10 years of age (slightly older than the average child with septic arthritis). The prognosis is excellent, and only supportive treatment measures are required. The perils of septic arthritis, on the other hand, make a timely and accurate distinction between these conditions a must. Given the potential long-term complications of a neglected septic hip, a high degree of suspicion is warranted at all times. Particularly in toddlers and slightly older children, how-ever, there are a number of clues that may be used to help differ-entiate these conditions. There are four well-studied factors that alone, or in combination, suggest the presence of a septic joint: fever (>38.5° C), history of refusal to bear weight, white blood cell count greater than 12,000, and erythrocyte sedimentation rate greater than 40. When none or only one of these criteria are pres-ent, only a small minority of children will have a septic joint. How-ever, if three or more are present, as many as 90% of such children will have septic arthritis. As illustrated in the patient just dis-cussed, however, young children (<1 year of age) may lack any or all of these criteria, and the threshold for aspiration should be much lower.

ADVANCED READING

Choi IH, Pizzutillo PD, Bowen R, Dragann R, Malhis T. Sequelae and recon-struction after septic arthritis of the hip in infants. J Bone Joint Surg Am 72:1150-1165, 1990.

Kocher MS, Zurakowski D, Kasser JR. Differentiating between septic arthri-tis and transient synovitis of the hip in children: An evidence-based clini-cal prediction algorithm. J Bone Joint Surg Am 81:1662-1670, 1999.

Matan AJ, Smith JT. Pediatric septic arthritis. Orthopaedics 20:630-635, 1997.

Morrissy RT. Bone and joint infections. In Morrissy RT, ed. Lovell and Win-ter's Pediatric Orthopaedics, 3rd ed. Philadelphia: Lippincott, 1990, vol 1, pp 539-561.

Shaw BA, Kasser JR. Acute septic arthritis in infancy and childhood. Clin Or-thop Relat Res 257:212-225, 1990.

10

Of Crime and Poodles

Keith J. Cannon

Mrs. Houlihan had been my patient for the greater part of 30 years. Now 60 years of age, she was a charming, handsome woman with whom I got along genuinely, all of which served to accentuate my frustration at not being able to arrive at a diagnosis. I had asked her to return to my office on a Friday, the day on which my longtime friend Holmes customarily called to invite me out for a bit of lunch. (Being myself of somewhat corpulent dimensions and enjoying indulgence in culinary delights, I seldom refused these invitations.) As for Holmes, he was by trade a detective, and he enjoyed dabbling at times in the more challenging aspects of the practice of medicine. He often chided me by saying that his training as a detective had better suited him for medical diagnosis than had all my costly years at university. Never did I grant him this point, but secretly I concurred.

While Mrs. Houlihan changed into her gown in the examination room, my nurse informed me that Holmes had arrived and awaited me in my office.

"Holmes, dear boy! How wonderful to see you. I trust that this past week has been kind to you."

"Indeed it has, Dr. Watson. And judging from the newly loosened position of your belt, I see it has been quite kind to you as well."

"Yes, quite. Ahem. Yes, well I wonder if I might persuade you to look in on a patient of mine."

I proceeded to describe Mrs. Houlihan's recent complaints. She had a daily custom of walking her two French poodles about the neighborhood. Over the past couple of months, she had experienced pain in her buttocks, thighs, and legs after walking. This was accompanied by a sense of "poor circulation" in the lower extremities that included a tingling and burning in her feet. She stated that her legs felt weak at times. She would stop walking for a spell, but it was only after sitting for some time that the symptoms would start to subside. The distance she could walk before having this difficulty varied greatly from day to day. At home Mrs. Houlihan had no trouble with daily activities, but she did complain of low back pain, which had caused her chronic suffering for 2 or 3 years. I had attributed it to age and disc degeneration.

"What were your initial thoughts in this case, Doctor?" Holmes was already pondering the information I had given him, as evidenced by the malodorous pipe he had lit up. I gently reminded him that this was a smoke-free clinic and that pipe smoking was extremely unhealthful.

"Frankly, Holmes, it seemed at first a clear-cut case of intermittent claudication secondary to vascular disease at the level of the iliac arteries. But what has puzzled me about the history is that Mrs. Houlihan needs to sit for relief, not merely to stop walking. In addition, she can walk several blocks virtually pain free on some days and then only one block or so on others. Her physical examination shows no evidence of peripheral vascular disease. She has normal distal pulses and capillary refill. There is no marked skin atrophy or hypertrophy of the toenails and no dependent rubor. It's a bewilderment."

"To be sure. Do you think our dear poodle fancier would oblige me a quick examination of my own?"

"I don't see why not. But do please refrain from using that ridiculous magnifying glass of yours."

I introduced Holmes to Mrs. Houlihan, who declared it a distinct honor not only to make the acquaintance of the renowned Mr. Holmes but to be scrutinized by his keen eye as well. Blushing almost imperceptibly, Holmes began to gather clues in his characteristically systematic fashion. Much to my surprise, he limited himself to a general back examination. I had learned in medical school to perform this examination on anyone presenting with low back pain. Holmes first observed Mrs. Houlihan as she stood. He assured himself that the iliac crests were level with each other and that the shoulders were even. He palpated along the spine and adjacent musculature. He then asked Mrs. Houlihan to bend forward as he looked for scoliosis and measured the distance from her fingertips to the floor. He completed his assessment of the range of motion by having Mrs. Houlihan bend backward and to either side. Holmes observed Mrs. Houlihan's gait and asked her to walk on her heels and tiptoes.

With Mrs. Houlihan sitting, Holmes conducted a neurologic examination, paying careful attention to the deep tendon reflexes, motor strength, and sensation in the lower extremities. He measured the circumference of the calves and thighs to rule out muscle atrophy. He palpated the pulses and performed a straight-leg raising test.

PHYSICAL EXAMINATION OF LUMBAR NERVE ROOTS:

Root	Motor	Sensory	Reflex
L4	Quadriceps, tibialis anterior	Medial calf	Knee jerk
L5	Extensor hallucis longus	Dorsum of foot, lateral calf	None
S1	Gastrosoleus	Lateral/plantar foot, posterior calf	Ankle jerk

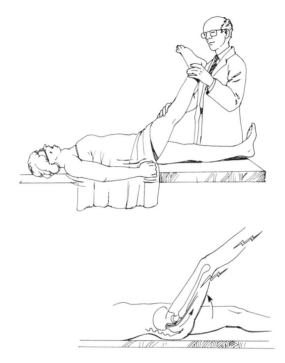

Flexing the hip with the knee extended draws the sciatic nerve distally. This maneuver causes radiating pain if nerve root irritation is present.

With Mrs. Houlihan lying supine, Holmes checked the range of motion of both of her hips and repeated the straight-leg raising test. Finally, he asked her to lie on her side and he applied pressure to the iliac crest to see whether she experienced pain with pelvic compression.

"Mrs. Houlihan, would you be so kind as to walk around the block until you experience symptoms and then return to the office?"

"Why, certainly, if it will help you solve this mystery. You know I've long been one of your ardent admirers, Mr. Holmes. Little did I know how charming you would be in person. Shall I go outside in this trifle of a gown?"

I suggested that my patient get dressed before taking her walk. Holmes readily agreed and then lingered in the examining room watching Mrs. Houlihan's feet behind the room divider as she dressed. Back in my office I inquired whether he had ascertained any useful information. "Well, Doctor, aside from some mild tenderness in the region of the lumbar spine, the results of our dear lady's examination were essentially normal. There were no neurologic abnormalities, no pain on straight-leg raising, and the pulses were normal."

P R I N C I P L E :   Observing a patient's movements during routine activities may reveal a problem not evident on a formal physical examination.

"Then we aren't any closer to a diagnosis than before."

"Not so, Dr. Watson. Given Mrs. Houlihan's history, the lack of physical findings at rest is very intriguing. I believe we shall have our diagnosis when the patient returns after exercise. In fact, I think I hear her now."

We returned at once to the examination room only to find a distraught Mrs. Houlihan standing stooped and steadying herself on the table. Holmes repeated part of his examination. Curiously, the patient's ankle jerk reflexes were nearly absent, whereas they had been normal before.

"Aha!" exclaimed Holmes. "We have our culprit. This is not a case of claudication at all, but rather pseudoclaudication—neurogenic claudication, if you prefer. Of course, we shall need an MRI or CT myelogram to be certain, but I believe that you suffer from lumbar spinal stenosis, Mrs. Houlihan."

"Dear me! Can anything be done? I don't know what my precious puppies would do if I couldn't take them out for their daily constitutional."

"Patience, madam. Allow me to explain what spinal stenosis is. By definition, it is the narrowing of the spinal canal and intervertebral foramina."

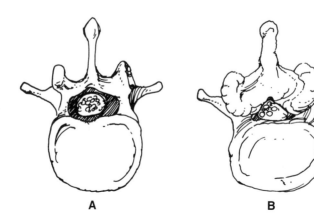

A, Spinal cord and nerve roots normally have sufficient space within the spinal canal.
B, Encroachment of osteophytes from facet joint arthritis into the canal and intervertebral foramen impinges on the neural structures in spinal stenosis.

A   B

A, Axial T2 MRI of the lumbar spine revealing normal canal space and cauda equina. **B,** Spinal stenosis at L4-5 secondary to facet osteophytes, intervertebral disc bulging, and hypertrophy of the ligamentum flavum. Note the narrowed space available for the cauda equina *(arrow)*.

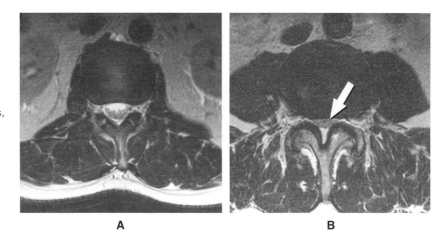

A　　　　　　　B

Sagittal MRI views of two different patients revealing multiple degenerative and bulging discs encroaching into the spinal canal (normal disc signal on T2-weighted images is bright). Notice the dark signal of the discs due to decreased water content.

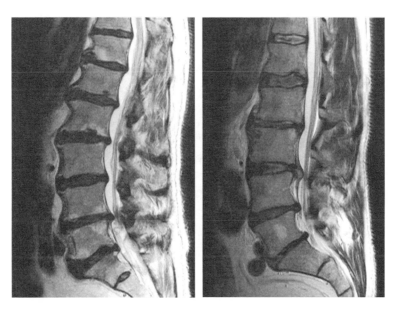

"In your case, this stenosis is likely due to degeneration of the intervertebral discs, along with arthritis and subluxation of the facet joints. As our discs begin to degenerate and lose height as we age, even in the absence of discrete herniation, they tend to bulge posteriorly and encroach on the spinal canal. And on the other side of the canal, as the facet joints degenerate, osteophytes form that narrow the intervertebral foramen and when severe, compress the canal contents as well. Finally, as the disc spaces begin to collapse anteriorly, the thick ligament coursing along the posterior aspects of the canal (the ligamentum flavum) is no longer pulled taught and tends to buckle forward, leading to further narrowing. Now all of this is made worse when you stand and exercise, because with extension of the lumbar spine, there is normally a narrowing of the intervertebral foramina. When this occurs in the presence of degenerative changes, as in your case, the narrowing is severe enough to cause symptoms. And as extension of the lumbar spine causes narrowing of the foramina, the converse is also true—flexion of the spine will tend to open the foramen. Just as you have already figured out on your own, you need to flex your back by stooping or sitting for relief."

At this point I assumed control of the conversation, feeling it necessary to translate Holmes's rather windy explanation into common parlance. I also explained the treatment options for spinal stenosis. I believed it unlikely that we could ever completely relieve Mrs. Houlihan's low back pain. Our treatment would be aimed at allowing Mrs. Houlihan to ambulate as much as possible with minimal symptoms. Elements of nonoperative therapy would include nonsteroidal antiinflammatory drugs, exercises for endurance and abdominal strength, a corset for lower back support, and possibly epidural steroid injections.

I also explained to Mrs. Houlihan that lumbar stenosis often has a chronic, progressive course. The narrowing becomes severe enough in some patients to cause symptoms even at rest, and with prolonged compression persistent dysfunction of the nerve roots could cause significant weakness in the legs. Also, the sacral nerve roots supplying bowel and bladder function could become disturbed in severe cases. In such cases, surgical decompression of the involved nerve roots is often considered. Although the return of nerve functioning after surgery is somewhat unpredictable, relief of pain, particularly leg pain, is often quite successful.

After arranging for an MRI, I bid Mrs. Houlihan a fond farewell. I then returned to my office to commune with Holmes, still hoping for a luncheon invitation.

"Splendid job, old man! How did it ever occur to you that Houlihan's back was the root of her problems?"

"Elementary, Watson. She was 60 years old and had a history of chronic low back pain. She reported claudicatory symptoms but showed no signs of vascular disease. Besides, why ever would a vascular surgery case appear in an orthopedic text such as this?"

"Quite right. You know, I see a lot of patients with low back pain. They say it affects 80% of all people at least once in their lives. I often wish I had your mind for deductive reasoning when I work up low back pain. The differential diagnosis is extensive, and it includes gynecologic, genitourinary, and gastrointestinal conditions. Of course, spinal stenosis is not the most common cause of low back pain."

"Most certainly not. Do you perchance recall 'The Case of the Corrupt Curator'? It was low back pain that landed that character behind bars."

How could I have forgotten that case? Holmes referred to a case in which certain priceless items of antiquity kept disappearing from the National Museum. There were never any signs of breaking and entering—a definite inside job. Our key contact was the museum's curator, who was coincidentally one of my patients. After the disappearance of a large Grecian urn, the curator came to my office complaining of low back pain and stiffness of acute onset. He had all the classic risk factors: obesity, faulty work habits, lack of daily exercise, cigarette smoking, poor muscle tone, and (unknown to the general public) on evenings and weekends, he was in the practice of wearing women's clothing, including high-heeled shoes. His back pain had come on suddenly when he lifted a heavy crate at work.

The physical examination showed no tenderness of the spine itself but marked tenderness and spasm of the muscles on the right side of his lower back. The curator's range of motion was limited, and bending his back away from the affected side produced severe pain. The neurologic examination of the lower extremities was completely normal, and straight-leg raising produced no pain. I was certain that acute muscle strain was the cause of the curator's back pain. Muscle strain is, by the way, the number one cause of low back pain.

The curator made the unfortunate error of mentioning his backache to Holmes during the course of the investigation. That was a tip-off that led Holmes to confirm his suspicions. The curator was himself guilty of stealing the missing relics. He should have stopped short of lifting a Grecian urn that was heavy enough to injure his back. After that, the muscular low back strain was the least of his problems. He was cast into prison, where he certainly received the standard treatment. I usually recommend strict bed rest for 2 days (but no more) with control of the pain and inflammation using nonsteroidal agents. I try to reduce muscle spasm with ice packs or a heating pad. Massage can also be helpful. Although muscle relaxants may be of benefit acutely, I try to limit their use to short-term courses only. The most important aspect of treatment, in my opinion, is a regimen of low back exercises that strengthen the back and abdomen and stretch and strengthen the muscles of the lower extremities. I also educate my patients on losing weight and being kind to their backs when lifting and performing other kinds of work. Fortunately, most of these cases resolve with this therapy. I have the patients return for follow-up in 4 to 6 weeks; of course in the case of the curator, he was otherwise indisposed by that time.

Holmes continued to reflect: "It's a wonder, Dr. Watson, that portly gentlemen such as yourself don't injure their backs more often. If you recall, you and I cooperated in another investigation that involved the second most common cause of low back pain. It was, if memory serves me, 'The Case of the Errant Heir Apparent.'"

"Right you are. I remember it well. That was the case in which an American came to England claiming to be the lost son of the recently deceased Duke of Cornwall and of course heir to the family fortune. The whole affair was an elaborate charade staged by the late Duke's young mistress. The impostor stated that his vocation back in the United States was that of bookkeeper, but he hadn't counted on clashing with the cunning of one Mr. Holmes."

"Well said, Doctor. The young man had a curious suntan that was conspicuously a deeper bronze on the left arm and face than on the right. Knowing as I did that you Americans drive on the wrong side of the road, I deduced that this presumed heir spent more time behind the wheel of a vehicle than one would expect of a bookkeeper. But I wasn't sure."

"Not sure until the young scoundrel came to my office with a complaint of low back pain."

I thought back to the time that the asymmetrically suntanned man had come to see me, unaware of my connection with Mr. Holmes. By chance he had come on a Friday, right before the lunch hour. The 35-year-old man reported that for just short of a year he had suffered a deep, aching pain in the lower back. Coughing and sneezing made it worse, and rest relieved it. The pain at times radiated to his left buttock. I asked when the pain bothered him most, and the man said that he was a lorry driver in his home country (or truck driver, as they say in the States) and that the pain was at its worst after he had sat behind the wheel for a prolonged period. For the past month or so, he had experienced an occasional shooting pain in his left leg and foot with noticeable tingling in the same area.

The physical examination showed that the Yankee had moderate tenderness on the left side of his lumbar spine. His forward flexion was quite limited, but extension and rotation were normal. In contrast with the corrupt curator, the young truck driver experienced pain on bending toward the affected side. He had difficulty walking on his heels. His deep tendon reflexes were all normal, but his left great toe was nearly numb. Straight-leg raising produced pain in both the sitting and recumbent positions. Several testing modalities were at my disposal, including CT, MRI, myelography, and electromyography; but based on the physical findings, I was fairly certain that the man had a herniated nucleus pulposus between the fourth and fifth lumbar vertebrae.

"Bookkeeper indeed! Fortunately for that fellow, the deceased Duke's attorney knew that the mistress was behind the whole scheme. He let the Yank return to his trucks in America on condition that he never again set foot in England. What sort of therapy do you suppose he received for his disc herniation, Doctor?"

I proceeded to enlighten Holmes on the topic. "The intervertebral discs consist of a semifluid nucleus and a surrounding fibrous anulus—something like a jelly doughnut. After age 30, the discs begin to change until by age 60 the gelatinous center has dried out and the fibrous anulus has lost most of its elasticity. The anulus can tear and allow the nucleus to herniate into the spinal canal. In the lumbar spine, this typically occurs in the posterolateral aspect of the disc, and the resultant herniation presses against the traversing nerve root just before or as it enters the neural foramen. This elicits both mechanical compression as well as an inflammatory reaction around the nerve root, leading to the characteristic back and leg pain. When severe, motor weakness may also be present. Ninety-five percent of the time this occurs below the fourth or fifth lumbar vertebra, affecting the L5 and S1 roots, respectively."

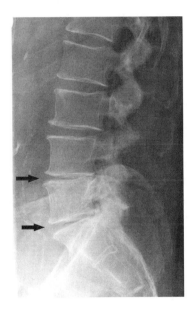

Degenerative disc disease with joint space narrowing at the L4-5 and L5-S1 levels *(arrows)*.

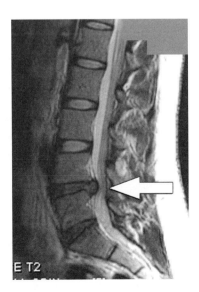

MRI showing large disc herniation at L4-5 *(arrow)*. What signs and symptoms would you predict based on this MRI?

"Conservative therapy is much the same as for muscular low back strain: strict bed rest acutely, nonsteroidal drugs, and an exercise regimen for the recovery period. Half of those so affected are better in 2 weeks and 90% in 2 months. If this therapy fails or if there are major or progressive neurologic signs, or if the patient is on the brink of economic catastrophe because of persistent symptoms, surgical decompression is warranted. If and when to operate is still a hotly debated subject, but most surgeons like to try conservative measures for at least 6 weeks. With the newer minimally invasive techniques, however, recovery after surgery is quite expedient, leading some to pursue earlier operative intervention. There is no debate, however, in the case of a large central herniation. This entity presents as cauda equina syndrome, which consists of saddle block anesthesia, bilateral leg weakness or paralysis, and sphincter disturbances or frank incontinence. This is a true surgical emergency because prompt decompression can avert lifelong paralysis."

At the conclusion of my discourse, Holmes prepared to leave, and I prepared to accept his invitation to dine. "Dr. Watson, as always you have broadened my knowledge of the field of medicine. All this talk about low back pain has given me a voracious appetite. If you'll excuse me, I have a luncheon date with a certain Mrs. Houlihan. Until next Friday then, good day."

ADVANCED READING

Arbit E, Pannullo S. Lumbar stenosis: A clinical review. Clin Orthop Relat Res 384:137-143, 2001.

Biyani A, Andersson GB. Low back pain: Pathophysiology and management. J Am Acad Orthop Surg 12:106-115, 2004.

Postachini F. Management of herniation of the lumbar disc. J Bone Joint Surg Br 81:567-576, 1999.

Saal JA, Saal JS. Nonoperative treatment of herniated lumbar intervertebral disc with radiculopathy: An outcome study. Spine 14:431-437, 1989.

Saal JA, Saal JS, Herzog RJ. The natural history of extruded disc herniations treated nonoperatively: An MRI follow-up study. Spine 15:683-686, 1990.

Sengupta DK, Herkowitz HN. Lumbar spinal stenosis. Treatment strategies and indications for surgery. Orthop Clin North Am 34:281-295, 2003.

Truumees E, Herkowitz HN. Lumbar spinal stenosis: Treatment options. Instr Course Lect 50:153-161, 2001.

11

The Closing Argument

"Ladies and gentlemen of the jury, after 2 days of testimony from multiple witnesses and the defendant, Dr. Goode, I will now summarize the sequence of events leading to the pain, misery, disfigurement, and severe disability that have become a fact of life for this poor young man sitting before you.

"Although Mackenzie Whitherspoon had a rough start in life, at 8 years of age he seemed to be adjusting well to his new foster home—that is, until one morning last year when he fell from the neighbor's tree while borrowing several apples. Typical for such a headfirst fall, the lad wisely extended his hands to protect himself. Unfortunately, because of this instinctive and highly judicious act, Mackenzie's right elbow was forced into hyperextension, causing the humerus to break distally. This is an injury the experts have told us is common in children and adolescents, and is best described as a supracondylar fracture. Two complications are well known: malunion with alteration of the carrying angle of the elbow, and compartment syndrome with devastation of the muscles in the forearm. We have found no fault with his neighbor's emergency aid: splinting the limb in an extended position with folded newspaper and masking tape, and once he explained to us Mackenzie's unwillingness to come to the hospital, we understood the reason for transporting him in the trunk of his car.

"The radiologist described to us the initial x-ray findings typical for this injury: a short oblique fracture of the distal humerus with proximal and posterior displacement of the distal fragment."

PRINCIPLE: Fractures and other conditions causing limb deformities are described as displacement of the distal portion with respect to an anatomically aligned proximal portion.

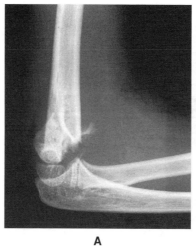 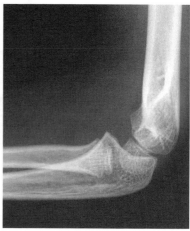

A, Posterior displacement and apex anterior angulation of distal humeral fracture just proximal to condyles—a supracondylar fracture. **B,** Opposite, uninjured side for comparison.

A   B

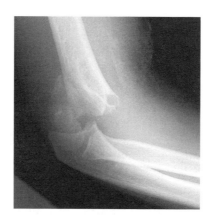

Example of a severely displaced supracondylar humerus fracture. Note the posterior translation as well and rotational malalignment of the distal fragment.

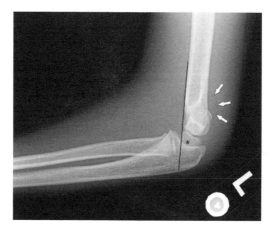

At times the radiographic presentation of a supracondylar humerus fracture is subtle, as seen here. Draw a line along the anterior aspect of the humerus toward the elbow. This line should intersect the middle of the capitellum *(asterisk)* on a true lateral view. Note the posterior displacement of the capitellum relative to this line. What is the semicircular area of lucency *(white arrows)* just posterior to this distal humerus seen on this view?

"From the anatomic sketches introduced earlier, it was obvious to everyone here that the sharp edge of the proximal fragment pressing anteriorly against the nearby brachial artery could easily compress, if not actually tear or cut it. Furthermore, swelling and hematoma from the injury could contribute to both arterial and venous occlusion."

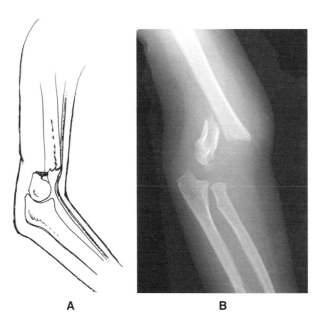

A, The bone end tents the brachial artery and may bruise or tear it. **B,** Severely displaced supracondylar fracture. Try to picture the course of the brachial artery with this deformity.

A   **B**

"Next we come to Dr. Goode's emergency room notes, sparse as they were. Let me reread Dr. Goode's initial evaluation."

Filthy urchin, screaming with elbow pain. Hyperextension deformity of the right elbow. No obvious breaks in skin. No other injuries apparent. X-rays show displaced supracondylar fracture. Will try for closed reduction and possible percutaneous pinning in the operating room under general anesthesia.

"Three experts reviewed this marginally legible note with us, and none could find any notation of this unfortunate lad's initial distal neurovascular status. Each emphatically stated that such an evaluation is the standard of care in all cases and critical in an injury such as this in which neurologic and vascular complications are well known."

> **NOTE:**   *Injury to the median, ulnar, and radial nerves, all of which course in close prox-*
> *imity to the elbow, have been described with supracondylar humerus fractures.*
> *The most common nerve palsy associated with this fracture, however, involves*
> *the anterior interosseous nerve (AIN), the distal motor branch of the median*
> *nerve in the forearm. The AIN supplies the flexor digitorum profundus to the*
> *index and long fingers, the flexor pollicis longus, and the pronator quadratus.*
> *An easy physical examination maneuver to test the AIN is to have the patient*
> *make an "OK" sign with his thumb and index finger.*

"Next, we have Dr. Goode's operative note. He was kind enough to read it to us in its entirety and to explain the medical terminology. Let me review several key sentences."

The little bastard bit the anesthesiologist during an otherwise routine induction. . . . Even with the elbow in complete flexion and hinging the distal fragment on the intact posterior periosteum and triceps, the fracture remained unstable and marginally reduced. Therefore I inserted several crossed Kirschner wires (K-wires) from the lateral and medial epicondyles to stabilize the fracture. At this point the radial pulse was noted to be absent. X-rays now revealed anatomic reduction of the fracture with one K-wire protruding slightly anteriorly. When this K-wire was withdrawn, the radial pulse could be palpated. . . . A long-arm splint was applied, and the patient left the operating room in satisfactory condition. He will be admitted for overnight observation.

"Now let me draw your attention to the meticulous notes Nurse Skylark made that night."

11:00 PM   Eight-year-old boy admitted from the recovery room after percutaneous pinning of right elbow fracture. Patient says elbow hurting more. Vital signs stable, right arm in splint. Left hand cooler than right; radial pulses equal. Sensation to fingertips intact. Full passive extension of digits causes mild discomfort at fracture site. Generally disheveled. Washed face. Told me he could curse in six languages.

2:00 AM   Patient complains of increasing pain. Vital signs stable; radial pulse intact. Gave prn acetaminophen dose twice; spat first dose out.

3:15 AM   Patient screaming with pain. Vital signs unobtainable due to lack of cooperation. Fingers held in flexed posture; efforts at passive digital extension cause agonizing pain. Fingers cool, capillary filling OK, diminished pinprick sensation on fingertips. Called Dr. Goode. He asked whether radial pulse was intact. I checked and it was. He prescribed codeine.

3:55 AM   Pain worse. Dr. Goode notified.

> 4:20 AM   Dr. Goode arrives. Boy is swearing and writhing in pain. Dr. Goode says he can feel radial pulse and not to worry. He splits outer portion of bandage. No change in pain. Orders Demerol. Medical student asks if she can do forearm compartment pressure study. Dr. Goode says OK.
>
> 4:30 AM   Medical student wakes Dr. Goode at nurses' station and reports forearm pressure of 85 mm Hg.
>
> 4:31 AM   Dr. Goode transfers patient to gurney himself and runs to operating room.

"Gentlemen and ladies, the rest is sad, yet straightforward. The experts have explained to us in detail compartment syndrome, but let's briefly review it. In the muscular compartments of the forearm, the enclosing fascia is unyielding. With significant swelling from trauma or bleeding from an arterial injury, the added volume increases the pressure within the compartment. When the pressure in the compartment exceeds the venous pressure, blood outflow is impaired. The accumulation of waste products and the lack of oxygenated blood triggers some of the early symptoms of compartment syndrome—pain and nerve irritability. Skeletal muscle responds to this ischemia by releasing inflammatory mediators such as histamine that increase vascular permeability. This further increases the edema within a compartment, compounding the problem. Ultimately, with increasing muscle ischemia and edema, tissue pressure exceeds capillary perfusion pressure in a tamponade-like effect. Untreated, the muscles and nerves within the compartment undergo ischemic necrosis."

"The forearm and leg are particularly vulnerable to this devastating condition because of the tight fascial restraints surrounding the muscles in these locations. The physical findings are easy to remember—the five Ps—pain, paresthesias, paralysis, pallor, and pulselessness. The first three are related to nerve ischemia and are early signs since the nerves are quite sensitive. Any movement of the muscles heightens the pain, an observation Nurse Skylark noted when she tried to straighten the digits. The last two signs, pallor and loss of pulse, occur late and only after the compartment pressure exceeds the systolic pressure. As you have learned, compartment pressure measurements are useful, particularly in comatose or otherwise uncooperative patients."

PRINCIPLE: The importance of pain as a clue to impending compartment syndrome cannot be overemphasized. In fact, some refer to the five Ps of compartment syndrome as pain, pain, pain, pain, and pain. Following traumatic injury to the extremities, any patient with notably increasing pain, pain unrelieved by narcotic medication, or pain with passive stretching of the muscles in a compartment must be presumed to have an impending compartment syndrome.

"As a temporizing measure, completely splitting all circumferential dressings to relieve any external compression may help, but emergency fasciotomy to allow for tissue swelling and restoration of capillary perfusion is critical. Split-thickness skin grafting several days later can then cover the swollen muscles. Unfortunately, when the fasciotomy is delayed, the prolonged ischemia and necrosis lead to permanent muscle and nerve damage, observations first noted by Dr. Volkmann as long ago as 1881.

"To Dr. Goode's credit, his operative management of the supracondylar fracture resulted in anatomic alignment, and this avoided the complication of a disfiguring malunion. The issue of a vascular complication, however, is a different matter. Dr. Goode admitted that his failure to perform and record an initial neurovascular examination while in the emergency room is defenseless. One can only surmise whether the subsequent vascular compromise was related to the fracture itself or to the manipulation and K-wire insertion in the operating room.

"Dr. Goode's adamant position has been that the radial pulse remained intact through the night, and therefore the boy's pain was just surgical and not ischemic. Intuition and our expert witnesses, however, tell us that distal pulses remain intact until the compartment pressure approaches the systolic pressure, but the damage begins long before—when the pressure exceeds capillary perfusion pressure. Dr. Goode, unfortunately, didn't recognize that pain is the most sensitive of the five Ps; and if he had heeded Nurse Skylark's initial warning about young Mackenzie's spiraling pain, this young man could have led a productive and fruitful life. Now forever maimed, who knows what other tragedies await him? I rest my case."

PRINCIPLE: Listen to the nurses. Read their notes.

ADVANCED READING

Culp RW, Ostennan AL, Davidson RS, et al. Neural injuries associated with supracondylar fractures of the humerus in children. J Bone Joint Surg Am 72:1211-1215, 1990.

Flynn JM, Sarwark JF, Waters PM, et al. The surgical management of pediatric fractures of the upper extremity. Instr Course Lect 52:635-645, 2003.

Hovius SE, Ultee J. Volkmann's ischemic contracture. Prevention and treatment. Hand Clin 16:647-657, 2000.

Lins RE, Simovitch RW, Waters PM. Pediatric elbow trauma. Orthop Clin North Am 30:119-132, 1999.

Kurer MHJ, Regan MW. Completely displaced supracondylar fracture of the humerus in children. A review of 1708 comparable cases. Clin Orthop Relat Res 256:205-214, 1990.

Minkowitz B, Busch MT. Supracondylar humerus fractures. Current trends and controversies. Orthop Clin North Am 25:581-594, 1994.

Volkmann R. Die ischfunischen Muskel Uihmungen und Kontarackturen [Ischemic muscle paralyses and contractures]. Centralb Coo 51:801-803, 1881.

◆ *Why is cubitus varus called a gunstock deformity?*

12

Crystals in the ER

Ira Zunin ✦ *Roy A. Meals*

Looking over his round belly and past his thick gold bracelet, Marcus Thompson searched for a reason behind the excruciating pain radiating from his thumb. Its base was red, hot, and swollen, but why? "Could I have sprained it at the Napa Valley Wine Auction banquet?" All he could recall was goose liver pate, baked scallops with truffles, and those splendid reserve wines. "You deserved to indulge a little," he reassured himself.

Just then, Marcus heard a moan. He squinted across the hall and saw his apparent twin: midsixties, gray, and balding. His tuxedo fit sharply, except that the new arrival had taken his cummerbund to make a sling for his left wrist. "Don't tell me," said Marcus. "You were out for a fabulous Saturday evening, and suddenly your wrist started killing you." Zachary Blake offered his remaining hand. The two men shook hands and smiled at the irony of their shared plights.

"It's hell getting old," Zach observed. The echo of approaching footsteps made him look up. A tall, dark physician wearing a long white coat approached. Half a step behind followed a young man with a five o'clock shadow. The pockets of his short white jacket bulged with dog-eared papers and booklets.

"Hello gentlemen; my esteemed medical student, Mr. Zunin here, has told me your stories and shown me your x-rays. Sounds like you both have acutely inflamed joints without any known injury." Both men nodded in agreement.

Dr. Godot continued: "I guess the bottom line is that we need to take some fluid out of those hot joints to confirm your diagnoses and start both of you on appropriate treatments. Are you ready?" The men exchanged weary glances and then slowly nodded.

"The joint fluid analysis and culture will rule out infection as a possible cause. But it is our good friend, the polarizing microscope, that will confirm my suspicions. I think one of you has gout and the other has pseudogout."

The men again looked at each other with wrinkled foreheads and then turned back to the doctor. Dr. Godot began, "Allow me to explain. On acute presentation, gout and pseudogout can be difficult to distinguish clinically. Both types of crystal arthritis tend to occur in men who are middle-aged and older, and suddenly affect a single joint, which makes weight-bearing impossible if the lower limb is affected. Attacks can be triggered by an injury, surgery, or drugs or they may just occur spontaneously." Both men nodded in agreement about the surprising, unexplained onset of their problems.

Dr. Godot turned to Mr. Zunin "I suspect the synovial fluid analysis will show an inflammatory reaction—the white blood cell count can be quite high, up to 50,000 or more. When fever, leukocytosis, and an elevated sedimentation rate are also present, these findings can be easily mistaken for septic arthritis. The definitive diagnosis of gout or pseudogout can be established only by a special microscopic examination of the synovial fluid. When properly aligned in polarized light, the urate crystals of gout are yellow and needle shaped. In contrast, the calcium pyrophosphate crystals of pseudogout are blue and rectangular in the proper orientation."

NOTE: *Don't be fooled by a laboratory report from a synovial fluid analysis that comments "no crystals observed." Talk to the laboratory technician or pathologist and make sure the specimen was analyzed under polarizing light (most often it was not), or whenever possible, look at it yourself.*

Dr. Godot held the x-rays up for all to see. "X-ray films are sometimes helpful," she said. Turning toward Marcus she explained: "In gout, discrete, punched-out periarticular defects in the bone may be present, and the big toe is frequently the first joint to act up." Directing her remarks to Mr. Blake, she continued: "In pseudogout, calcifications of cartilage are present; and large peripheral joints such as the wrist, knee, and ankle are more likely to be. . . ."

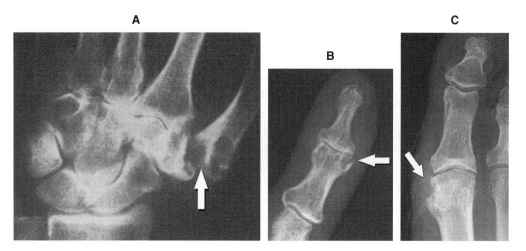

Gout causes punched-out lytic bone defects with characteristic overhanging borders adjacent to joints. **A,** Note the lesions at the base of the thumb metacarpal and trapezium. **B** and **C,** Periarticular punched-out lesions at the distal **(B)** and proximal **(C)** interphalangeal joints of the great toe.

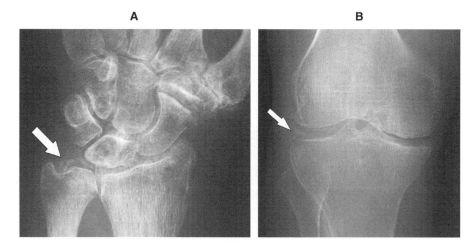

Pseudogout can be distinguished from osteoarthritis on x-ray films if calcification of cartilaginous structures is present. **A,** In this radiograph of the wrist, the triangular fibrocartilage in the ulnocarpal interval shows such changes. **B,** Note the faint calcification of the lateral meniscus of the knee, as well as the early degenerative changes including joint space narrowing and marginal osteophyte formation.

"Hey, I resent being called a pseudo," interrupted Mr. Blake. "It's not like I'm faking all this."

"Well, doctors have known about gout for hundreds of years. It has a genetic tendency. But only more recently have we understood that other types of crystal deposits can cause a gout-like picture. If you prefer, pseudogout can be called calcium pyrophosphate deposition or chondrocalcinosis."

"I like that better," Mr. Blake replied.

With the joint fluid specimens in hand, the doctor and the medical student headed for the laboratory. Dr. Godot continued, "Uric acid is formed by the oxidative degradation of purine bases, but unfortunately it has a relatively limited solubility. At serum concentrations above 7 mg/dl, crystals can precipitate. People over the age of 30 with chronically elevated levels of 10 mg/dl or greater have more than a 90% likelihood of developing gout. There are basically two ways that levels can get that high—overproduction or underexcretion or uric acid—although the latter is most often responsible.

Overproducers usually have heritable disorders of purine metabolism but may have increased nucleic acid turnover caused by conditions such as chronic hemolysis, leukemia, or multiple myeloma. More common, however, is an underlying underexcretion of uric acid due to renal insufficiency. There are also several drugs that impair renal excretion of uric acid, including aspirin, thiazide diuretics, niacin, and of course our favorite, ethanol. Purine-rich foods such as red meat, certain organ meats (most notably liver), game fowl, and seafood can trigger attacks as well. And just to confuse things, it is not uncommon for a patient to recall some type of trauma to the affected joint prior to the acute attack. In any case, the precipitated urate crystals are engulfed by leukocytes, which then incite an intense inflammatory response."

"So why can't we just measure a serum uric acid level?"

"Well, we can, but the information it provides is often not very useful, at least in the acute setting. Although the magnitude and duration of hyperuricemia do correlate with the development of gouty arthritis, fewer than 25% of hyperuricemic patients ever develop gout. Conversely, as many as 10% of patients will have normal uric acid levels at the time of the attack. So, as we will talk about, uric acid levels are helpful in following a patient's response to treatment, but they don't offer much in terms of acute diagnosis.

"Asymptomatic hyperuricemia classically precedes by 20 or 30 years the first acute attack, which may affect the synovial fluid in either a joint or a bursa. Classically it's the metatarsophalangeal joint of the great toe that is first affected. The pain is characteristically described as so intense that even the weight of a simple bed sheet on the toe is unbearable. Some patients never have a second attack, and some will progress immediately to chronic tophaceous gout. The vast majority of patients, however, will recover fully after days to weeks—even without treatment—to have a second episode within a year. Eventually, chronic polyarticular urate deposits known as tophi develop, and kidney stones and other forms of renal dysfunction become problematic."

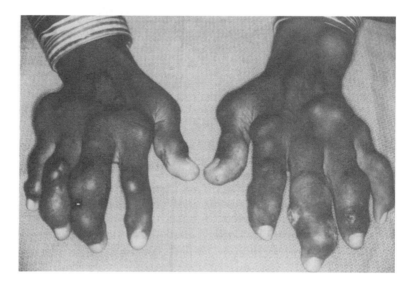

Example of long-standing tophaceous gout. Urate deposits have accumulated around multiple joints as well as in tenosynovial locations.

"So what about pseudogout?" queried the medical student.

"It's a disease of later life that is characterized by the deposition of calcium pyrophosphate crystals in the soft tissues, most notably hyaline cartilage, synovium, and menisci. Although the etiology remains unclear, it is often attributed to degradation of phosphate compounds in association with physical and biochemical changes of the aging cartilage. In most cases the natural history is that of progressive arthritis, virtually indistinguishable from osteoarthritis. X-rays showing calcification of the fibrocartilage in the wrist, symphysis pubis, or knee menisci are pathognomonic, however. In addition to this chronic degeneration, acute attacks can also occur, and that is when analysis of joint fluid may be necessary to differentiate it from gout or septic arthritis. Let's go talk to these men."

"How are we going to treat them? They both seem pretty miserable."

"If their stomachs are up to it, a short course of nonsteroidal antiinflammatory medication usually suffices for both conditions.

If not, a cortisone injection into the joint can calm things down. Colchicine can also be helpful should nonsteroidal antiinflammatory drugs or steroids be contraindicated, although its use can be limited by the nausea and vomiting it often causes."

PRINCIPLE: Begin treatment with modalities that have the highest benefit-to-risk ratio.

"Any other way to prevent future attacks?"

"Not much can be done for calcium pyrophosphate deposition disease, but for gout we can reduce production, increase excretion, or both. That type of management falls outside the expertise of most orthopedists, but it basically includes institution of a low-purine diet, avoidance of heavy alcohol intake, and drug management, if necessary."

"I remember now from pharmacology that allopurinol blocks purine metabolism, so less uric acid is formed. And don't drugs like probenecid prevent uric acid reabsorption in the renal tubules?"

"That's right. Glad to see you applying information like that. But it's also important to remember that treatments to lower serum urate levels can somewhat ironically trigger additional attacks, at least in the short term. It seems that changes in the serum level, rather than the absolute level itself, are what often precipitate acute episodes. For this reason it is best not to start these medications until after an acute flare has resolved."

"Gentlemen, we're back and we have answers. Mr. Zunin will tell each of you about your condition, and I will get a prescription pad. My crystal ball tells me you both will feel much better in the morning."

SYNOVIAL FLUID ANALYSIS IN COMMON FORMS OF ARTHRITIS:

	Normal	Noninflammatory (osteoarthritis)	Inflammatory (crystal arthritis)	Septic arthritis
Color	Clear	Light yellow, clear	Yellow, translucent	Brown, opaque
Viscosity	High	High	Low	Low
WBC/mm^3	<200	200-3000	3000-50,000	>50,000
PMNs	<25%	<25%	>50%	>75%
Gram stain	(−)	(−)	(−)	Often positive
Crystals			(+) in gout/pseudogout	

WBC = white blood count; PMNs = polymorphonuclear lymphocytes.
Modified from Munoz G, Raycraft EW. Septic arthritis. eMedicine Clinical Knowledge Database, 2003.

ADVANCED READING

Cardenosa G, DeLuca SA. Radiographic features of gout. Am Fam Physician 41:539-542, 1990.

Concoff AL, Kalunian KC. What is the relation between crystals and osteoarthritis? Curr Opin Rheumatol 11:436-440, 1999.

Roubenoff R. Gout and hyperuricemia. Rheum Dis Clin North Am 16:539-550, 1990.

Ryan LM. Calcium pyrophosphate dihydrate crystal deposition. In Klippel JH, ed. Primer on the Rheumatic Disease, 11th ed. Atlanta: Arthritis Foundation, 1997.

Sack K. Monarthritis: Differential diagnosis. Am J Med 102:30S-34S, 1997.

Swan A, Amer H, Dieppe P. The value of synovial fluid analysis in the diagnosis of joint disease: A literature survey. Ann Rheum Dis 61:493-498, 2002.

Terkeltaub RA. Clinical practice. Gout. N Engl J Med 349:1647-1655, 2003.

◆ *How can some people with arthritic joints or healed fractures recognize an impending change in the weather?*

13

The FOOSH Family

After an unexpected ice storm, four patients in the emergency room, ages 6, 11, 17, and 70, give precisely the same history. Each slipped while walking across a parking lot and **F**ell **O**nto his or her **O**ut**S**tretched **H**and—FOOSH! Each notes wrist pain and limited motion. The 17-year-old landed equally hard on both wrists and complains of pain bilaterally. Is it likely that they all have the same type of injury?

The distal neurovascular status of each is normal. You note tenderness in the wrist area of each patient. The following x-rays are available.

Wrist fracture patterns characteristic of individuals of different ages. Large arrow indicates the fracture line. Small arrows indicate active growth plates. **A,** Torus fracture: Young children. **B,** Epiphyseal plate fracture: Older children. **C,** Scaphoid fracture: Young adults.

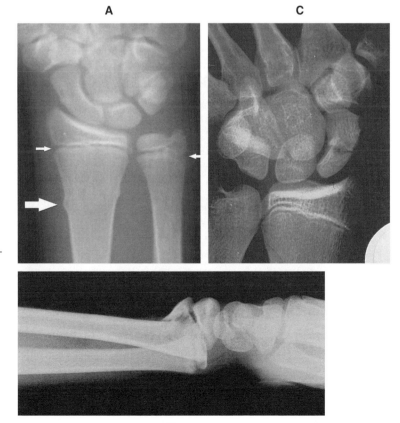

A   C

B

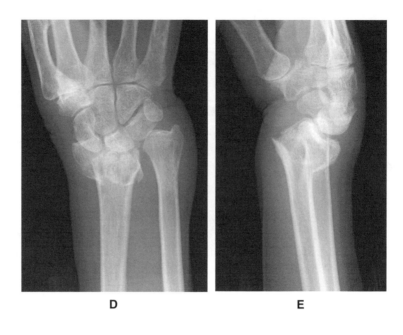

D and **E,** Distal radius fracture: Elderly adults.

D   E

✦   ✦   ✦

Despite a similar mechanism, each patient sustained a different type of skeletal injury because the "weak link" in the skeleton varies with age.

P R I N C I P L E :   The same injury mechanism may well produce age-specific injuries.

In young children the joint capsule is lax and supple, and the cartilaginous epiphyseal growth plate is stronger than the bone. Bone at this young age is somewhat supple, so an angularly direct-ed force such as in a FOOSH injury merely buckles one side of the bone, resulting in a torus fracture (known aliases: greenstick frac-ture, buckle fracture). Bones in this age group can also undergo what is referred to as plastic deformation. Exactly as it sounds, the bone can literally bend during loading without fracturing, and when the injury is severe, the bone will stay bent after the injury.

In older children the epiphyseal plate is weaker than the bone. FOOSH injuries now cause skeletal disruption through the growth plate. Five general patterns of epiphyseal injuries are recognized.

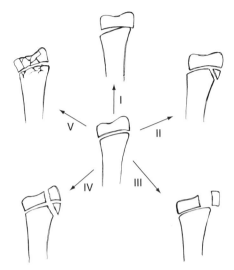

Patterns of fractures involving the physes (growth plates) at the ends of immature bones. Which type is evident on the radiograph (overleaf) of the 11-year-old?

It is also important to realize that the ligaments surrounding joints in children are much stronger than both the growth plate and surrounding bone. This is true throughout the immature skeleton. Thus it is far more likely for a child to sustain a fracture through a growth plate than to sustain a ligamentous injury, which is common in adults. Thus a diagnosis of a ligament sprain in a child should be viewed with skepticism, and further investigation for occult fracture should be undertaken.

The epiphysis of the distal radius closes in girls at about age 16 and in boys several years later. The radius becomes stronger, and the adjacent scaphoid is now the weakest link, so a FOOSH injury can occur here in teenagers and young adults. Scaphoid fractures are not always easy to see on x-ray examination because the scaphoid lies obliquely to the planes of both posteroanterior and lateral wrist x-rays and because the fracture line through the scaphoid may lie in yet another plane.

Not every impact on the heel of the hand results in a fracture, of course. Ligamentous disruptions occur, especially in young adults when the bone is strongest. Minor tearing of the supporting capsule is what is commonly known as a sprain. Major ligamentous disruptions may result in a perilunate dislocation in which many or all of the ligaments between the carpal bones and lunate are disrupted. Intervening degrees of disruption, however, may be difficult to diagnose and require special studies such as MRI and arthroscopy. Most commonly, injury to the scapholunate ligament occurs. Although in its more severe forms, this injury can be diagnosed rather easily on x-rays by a widening of the space between the scaphoid and the lunate, its less severe forms have more subtle presentations. In fact, it is not uncommon for a young adult to sustain a ligamentous injury that causes only a dynamic instability—that is, it does not appear on static x-rays but causes instability with wrist motion or loading. Somewhat analogous to a scaphoid fracture, these injuries can disrupt the normal patterns of carpal motion, causing abnormal loading patterns within the wrist joints and premature degenerative arthritis.

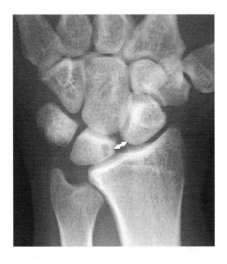

Scapholunate dissociation. Note the widened interval between the scaphoid and lunate *(arrow)*, which is indicative of this ligamentous injury.

With advancing age, osteoporosis gradually reduces the bone density of the distal radius, again rendering it the most vulnerable site in a FOOSH injury. This fracture of the distal 1 inch of the radius with apex palmar angulation was first described by Abraham Colles in 1814 and bore his name for many years. With recognition of numerous other slightly different fracture patterns at the distal radius, the eponym "war" became so furious that the trend now is just to call them all distal radius fractures and describe the exact pattern of the fracture lines.

Treatment of the greenstick fracture consists of casting to protect the limb from additional injury during the time required for healing. At this age, growing bone heals quite rapidly, and if there is no tenderness at the fracture site at 3 weeks, the cast may be left off.

PRINCIPLE: Tenderness at the site of a healing fracture is an excellent clinical sign of persistent inflammation, hence incomplete healing. Thus the presence of fracture-line tenderness usually dictates further protection of the limb.

Most physeal fractures of the distal radius are type I or II. The desire for anatomic reduction must be balanced against the risk of further damage to the growth plate and possible growth arrest caused by multiple manipulations. With muscle relaxation and analgesia, longitudinal traction and wrist flexion can achieve anatomic or near-anatomic reduction. A long-arm cast (from axilla to mid-palm) worn for 4 weeks usually suffices. Residual angular deformity adjacent to an open growth plate will remodel with further growth when the deformity is in the plane of major motion of the adjacent joint. Deformities in the two planes perpendicular to the motion will not correct as well with remodeling. In this patient, any slight undercorrection of the anterior apex will correct with further growth, so here it is safer not to struggle for a perfect reduction.

PRINCIPLE: Perfect is the enemy of good.

The scaphoid serves as an important link between the proximal and distal rows of carpal bones. With injury to this link, the resulting abnormal carpal motion gradually results in degenerative arthritis. Since scaphoid fractures occur in young adults, anatomic reduction and healing are important, not so much for short-term function, but to preclude degenerative arthritis 10 to 20 years later. The scaphoid is covered on nearly all surfaces by cartilage, and its nutrient arteries are sparse. Consequently the blood supply to the proximal pole may be disrupted after fracture, resulting in an avascular necrosis and possibly collapse of the proximal aspect of the scaphoid. Ninety-five percent of scaphoid fractures will eventually heal, but prolonged immobilization may be required because of the poor blood supply. Twelve to 16 weeks in a thumb spica cast may be required for healing. (Irrelevant fact: Spica means "ear of wheat" in Latin, and some poet saw the resemblance of the overlapping layers in a spica cast to a head of wheat.)

PRINCIPLE: Bone is living tissue despite its hard and somewhat inert appearance. It has a blood supply that is critical to its health and healing capacity.

Rigid screw fixation for undisplaced fractures probably does not significantly reduce the healing time, but it does allow the patient to go without a cast, which would be particularly important to surgeons and dentists. When a scaphoid fracture is displaced or angulated, operative intervention is routinely advised to achieve anatomic reduction, promote healing, and minimize the risk of degenerative arthritis.

Distal radius fractures in elderly adults disturb the normal alignment of the hand on the forearm, a deformity likened to the curve of a fork. (It is called the "silver fork deformity," although steel and plastic forks are shaped identically.) Not only is the deformity unsightly, but wrist flexion and consequently a large portion of hand function can be lost. Thus anatomic reduction and healing are sought, even more so when the fracture is comminuted with irregularity of the articular surface of the distal radius. This goal is frequently achieved by closed manipulation and splinting followed in several days by casting after local swelling has subsided. Premature placement of circumferential plaster risks vascular compromise from associated soft tissue swelling. At times percutaneous pinning, external fixation, or open reduction with internal fixation may be required to achieve and maintain the desired reduction. Open reduction and rigid internal fixation allow for early wrist motion and, providing that the fixation holds the osteoporotic bone fragments securely, complications of immobilization are obviated. Complications after Colles' fractures abound and include malunion; restricted forearm, wrist, and finger joint motion; median nerve compression; reflex sympathetic dystrophy; and loss of forearm rotation due to disruption of the distal radioulnar joint. Despite the layman's impression that "it's just a wrist fracture," most persons with Colles' fractures are left with some residual dysfunction.

Follow-up Note: Despite enforced hand elevation and loosening of the splint applied after reduction in the emergency room, the 70-year-old woman with the distal radius fracture complains of increasing pain and decreasing sensation in the fingertips. Repeat sensory examination shows loss of two-point discrimination in the median nerve distribution, a distinct change from the original neurovascular check. Emergency carpal tunnel release is required to relieve the progressive median nerve compression.

The 17-year-old was initially placed in bilateral thumb spica casts for an obvious scaphoid fracture on the right side and a possible scaphoid fracture on the left. On examination 3 weeks later with the cast removed, the left scaphoid area is entirely nontender, and x-rays show no fracture. Thus, by process of elimination, this patient had a wrist sprain on the left, which healed with 3 weeks' immobilization. The scaphoid fracture on the right side took 14 weeks to heal.

The two children were out of their casts and back to full activities within a month.

From sharing their common adversities, these four patients became friends. Now, 6 months later, they invite you to a roller skating party.

ADVANCED READING

Barton NJ. The late consequences of scaphoid fractures. J Bone Joint Surg Br 86:626-630, 2004.

Colles A. On the fracture of the carpal extremity of the radius. Edinb Med Surg J 10:182-186, 1814.

Cooney WP III. Scaphoid fractures: Current treatments and techniques. Instr Course Lect 52:197-208, 2003.

Crawford AH. Pitfalls and complications of fractures of the distal radius and ulna in childhood. Hand Clin 4:403-413, 1988.

Flynn JM. Pediatric forearm fractures: Decision making, surgical techniques, and complications. Instr Course Lect 51:355-360, 2002.

Noonan KJ, Price CT. Forearm and distal radius fractures in children. J Am Acad Orthop Surg 6:146-156, 1998.

Ruch DS, Weiland AJ, Wolfe SW, et al. Current concepts in the treatment of distal radial fractures. Instr Course Lect 53:389-401, 2004.

Simic PM, Weiland AJ. Fractures of the distal aspect of the radius: Changes in treatment over the past two decades. Instr Course Lect 52:185-195, 2003.

✦ *Could you manage perineal hygiene if your wrist was stiff in a 60-degree extended position? Is your grip strength greater with your wrist extended or flexed? Why? If you had to have your wrist fused, what position would be best?*

14

Lunch

"Sure you can sit here. Most people take one look at me in my wheelchair with my hand jerking around, and zoom, off they go. Sometimes I'm treated with condescension, hollered at like I don't understand English, or shunned like I'm contagious. Intolerant strangers on the phone have rudely told me to call back when I was sober, but I'm told that with a little effort anybody can understand me. You know, there's a sensitive human being trapped here inside this body with bad wiring. While you eat your lunch, let me tell you what it's like to have cerebral palsy (CP). It will make you a better doctor.

"As you may know, CP is the most common physical disability of childhood onset. For every 1000 children, there are two or three of us. The primary symptom—you can't miss it—is the movement disorder. It results from nonprogressive damage to the immature central nervous system. The list of potential causes is quite long, but most often the actual cause is unknown. Prenatal or neonatal hypoxia is frequently thought to be contributory, as is prematurity itself. For instance, I weighed 2 kg at birth; and for all premature infants, the lower the birth weight, the higher the risk of CP.

"Of course, Mom didn't know that at the time, and her first concern wasn't until I was 9 months old and was still having trouble sitting unsupported. Dr. Eldridge had noted my floppiness, persistent infantile reflexes, and delayed motor development much earlier but didn't want to alarm Mom until she was sure, because initial neurologic abnormalities sometimes resolve. The floppiness was gradually replaced by spasticity, and by my first birthday Mom noted rigidity in my limbs when she was bathing and dressing me. By age 3 I could finally sit independently, and Mom remembers that I never crawled on my hands and knees but instead kept my trunk on the floor and sort of rowed with my limbs. When I finally started walking at about 6 years of age, I walked on my tiptoes with my knees banging. I would quickly wear out the toes of my shoes and the inside knee area on my trousers from all the scraping and rubbing.

"People call it a lurching, drunken gait. But that's the way I've always walked. It isn't painful, so I don't think anything about it. I walk normally as far as I'm concerned, just like I'm sure you think you walk normally too, though I do get winded easily. Dr. Eldridge says my gait requires great energy expenditure, so as I've gotten older, I rely on my electric wheelchair if I'm out of the house.

"The electric wheelchair and Velcro hook and loop fasteners are the two greatest inventions as far as I'm concerned. You should see me wrestle shoestrings or try to button a collar. With Velcro I can completely dress myself.

"I have the common spastic form of CP. A spastic muscle is one that tightens up rather than relaxes when it's stretched because of an exaggerated muscle stretch reflex. This results from an imbalance of inhibitory and facilitory centers in the midbrain and brainstem. Ironically, when I want to show my best behavior, my limbs totally fly out of control. Other times, when I couldn't care less, they can be quite relaxed and steady. Spastic quadriplegia means that all of one's limbs are affected, hemiplegia involves an arm and a leg on one side only, and diplegia affects just the lower limbs.

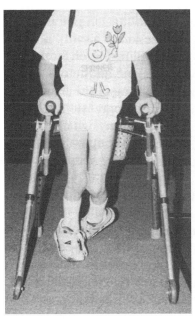 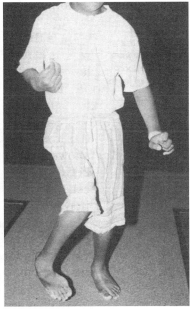

Which patient has the spastic, diplegic form of cerebral palsy, and which one has spastic hemiplegia?

"In the athetoid form of CP, the affected person has constant, uncontrollable movements; fortunately this form is now much less common because preventive treatments for neonatal isoimmunization and bilirubin encephalopathy are available.

"Some people with CP are mentally retarded, but the rest of us are not. And regardless, all of us have aspirations, just like you. Strong family support and personal determination can help anyone, but those of us with CP also benefit from care by a specialty team with expertise in pediatrics, orthopedics, neurosurgery, physical, occupational, and speech therapies, vocational counseling, and so forth. Specialists now have even more expertise and more sophisticated techniques than when I was growing up, so the development of progressive joint contractures and painful dislocations can usually be prevented.

"If spastic muscles, such as elbow and wrist flexors, hip adductors, and knee and ankle flexors, aren't regularly and systematically stretched, particularly during the rapid growth phases of childhood, the bones outgrow them. This further tightens already spastic muscles and can result in fixed joint contractures.

"Physical therapy and nighttime splinting can help keep muscles stretched and joints supple, but often tendon division, elongation, or transfer is necessary to provide lasting benefit. For instance, I had my Achilles tendons lengthened so I could put my feet flat on the ground. Before resorting to surgery, however, many doctors will try casting with muscles in a stretched position. Some are using botulism toxin—you know, botox. Yeah, that same stuff all the Hollywood types use to look pretty. Well, it can be put to real use for our spastic muscles. A couple of injections can relax our muscles enough so that the physical therapists can work out developing contractures before they become fixed deformities.

"There are other medications that people have been trying to help relieve severe spasticity—baclofen is probably the most common. It is certainly not a cure-all, but it does help. The problem is that it tends to have some pesky side effects at the high doses we need to loosen our muscles. Some doctors are now actually implanting small pumps to deliver the baclofen right where it is needed in the spinal fluid. That way they can achieve very high local doses without the systemic side effects.

"When it does come to surgery to treat spastic contractures and improve gait, a systematic approach is helpful. Sometimes, as in my case, it's pretty simple and there are only one or two spastic muscles that need to be lengthened. However, it can get complicated pretty quickly when you have spastic contractures in several joints involving multiple muscle groups. Now preoperative gait analysis using electromyography and computers with specialized three-dimensional motion analysis software has been developed to facilitate surgical planning. These sophisticated techniques allow the doctors to determine precisely which muscles are most involved and to identify muscles that contract asynchronously and disrupt gait. Correcting the abnormalities at all joints in the lower limbs at one surgical session greatly enhances the rehabilitation potential. For ambulatory individuals this means correction of abnormal posture and gait, which results in more efficient walking. Even for those who are nonambulatory, timely release of spastic hip flexors and adductors, possibly along with osteotomies to ensure firm seating of the femoral head in the acetabulum, precludes the natural progression to a painful hip dislocation.

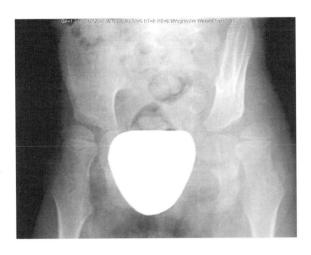

Pelvic radiograph of a patient with spastic diplegic cerebral palsy. Note the lateral subluxation of the left hip and, to a lesser extent, the right hip. Early release of spastic hip flexors and adductors may prevent these deformities.

P R I N C I P L E :   Since many muscles cross more than one joint, rebalancing the forces at one joint has implications for control of joints proximally and distally.

"Selective posterior rhizotomy, which means partial sectioning of the dorsal sensory rootlets to the spinal cord, is a more invasive procedure that can significantly reduce spasticity in some patients. It improves the balance between the facilitory and inhibitory control of the anterior horn cells, and apparently because of substantial overlap in the distribution of sensory nerves, no sensibility is lost.

"That's all pretty technical, and certainly concerns with physical disabilities are important, but so are emotional and social needs. A variety of educational, recreational, and social activities helps all of us develop confidence, self-image, social skills, and emotional resiliency. So if you choose orthopedics, you'll need help from other specialists to treat the patient with CP as a whole.

"And you *have* been a patient listener. One more thing: this fork is too dangerous for me. If you could pass me that spoon, I'll eat my lunch, and you can tell me about yourself."

ADVANCED READING

Brown C. My Left Foot. London: Mandarin Press, 1989.

Davids JR, Ounpuu S, DeLuca PA, et al. Optimization of walking ability of children with cerebral palsy. Instr Course Lect 53:511-522, 2004.

Gray D. On My Own Feet. The Autobiography of a Spastic. London: Max Parrish, 1964.

Karol LA. Surgical management of the lower extremity in ambulatory children with cerebral palsy. J Am Acad Orthop Surg 12:196-203, 2004.

Koman LA, Smith BP, Shilt JS. Cerebral palsy. Lancet 363:1619-1631, 2004.

Little WJ. On the influence of abnormal parturition, difficult labours, premature birth, and asphyxia neonatorum on the mental and physical condition of the child, especially in relation to deformities. Trans Obstet Soc Lond 3:253, 1862.

Manske PR. Cerebral palsy of the upper extremity. Hand Clin 6:697-709, 1990.

Osler W. The Cerebral Palsies in Children. London: HK Lewis, 1889.

Pidcock FS. The emerging role of therapeutic botulinum toxin in the treatment of cerebral palsy. J Pediatr 145:S33-S35, 2004.

✦ *Is your leg the same as your lower limb? Is your arm the same as your upper limb?*

15

The Long Fly Ball

Karl Christoffersen ✦ *Scott A. Mitchell* ✦ *Roy A. Meals*

"Leanne Ray! You again? Let me guess, knee or shoulder?"

"Knee, but don't worry; it's not the one you operated on. It's the right one this time. I was playing softball on the Fourth with the new residents. Radiology residents are supposed to be multidimensional, you know, so I really dug in at the plate, and on the first pitch, I gave it all I had. As my body came around with the bat, I felt a sharp pain in my right knee. Didn't really feel a pop like last time, though, and it didn't swell up right away either. But good thing I hit it into the woods because it was all I could do to hobble around the bases. I managed to finish the game but definitely at half speed. The knee gradually swelled up over the next several days, but it hasn't been particularly painful. Now and then it catches just for a second, but other than that, the movement has been OK."

"I wish everyone could give me such a good history: exact mechanism of injury, level of subsequent disability, degree of pain and swelling, other findings. Have you had any trouble with the right knee before?"

"No, but you remember the left: anterior cruciate ligament, medial meniscus, and medial collateral ligament—ended my intramural football career."

"Any other injuries or problems with your health?"

"Just my shoulder dislocation from rugby. That doesn't bother me at all now, but it took 2 years. What do you think is wrong with my knee?"

"Let's have a look. I'll tell you what I'm doing in case you come to your senses and decide to do an orthopedic residency when you finish radiology. See the effusion? I can push it back and forth under the patella from one side to the other. Also, see how the effusion has lifted the patella off the femoral condyles when your leg is straight? I can push right on the patella and feel it bob up and down—kind of like it's floating from the effusion. Looks like you may already have a little quadriceps atrophy too. That can come on really quickly after a knee injury. I'll measure your thigh circumferences in a minute. As I recall, you fully regained the strength in your left quadriceps after the surgery."

"Finally. It took about 8 months. Ouch! That hurts."

"It seems like the most tender area is right at the joint line medially. The collateral ligaments aren't tender . . ."

"Wait, how can you tell that the collaterals aren't tender if there is joint line pain medially or laterally? That is right where they cross."

"Sometimes it can be a little tough, but remember the collaterals originate from the femoral condyles and insert distally onto the tibia and fibula. Usually if they are injured, there will be tenderness just above and below the joint line over these attachments as well. Now of course with severe collateral ligament injury, the knee will begin to open up with varus or valgus stress. In your case, though, the collaterals are stable to stress, even with the knee flexed a little."

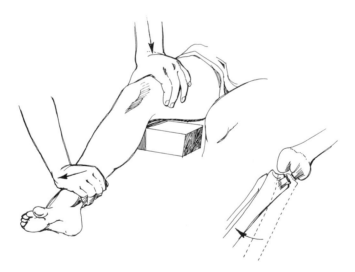

Test the stability of the medial collateral ligament with the knee flexed 20 degrees.

"What does that mean?"

"I guess you don't remember what happened with your other injury. Even with your medial collateral ligament out, your knee was stable to medial and lateral stresses when it was fully extended. Only with 20-degree knee flexion was the ligament instability evident. That's because in full extension the posterior capsule and cruciate ligaments are tight and mask the medial collateral ligament deficiency. OK, let's check the other two major supporting ligaments of your knee."

"The cruciate ligaments. I remember from before. With my knee partially flexed, you could practically pull my tibia right out from under the condyles of my femur. That sure felt weird."

"Right; and with the less common posterior cruciate tear, the tibia subluxes posteriorly on the femoral condyles. The drawer test, both at 20 and 90 degrees, looks fine.

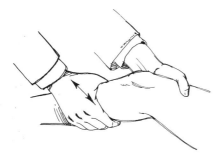

Test the integrity of the anterior and posterior cruciate ligaments with the knee flexed 20 degrees.

"If your anterior cruciate was torn, I'd check next for associated capsular injury by doing the pivot shift test. I'll show you. With your knee extended and straining the medial collateral ligament with a valgus stress, I internally rotate your tibia on your femur to try to get the tibia to sublux anteriorly. Then I slowly flex your knee. Ah, good, nothing happens.

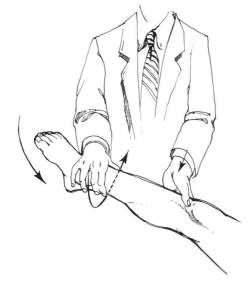

The pivot shift test starts with the knee extended and valgus and internal rotation stresses applied. A palpable clunk during knee flexion denotes laxity of the anterior cruciate ligament and joint capsule.

"If you had anterolateral instability, the subluxed tibia would reduce on the lateral femoral condyle with a clunk at about 20 to 40 degrees of knee flexion."

"What are you doing now? Ouch! I felt something pop."

"That's McMurray's test—extending the flexed knee with an internal or external rotational force on the tibia, almost the opposite of the pivot shift test—but this one's looking for meniscal tears.

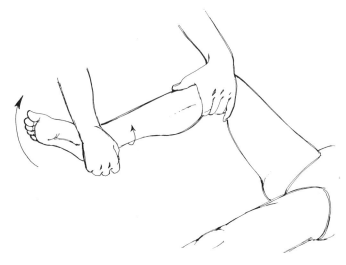

McMurray's test for meniscal tears axially rotates the tibia on the femur during knee extension.

Modified from the American Orthopaedic Association. Manual of Orthopaedic Surgery, 6th ed. Chicago: American Orthopaedic Association, 1985, p 89.

"The maneuver tries to momentarily catch the corner of a torn meniscus between the tibial and femoral joint surfaces, and it clicks when it pops out. Now most meniscal tears won't produce that classic click; rather the patient will just experience discomfort. But if you do feel a click, you can be pretty certain there is a meniscal tear. Now a bucket-handle tear. . . ."

"Ooh, I remember now. I've seen bucket-handle tears on MRI; they can get caught between the femoral condyle and the tibial plateau and keep the knee from reaching full extension."

"Precisely. We call that 'locking.' That doesn't seem to be your problem though. Your four major ligaments are stable, your only tenderness is right over the medial meniscus, and McMurray's test is positive. Now the best way to truly confirm a meniscal tear is by diagnostic arthroscopy. That's fairly invasive, though, so we usually don't like to jump to that right away. We have used arthrography for years to identify meniscal tears because injected dye will leak into any defects. It does require an injection and a few people are allergic to the iodine in the radiopaque dye. MRI has largely replaced it—no injection is required, and cuts at various levels through the knee improve visualization of many types of soft tissue pathology. It reliably predicts most meniscal tears, although it is by no means perfect. In your case, though, I think it's the logical next step."

Examples:
Sagittal **(A)** and coronal **(B)** MRI views revealing a tear through the posterior horn of the medial meniscus. The normal meniscus should appear uniformly black on MRI images. Note the linear streak of higher signal intensity in the region of the tear.

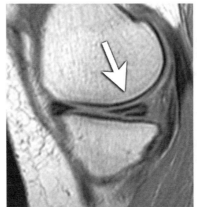 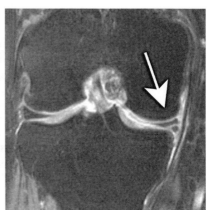

A   **B**

Peripheral tear of the posterior horn of the lateral meniscus. On a sagittal cut through the knee, how can you tell if you are looking at the medial or lateral compartment? Think about the different shape of the medial and lateral tibial plateaus.

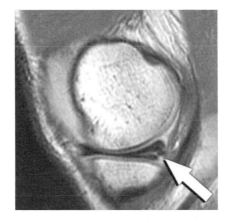

Complex degenerative tear of the posterior horn of the medial meniscus. Note the abnormal streaks of high signal extending throughout the posterior horn.

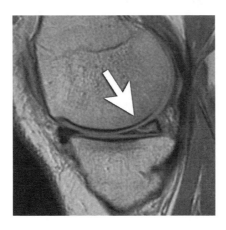

One Week Later

"Well, it looks like we were right. MRI shows a radial tear through the anterior aspect of the medial meniscus."

"Yeah, that's what I thought. I sneaked a look at the images as they were coming up on the computer right after I finished the scan. Of course I still wanted to get your professional opinion."

"Thanks, I think."

"So what's next?"

"Well, there are a couple of things I should tell you about meniscal tears before we decide on the best way to proceed. As I'm sure you know, the menisci are semilunar wedges of fibrocartilage covering approximately two thirds of the medial and lateral tibial plateaus. They increase the conformity between the rounded femoral condyles and the relatively flat tibial plateau, and they play a crucial role in shock absorption, load distribution, joint gliding, and stability. They are also important for the transmission of loads across the knee joint—as much as 50% with the knee in extension and even more in flexion. So you can probably guess that the best thing to do is preserve the meniscus, something that orthopedists have slowly come to realize. Unfortunately, however, it's not quite that simple."

"No surprise there. You guys like to complicate things even more than radiologists like to hedge."

"Point taken, but just indulge me a bit longer. As I was saying, the majority of the meniscus is avascular, and like articular cartilage depends on diffusion and mechanical pumping to provide an influx of nutrients. However, the peripheral margins of the meniscus (approximately 25%) are well vascularized. This vascularity is the primary determinant of the healing capacity of meniscal tears and serves as the basis for treatment decisions. Tears that occur in the poorly vascularized central regions have very limited healing capacity and are best treated by a simple debridement. Peripheral tears, however, have a greater chance of healing because they have a blood supply, so they are often amenable to some type of repair.

"I should also add that not all meniscal tears will require surgery, and certainly a trial of conservative treatment with activity modification, antiinflammatory medications, and a course of physical therapy to maintain strength and motion is justified. If a tear becomes asymptomatic with these measures, then it is best left alone. If, however, symptoms persist, or in the case of some elite athletes where a period of observation may be unacceptable, then arthroscopy is the next step. At that point, the tear pattern can be assessed and a debridement or repair as indicated can be performed."

"So let's go for it. I've got my softball career to think about."

PRINCIPLE: Except in a few emergency situations, nonoperative treatment should always be considered first in orthopedics.

Follow-up Visit

"So what did you find, Doc?"

"Just what we expected. You had an anterior horn tear of your medial meniscus—classic for your injury mechanism and your physical examination. With the scope I also had a good look at your lateral meniscus as well as the cartilage on your femoral condyles and tibial plateau. The good news is those looked perfectly healthy. Your tear was in the central avascular zone, so a repair wasn't feasible. I trimmed away the torn tissue and contoured the remaining meniscus to a stable rim, preserving as much healthy tissue as possible. So I can't say that you have a completely normally functioning meniscus, but at least your pain and mechanical symptoms should be taken care of.

Before we figured out how important the menisci were for load transmission and stabilization, torn menisci were routinely removed completely. In fact, I had my medial meniscus removed 30 years ago, and I'm beginning to get some degenerative changes. Techniques for meniscal transplantation have been developed, and even meniscal replacement with engineered tissue is in the investigational stages, but in either case the medial side of my knee is probably too far gone already for such things to help. But I digress. It's time for you to begin your quadriceps rehabilitation. Let's see a straight-leg raise; then you can go home."

"That's easy. Quite a change from when you operated on my left knee."

"Well, that side was more severely injured, and at the time the techniques for anterior cruciate reconstruction through the scope weren't so well worked out. Clearly, rehabilitation after an open arthrotomy is much longer than rehabilitation after arthroscopic surgery. Your motion on the right should be fine."

"Great. You warned me about the risk of some lost motion on the left, and I eventually recovered 120 degrees of flexion. Other than not being able to squat, it doesn't bother me, and I was never much of a catcher anyway. Do you think I'll be ready for some softball on Labor Day?"

"Should be, if you do your exercises and don't break your neck or something in the meantime."

ADVANCED READING

Arendt EA, ed. Orthopaedic Knowledge Update: Sports Medicine 2. Rosemont, IL: American Academy of Orthopaedic Surgeons, 1999.

Boyd KT, Myers PT. Meniscus preservation: Rationale, repair techniques, and results. Knee 10:1-11, 2003.

Greis PE, Holmstrom MC, Bardana DD, et al. Meniscal Injury: I. Basic science and evaluation; II. Management. J Am Acad Orthop Surg 10:168-187, 2002.

McMurray TP. Robert Jones Birthday Volume. London: Oxford University Press, 1928, p 305.

Noyes FR, Grood ES, Torzilli PA. Current concepts review. The definition and terms for motion and position of the knee and injuries of the ligaments. J Bone Joint Surg Am 71:465-472, 1989.

Woo SL, Vogrin TM, Abramowitch SD. Healing and repair of ligament injuries in the knee. J Am Acad Orthop Surg 8:364-372, 2000.

◆ *Can you sit in most theater seats with your knee fully extended? Could you walk efficiently with your knee fixed in 60 degrees of flexion? If you had to have your knee fused, what position would be best?*

16

Ruby

I heard a while back that Ruby Malinewski had suffered a mild stroke, but despite some left-sided weakness, she was still living by herself and getting around OK. This morning, however, she stumbled on one of her cats and crumpled to the kitchen floor—fortunately, not far from the phone. She requested that I see her as soon as the paramedics got her to the emergency room.

Obviously quite elderly now and more osteoporotic than ever, she was lying calmly on a gurney in the hallway outside of radiology. Her left hip didn't hurt too much, she said, as long as nobody tried to move it. Her left thigh rested in an abducted and externally rotated position, making her left lower limb appear shorter than her right.

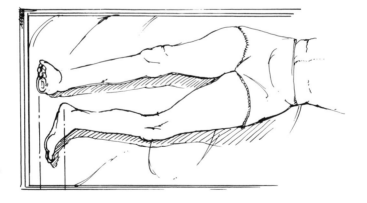

Typical shortened, externally rotated, and slightly flexed posture of the left lower limb after hip fracture.

Pulses and sensation in her feet were normal, and except for a couple of bruises, everything else checked out. The only thing left for the x-ray to show me was the level of the hip fracture, whether it was in the femoral neck or the intertrochanteric area. Fractures occur in these areas with nearly equal frequency in the elderly. A fracture in the subtrochanteric area can also occur, albeit somewhat less frequently, but it disconnects the femoral shaft from the psoas muscle, so the thigh doesn't rest in an externally rotated position.

103

Hip fractures occur more often in women than men, and Ruby's osteoporosis was certainly a contributing factor. When women reach their nineties, one third of them have had a hip fracture. When unsteadiness from a variety of causes—aging, inebriation, sedative medications, senile dementia, cardiac arrhythmias, muscle weakness, loss of close-up vision, and so forth—is added to environmental hazards such as throw rugs, bathtubs, dark hallways, glaring lights, and steps with worn carpet, it becomes a potentially lethal combination.

Knowing that the mortality rate during the first year after hip fracture is 20% and that falls are the leading cause of death due to accidents in people 75 years of age and older, I called Ruby's internist even before I had seen the x-rays. Although operating on frail, elderly people is certainly not without its risks, treating the fracture with prolonged bed rest not only ensures further wasting of muscles and bone but also heightens the chances of pressure sores, pneumonia, deep venous thrombosis, pulmonary embolism, and other complications, not to mention malunion or nonunion of the fracture itself. With modern means of internally fixing hip fractures, the goals are to operate as soon as the patient is medically stable and to mobilize the patient quickly after surgery.

Although the two most common types of hip fractures—intertrochanteric and femoral neck—occur within a few centimeters of one another, they are profoundly different from biological and biomechanical perspectives. The blood supply to the femoral head arises predominately from branches of the medial circumflex femoral artery. This artery wraps around the posterior aspect of the femoral neck before diving into the capsule of the hip joint and passing up the neck into the femoral head. With fractures through the trochanteric region, these branches are typically well preserved. However, because of this retrograde blood supply, fractures across the femoral neck, particularly displaced fractures, can disrupt these vessels, resulting in avascular necrosis of the femoral head. Further, intertrochanteric fractures occur through the broad femoral metaphysis—a region of well-vascularized cancellous bone—and are quick to heal. Femoral neck fractures, on the other hand, occur through a relatively narrow region comprised of sparsely vascularized cortical bone, which heals at a much slower rate than cancellous bone. Thus neck fractures have an inherently higher risk of nonunion in addition to the potential for avascular necrosis.

There is general consensus for surgical fixation of intertrochanteric fractures because of the high likelihood of successful union. The management of femoral neck fractures, however, remains controversial. In young patients an attempt to save the femoral head should be made by reducing and internally fixing the fracture as soon as possible in hopes of preserving any remaining blood supply. In elderly patients with a displaced fracture through the femoral neck, prosthetic replacement of the femoral head or even total hip arthroplasty is justified. This precludes the need for a second major operation should nonunion or avascular necrosis occur after fracture fixation. What defines a young versus an elderly patient remains nebulous, however. Additionally, a nondisplaced fracture through the femoral neck poses less risk of avascular necrosis or nonunion, and most surgeons prefer internal fixation regardless of age in this situation.

Needless to say, amidst all of the controversy, I was relieved that Ruby's x-rays showed an intertrochanteric fracture.

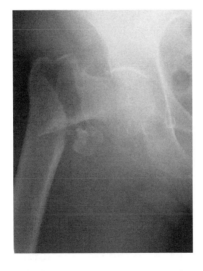

Intertrochanteric fracture of the right hip. Note the displaced lesser tuberosity fragment— an unstable fracture pattern.

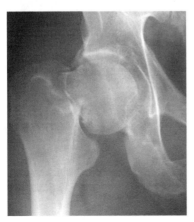

Displaced right femoral neck fracture.

Ruby's internist checked her carefully and reported that neither had she suffered another stroke nor were there any cardiac abnormalities that would preclude early surgery. I knew from dealing with Ruby before that she would have a million questions about the fracture pattern, the devices used for fixation, their biocompatibility, the need for secondary surgery, and so forth. Since the word "doctor" is derived from the word for teacher, I reserved plenty of time for our preoperative discussion so I wouldn't begrudge her any information.

I showed Ruby a sliding screw-plate device designed to stabilize intertrochanteric hip fractures. The screw threads get a firm purchase in the femoral head. The screw shank slides through a sleeve on the upper end of the plate, which fixes rigidly to the femoral shaft. Thus the device not only restores the normal varus-valgus relationship of the proximal femur, it also hastens fracture healing by allowing impaction of the fracture fragments as the screw shank slides distally and laterally through the sleeve during weight bearing. Ruby liked the idea that this concept of fixation is known as "load sharing," since some weight-bearing forces are taken up by the hardware and some by the bone. Load-bearing implants, on the other hand, take up all of the load and consequently tend to cut right out of osteoporotic bone.

PRINCIPLE: Impacted fracture fragments heal faster than bones with large gaps between the fracture fragments.

Ruby's hardest question concerned when she could go home. Of course, we were planning to begin ambulation just days after surgery, but statistics indicate that only slightly more than half of patients regain their prefracture ability to walk within a year and only a third will ever regain their prefracture level of independent living. Particularly as our population continues to age, the hospital and nursing home resources needed to deal with this injury will become a monumental public health concern.

Ruby's surgery is scheduled for first thing in the morning, and I told her I'd go feed her cats on the way in, so I'll stop for now.

A D V A N C E D   R E A D I N G

Lin JT, Lane JM. Prevention of hip fractures: Medical and nonmedical management. Instr Course Lect 53:417-425, 2004.

Lindskog DM, Baumgaertner MR. Unstable intertrochanteric hip fractures in the elderly. J Am Acad Orthop Surg 12:179-190, 2004.

Lorich DG, Geller DS, Neilson JH. Osteoporotic pertrochanteric hip fractures: Management and current controversies. Instr Course Lect 53:441-454, 2004.

Masson M, Parker MJ, Fleischer S. Internal fixation versus arthroplasty for intracapsular proximal femoral fractures in adults. Cochrane Database Syst Rev 3:CD001708, 2003.

Schmidt AH, Swiontkowski MF. Femoral neck fractures. Orthop Clin North Am 33:97-111, 2002.

17

A Cruel Poet's Curse

"Dr. Goode! There's an infant in the newborn nursery you need to see. Really strange feet."

"What do the boy's feet look like?"

"Well, it's hard to describe. It's . . . like . . . if he were old enough to stand up, the first part of his foot to touch the floor would be the outside of his little toe.

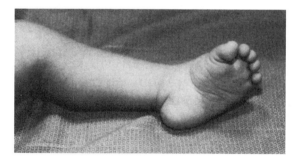

"How'd you know it's a boy, anyway?"

"Just a hunch. Let's say his feet were left as they are; how would it be walking on them?"

"Impossible. He'd never get the soles of his feet on the ground."

"Not impossible. Somerset Maugham and others have gotten by, but basically it's avoidable if treated promptly. Remember what another English author said, 'Just as the twig is bent, the tree is inclined.' We don't have much time to lose. Get some plaster so we can start bending those twigs. What do you know about his family and developmental history?"

"His family history is negative except that his father had a couple of surgeries on his right foot when he was in grade school and has always had trouble finding shoes that fit. Gestationally, both mom and the infant did fine. No known risk factors, born full term, uncomplicated delivery, weighs 8 pounds even, Apgar score of 10."

"Is this the lad? How are the results of his musculoskeletal examination overall?"

"Everything checks out except his feet. Twenty digits, symmetrical limbs and skin contours, full passive motions, hips abduct fully, and I've seen him move all his joints, but look at these feet. It looks like they got all scrunched up inside the uterus."

PRINCIPLE: Always perform a complete musculoskeletal examination in infants with any limb anomaly. There may be others.

Embryologically, limb formation occurs concurrently with multiple organs such as the heart and kidneys. Thus limb anomalies should arouse suspicion of coexisting internal anomalies.

"Fetal positioning may contribute; but remember, nearly every infant is folded up inside the same way, and clubfoot occurs only once in a thousand infants. But you do have a point, as clubfoot is commonly associated with other so-called 'packaging problems' such as developmental dysplasia of the hip and tibial torsion in which uterine positioning is thought to contribute. It isn't quite that simple though, and at one time or another, nearly every tissue in the foot has been implicated as causative, but the true cause remains enigmatic."

"You called it clubfoot. Is that like club sandwich?"

"No. I'm afraid some poet saw a likeness to a caveman's wooden club. It's rather cruel, but I think we're stuck with it. The Latin name is even worse—talipes equinovarus, which literally translates as ankle-foot-horse-turned-in."

"So what does it all mean, and how did you know this kid was a boy before I told you about him?"

"Clubfoot is twice as common in boys as in girls, so I went with the odds. You also mentioned that his family history was negative except for his father's foot problem. That might, in fact, be relevant since there is a familial tendency for the condition. It sounds like Dad may not have had a complete correction in infancy, and some palliative surgery was done later. Do you have a pen? I'll sketch the three parts to clubfoot.

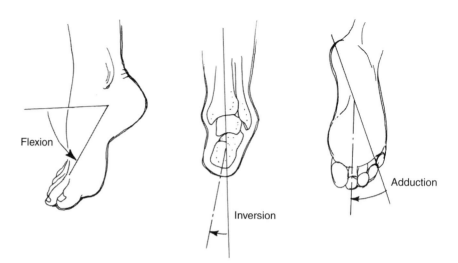

The three components of clubfoot.

"First, the ankle is held in complete plantar flexion or equinus, so called because horses walk on their toenails with their ankles completely flexed. Second, the subtalar joint is turned in, inverted, supinated, or in varus—they all essentially refer to the same thing, so the foot is under the medial malleolus. Then the midfoot is adducted, or deviated medially, and supinated. Finally, there is an increased height of the longitudinal arch of the foot, referred to as a cavus deformity. With all these different terms being thrown around, many of which are a bit redundant, I find it nice to use a simple mnemonic that one of my own professors taught me. Just think of the word 'cave.' C for *cavus,* A for *adductus* of the mid- and forefoot, V for *varus* of the hindfoot, and finally E for *equinus* of the ankle."

"What's the plaster for? Aren't you going to operate?"

"Watch. By firmly grabbing the heel and stabilizing it, I can gently push the forefoot laterally out of its adducted position. Then, by pushing up on the midfoot and rotating the heel outward, I can begin to correct the supination and varus. Now all we have to do is hold it with an artfully applied cast. Don't worry too much about the equinus for now—that comes later. First we want to stretch the foot into a better position; then we'll address the ankle. Because these little limbs are so well padded with baby fat, the casts have to go above the knee to maintain corrective forces on the feet. Also, these little ones are escape artists—they can wriggle themselves out of virtually anything that doesn't come above the knee. We change the casts weekly at first, then biweekly, gaining a little more correction each time."

"That's easier than I thought."

"Usually. Depending on whom you ask, serial casting corrects about 50% of clubfeet. Many of these patients will ultimately require minor surgery such as heel cord lengthening to fully correct the deformity. And sometimes the deformity simply defies meticulous casting, and more extensive surgery is required. This is usually reserved until the child is about 6 to 9 months old. The distorted anatomic structures are easier to identify then, and the child has a corrected foot on which to stand and walk a few months later. Numerous soft tissue release procedures have been devised to correct a resistant clubfoot; surgeons have their favorites, but the procedure chosen must meet the needs of that particular foot."

"I see an unsettling consistency here. For as common as the condition is, its names are neither generous nor fully descriptive, and the etiology, pathologic anatomy, classification, and surgical treatments are all controversial."

"You're right. The goals of treatment, however, are well accepted: to correct all aspects of the deformity and leave a supple, normally contoured foot that will painlessly support weight bearing. If complete correction is delayed beyond infancy, the growing tarsal bones become permanently misshapen, and then even bony surgery cannot completely achieve the goals."

"I doubt his parents will be thrilled about big, hulking casts on their newborn, but it sure beats the prospect of hobbling around on sore feet in ill-fitting shoes. I'll write a note in the chart. May I have my pen back?"

ADVANCED READING

Cummings RJ, Davidson RS, Armstrong PF, et al. Congenital clubfoot. J Bone Joint Surg Am 84:290-308, 2002.

Little WJ. A treatise on the nature of club-foot, and analogous distortions; including their treatment both with and without surgical operation. London: Longmans, 1839.

Maugham WS. Of Human Bondage. New York: Doubleday, Doran, 1929.

Noonan KJ, Richards BS. Nonsurgical management of idiopathic clubfoot. J Am Acad Orthop Surg 11:392-402, 2003.

Roye DP Jr, Roye BD. Idiopathic congenital talipes equinovarus. J Am Acad Orthop Surg 10:239-248, 2002.

◆ *Could you walk in high-heeled shoes if your ankle was stiff in neutral? Can you walk efficiently if your ankle is fixed in 30 degrees of plantar flexion? If you had to have your ankle fused, what position would be best?*

18

The Hill Twins

James H. Lubowitz ✦ *Roy A. Meals*

The Hill twins ran faster than any other kids on the cross-country team. They were, in fact, by far the finest junior high athletes in town. Unfortunately, although they led their respective undefeated basketball teams in points, rebounds, and assists, each complained of knee pain every night.

Jack first noticed his left knee pain 3 months before the basketball season. It bothered him while he was riding his bike, but basketball, especially getting down low on defensive drills, really made it ache; and kneeling was sheer agony. His coach recommended aspirin, but it didn't help a bit. Grandmother Hill came for a visit and noticed a bump below his kneecap, but Jack's parents thought she was seeing things.

PRINCIPLE: **Listen to your patients' grandmothers. They are observant and experienced caregivers.**

Jill complained of pain in both knees. She wasn't really sure when it started, but basketball definitely made it worse. The dull, throbbing pain bothered her after practice, especially on cold days. Sometimes the whole knee ached, sometimes just the front. Climbing stairs hurt, and so did sitting with her knees flexed. She had to sit in the front seat of the car and in an aisle seat at the movies; otherwise she couldn't straighten out her aching joints. Jill's coach also recommended aspirin, and it helped a great deal.

Finally, Grandmother Hill took Jack and Jill to Dr. Godot. Both children had full range of motion of their knees and good stability of their ligaments in both the mediolateral and anteroposterior directions. Neither had an effusion. Jack's only positive physical finding was a tender and prominent left tibial tubercle.

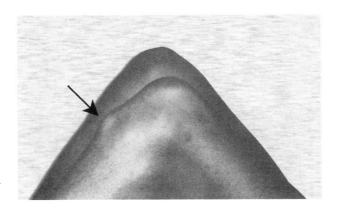

Bony prominence at the insertion of the patellar ligament on the left tibial tubercle.

His grandmother smiled knowingly, but she was confused when the doctor also carefully examined the youth's back and hips. Dr. Godot was not about to be fooled. She knew that knee pain may be referred from disease in the hip or low back.

Findings from Jill's back, hip, and knee examinations were *entirely* normal—not even a bump. Dr. Godot spent a long time with Jill's kneecaps. With Jill's knees extended and quadriceps relaxed, she tried to push them medially and laterally, but they didn't go very far, and trying didn't bother Jill a bit. A sudden look of apprehension might have implied that the joint was in a precarious position on the brink of a painful subluxation or dislocation. Dr. Godot then slipped her fingers behind the edges of each kneecap but found no tenderness on either the lateral or medial facet. Compressing the patella firmly against the femoral condyles with the knee in slight flexion also caused no pain. She carefully inspected Jill's quadriceps muscle bulk and tone but found no evidence of atrophy. Finally, she checked for any rotational malalignment of Jill's lower extremities. No problems there either.

PRINCIPLE: Keep an eye on the patient's face during the examination.

Dr. Godot sent Jack and Jill for x-ray examinations to confirm her working diagnoses. In addition to routine x-rays, which would rule out a bone tumor or an indolent infection, she ordered a special sunrise view of Jill's kneecaps to observe the patellofemoral joint space. Jack's lateral view showed enlargement of the tibial tubercle with fragmentation of the apophysis. There was also a region of new bone formation at the insertion of the patellar tendon, exactly at the spot where his grandmother had noted the bump.

Jill's x-rays were entirely normal. The sunrise view did not show any lateral tilt or shift of the patella. Because the family seemed interested, for comparison Dr. Godot showed them the x-ray of another patient with advanced patellofemoral arthritis.

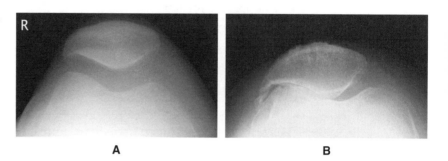

A, A normal patello-femoral relation-ship seen on a sunrise view. **B,** For comparison, cartilage loss with peripheral osteophyte formation is visible in an arthritic patellofemoral joint.

A   B

NOTE: *The patella is the largest sesamoid bone in the body. What is the name of the lesser known sesamoid bone located posterior to the knee joint?*

The doctor then told Jack and Jill what they had. She started with Jack because, although traction apophysitis or Osgood-Schlatter disease sounds bad, it is easy to explain. She described the physes—growth plates at the ends of bones that make them longer. Apophyses are also cartilaginous growth plates, but they occur on the sides of certain bones rather than the ends, making bony prominences where tendons attach. The proximal tibia is relatively unique in that the physis is continuous with the anteriorly situated apophysis. This apophysis extends distally down the tibia to form the tibial tuberosity at the site of insertion of the patellar tendon. With repetitive traction on the immature bony tubercle of the tibia from the pull of the patellar tendon, the apophysis becomes inflamed and sometimes even partially avulsed. This generates tenderness as well as new bone formation. It's a malady mainly of 10- to 14-year-old boys, and it occurs bilaterally in some adolescents. The pain typically resolves spontaneously in a year or two as the apophysis consolidates and fuses to the proximal tibia, so the patient's symptoms can serve as a guide to his activity level. Dr. Godot suggested that Jack ease off on his cycling and squatting drills but said he could continue to play basketball as hard as he wanted. Also, wearing knee pads would ease the pain of a direct blow.

The orthopedist then looked at Jill, took a deep breath, and sighed. She explained that anterior knee pain was very common in teenage girls and that the cause was usually not evident. Although her coach had labeled it "chondromalacia patellae," Dr. Godot told the twins and their grandmother that "soft kneecap cartilage" was often an improperly applied term. Most patients with anterior knee pain in actuality have perfectly normal cartilage in their patellofemoral joints, even when inspected arthroscopically. Patients with true chondromalacia patellae, however, most likely have a knee joint effusion, tenderness on the deep surface of the patella when it is drawn to one side, and palpable crepitation behind the kneecap when the knee is forcefully extended, as when rising from a squatting position. Jill had none of these findings, and, in fact, a paucity of physical findings is the rule with this type of anterior knee pain. Consequently, many physicians now tend to label Jill's type of symptoms as patellofemoral syndrome, or simply anterior knee pain, when no identifiable pathology is present. Because of the variable nature of patient complaints and the lack of objective pathologic causes in most cases, diagnosing and treating this condition can be frustrating for patients and physicians alike.

N O T E: *The articular cartilage of the patella is among the thickest in the body, partly because of the stress imparted on the patellofemoral joint during resisted knee flexion. However, by increasing the lever arm of the extensor mechanism, the patella acts as a fulcrum to increase knee extension strength by as much as 50%.*

Although in most cases the etiology of patellofemoral pain is multifactorial, Dr. Godot also explained that sometimes patients will develop pain from a malalignment of the extensor mechanism (quadriceps, patella, and patellar tendon) relative to the underlying bony anatomy. This can result in maltracking of the patella within the trochlear groove with knee flexion, leading to anterior knee pain, patellar instability, or both. Predisposing factors include varus, valgus, or rotational malalignment of the lower limb anywhere from the hips down to the feet. Additional physical findings could include an increased Q angle (angle formed between a line drawn from the anterior superior iliac spine to the midpatella and from the midpatella to the tibial tuberosity), restricted patellar mediolateral tilt or glide from a tight retinaculum, and a positive "J" sign in which the patella glides proximally with quadriceps contraction and then deviates laterally as it clears the trochlear groove.

Dr. Godot then told the trio that treatment for Jill's condition also was nonoperative. Aspirin or other nonsteroidal antiinflammatory drugs sometimes help, at least with the pain if not with the underlying disease. She showed Jill how to do isometric quad sets and straight-leg raises to strengthen her quadriceps muscle while only minimally compressing the patellofemoral joint. She cautioned Jill against doing deep knee bends, which accentuate patellofemoral problems by forcing the kneecaps against the femoral condyles. She added that although many surgical procedures have been devised to treat this common problem, the results, particularly in the absence of discrete pathologic findings, have been almost universally disappointing. This made Jill even more committed to her exercise program.

PRINCIPLE: Operations can make people worse.

Dr. Godot concluded the consultation by washing her hands and attempting a hook shot into the wastebasket with the crumpled paper towel. It was deftly blocked by three hands.

ADVANCED READING

Baker MM, Juhn MS. Patellofemoral pain syndrome in the female athlete. Clin Sports Med 19:315-329, 2000.

Fulkerson JP. Diagnosis and treatment of patients with patellofemoral pain. Am J Sports Med 30:447-456, 2002.

Fulkerson JP, Shea KP. Current concepts review. Disorders of patellofemoral alignment. J Bone Joint Surg Am 72:1424-1429, 1990.

Kelly MA, Insall JN. Historical perspectives of chondromalacia patellae. Orthop Clin North Am 23:517-521, 1992.

Kraus BC, Williams JP, Catterall A. Natural History of Osgood-Schlatter Disease. J Pediatr Orthop 10:65-68, 1990.

Osgood RB. Lesions of the tibial tubercle occurring during adolescence. Boston Med Surg J 148:114-117, 1903.

19

Terminal Diseases

While attempting to catch a softball at the company picnic, a 49-year-old data entry specialist sustained a forced flexion injury to her dominant index finger. It is mildly painful, and she fears that her inability to extend the distal interphalangeal joint might jeopardize her career at the computer keyboard.

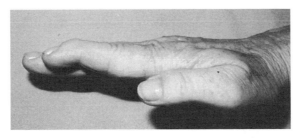

Injury resulting from forced flexion of a rigidly extended distal interphalangeal joint.

Your examination shows normal sensibility, color, and capillary refill in the fingertip, with mild swelling and tenderness at the distal interphalangeal joint. The joint rests in a 40-degree flexed position. She is unable to actively extend the distal phalanx, although passive extension is full. Active flexion is present. Collateral ligaments are stable. Active motion at the proximal interphalangeal joint is full. An x-ray was obtained in the emergency room.

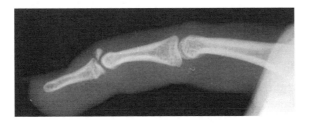

What is the diagnosis? What treatment do you recommend?

✦   ✦   ✦

She has a mallet finger, an abnormal flexion posture of the distal interphalangeal (DIP) joint caused by isolated loss of active terminal extension. It is also known as drop finger because of the incomplete extension or baseball finger because that is a common cause. It is hard to understand why someone thought it resembled a mallet. Anyway, mallet fingers are sustained when the rigidly extended DIP joint is suddenly forced into flexion, with disruption of either the extensor tendon or avulsion of its bony attachment from the base of the distal phalanx. The lateral x-ray distinguishes between the two and determines the length of treatment required inasmuch as cancellous bone heals faster than tendon (4 versus 6 weeks). Splinting the DIP joint in full extension allows the disrupted tissue to heal at its normal anatomic length thereby restoring continuity to the extensor mechanism.

You stress to the patient that a step-off of the articular surface on the distal phalanx does not forebode early degenerative arthritis. Minor incongruities of the joint surface are far better tolerated here than in weight-bearing joints, where the intensity and duration of compressive forces are far greater and anatomic restoration of the joint surface is de rigueur. So the risks of surgery are best avoided. Without splinting, however, an untreated mallet finger may result in a chronic swan-neck deformity, characterized by hyperextension of the proximal interphalangeal (PIP) joint in addition to the flexion deformity at the DIP joint. This occurs because the force of lateral bands of the extensor mechanism, which normally act to extend both the DIP and PIP joints, is concentrated on the PIP joint after detachment of the insertion onto the distal phalanx. This limits flexion of the PIP joint to produce a cosmetic as well as functional deformity.

PRINCIPLE: The rapidity with which a tissue heals is greatly dependent on the quality of its blood supply. Thus a disruption of poorly vascularized tendon requires a longer healing time than a fracture through well-vascularized cancellous bone.

This abnormally flexed posture at the DIP joint also could result from paralysis of the muscles responsible for extension, but because the intrinsic muscles simultaneously extend the DIP and PIP joints and flex the metacarpophalangeal joints, intrinsic paralysis would cause a claw deformity. This is an abnormal posturing of the digit at all three joints in a position exactly opposite the function of the intrinsic muscles (i.e., hyperextension at the metacarpophalangeal joint and flexion at the interphalangeal joints).

NOTE: *What is the primary function of the extensor digitorum communis? As already noted, it is the intrinsic muscles (interossei, lumbricals) that are primarily responsible for interphalangeal joint extension (as well as metacarpophalangeal joint flexion). How could you isolate the function of the long digital extensors on physical examination?*

Follow-up Note 1:   After 5 weeks of continuously splinting the DIP joint in extension, the patient returns with restoration of full active DIP extension and absence of tenderness. Based on these findings and the knowledge that the fracture has had plenty of time to heal, you decide to remove the splint. Do you need a follow-up x-ray?

P R I N C I P L E :   Obtain an x-ray only if you anticipate that the findings may affect treatment.

When she attempts to make a fist, her index finger DIP joint flexes only 20 degrees. She realizes in a panic that this too could interfere with her keyboarding skills. You remind her that stiffness after immobilization is quite common and can be overcome with some timely therapy. You show her active and passive exercises to mobilize the stiff joint and tell her that the exercises are best done under warm water because warmth actually makes the tissues more supple. Also, the warmth floods the brain with pleasurable sensations and suppresses painful sensations during the stretching exercises—the gate control theory of pain.

P R I N C I P L E :   Distraction and counterirritation are both worthy methods of pain control.

The next month she returns with a 3-day history of increasing pain, swelling, and redness around the nail fold of the same digit.

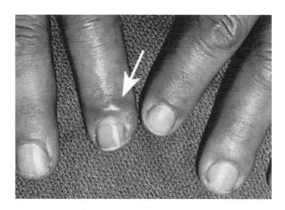

Inflammation around the nail fold, a paronychia, stems from a breakdown of the cuticle from nail biting or contact with caustic agents.

She recalls pulling out a hangnail with her teeth last week at work. This has not responded to several doses of ampicillin that she found in the back of her medicine cabinet.

Examination shows acute inflammation and palpable fluctuation along the nail fold without streaking or regional node tenderness. Do you double her ampicillin dose and have her begin soaking her hand again?

By pulling out a hangnail, she broke down the cuticle barrier of keratin that normally seals off the nail fold from the outside world. Bacteria enter this poorly vascularized space, first causing cellulitis and then abscess. Because it is next to the nail and because doctors like to speak Latin to impress everyone, it is called paronychia. Early on, the cellulitis can be treated with a penicillinase-resistant antibiotic (*S. aureus* is the most common offending agent) and warm soaks to improve local circulation, but when palpable fluctuation (i.e., pus) is present, surgical drainage is required. In the office after administering an intermetacarpal anesthetic block, you can lift the nail fold away from the nail with a semisharp instrument, allowing the entrapped pus to escape. Partial or complete removal of the nail is only occasionally required to totally externalize the abscess.

P R I N C I P L E :   Always drain pus.

Follow-up Note 2:   She comes back 8 years later, having just slammed a car door on the same digit. She is crying from the severe pain. There are superficial abrasions around the nail fold. After borrowing some nail polish remover from your secretary to clean the patient's nail, you note a large subungual hematoma.

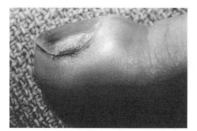

A large undecompressed subungual hematoma has lifted the nail base away from the underlying phalanx.

No other injuries are apparent, and x-rays are negative for distal phalanx fracture. Is this a good time to ask why she didn't come back to have her paronychia checked?

Being the humanitarian you are, you tell her you can drain her hematoma by making a hole in the nail with either a red-hot paper clip or a hypodermic needle. Once she regains consciousness, you quickly add that although conceptually agonizing, neither method causes any pain. The nail itself is nonliving keratin and is lifted away from the nail bed by the hematoma. She chooses the nonthermal method, and you adroitly spin a 20-gauge needle between your fingers until the hematoma is decompressed. Instantly, her pain is greatly relieved, and her repeated praises begin to nauseate your nurse. Rarely in medicine does such a simple, quick intervention yield such immediate and overwhelming gratification. Savor the moment. You caution her that the current nail will likely fall off in the coming months. As long as the proximal germinal matrix has not been severely injured, however, a new nail will grow.

Follow-up Note 3:   She next appears 7 years later. Now 64 years old and still entering data, she complains of a tender mass at the base of her left index fingernail. Present for about 6 months, it intermittently flares up and interferes with pinch activities like applying paper clips and turning keys. The mass is spherical, 3 mm in diameter, and fixed to the deep tissues just off the dorsal midline near the DIP joint. The overlying skin is thinned, giving the mass a faint bluish tinge. The nail has a shallow, longitudinal, concave trough in line with the mass.

A, Pressure from a mucous cyst causes a scalloped, longitudinal nail deformity. **B,** The underlying disease is osteoarthritis at the distal interphalangeal joint, seen here as joint space narrowing, sclerosis, and osteophyte formation *(arrows)*.

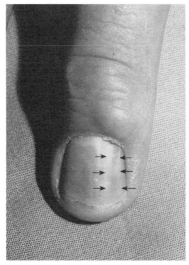

A

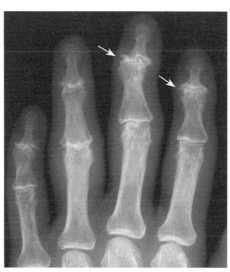

B

Heberden's nodes are present at multiple DIP joints on both hands. X-rays confirm osteoarthritis, characterized by joint space narrowing, bone sclerosis, and osteophyte formation at several DIP joints. You begin to explain to her that (1) the groove in the nail is caused by the mass pressing on the nail bed, (2) the mass is a mucous cyst caused by an osteophyte irritating the joint capsule, (3) the osteophyte comes from osteoarthritis, (4) osteoarthritis comes from living a long time, and (5) . . .

She interrupts to ask whether her problem is related to your treatment of her previous fingertip conditions. You check your chart and remind her that the other problems were on her right index finger. Aren't you glad you always make good office notes and keep them forever?

You start again and explain to her that the mucous cyst is like a ganglion and that the important step in surgical treatment is not so much removal of the mass itself but rather removal of the underlying irritable focus—the osteophyte, in this case. She interrupts again to ask whether her work entering gigabytes of data over the years caused the osteoarthritis. It might be plausible except that the Heberden's nodes on the interphalangeal joint of her left thumb are as large as those elsewhere in her hands, and this digit has largely been spared the keyboard all these years.

Later, with the patient under digital block anesthesia, you remove the offending osteophyte, which allows the mucous cyst and nail deformity to subside. She retires to Tahiti but says she will come back to see you, her fingertip doctor.

ADVANCED READING

Brzezienski MA, Schneider LH. Extensor tendon injuries at the distal interphalangeal joint. Hand Clin 11:373-386, 1995.

Gonzalez-Serva A. Structure and function. In Nails, Therapy, Diagnosis, Surgery, 2nd ed. Philadelphia: WB Saunders, 1997, pp 12-31.

Heberden W. Commentaries on the History and Cure of Diseases. London: Payne, 1802, pp 148-149.

Rizzo M, Beckenbaugh RD. Treatment of mucus cysts of the fingers: Review of 134 cases with minimum 2-year follow-up evaluation. J Hand Surg Am 28:519-524, 2003.

Seaberg DC, Angelos WJ, Paris PM. Treatment of subungual hematomas with nail trephination: A prospective study. Am J Emerg Med 9:209-210, 1991.

Wang QC, Johnson BA. Fingertip injuries. Am Fam Physician 63:1961-1966, 2001.

Wehbe M, Schneider L. Mallet fractures. J Bone Joint Surg Am 66:658-669, 1984.

Zook EG. Nail bed injuries. Hand Clin 1:701-716, 1985.

Zook EG, Brown RE. The perionychium. In Green DP, ed. Operative Hand Surgery, 4th ed. New York: Churchill Livingstone, 1999.

20

Pool Party

Michael C. Stephen ✦ Viet K.P. Le ✦ Roy A. Meals

"Tom, what did the dispatcher say?"

"Bad news, Dr. Jefferson. A 22-year-old dove into a half-empty swimming pool. Unable to move his legs at the scene. They think he's got a C-spine injury."

"Oh dear. We'll have our hands full when he arrives, so let's review some key points. What are you going to do first?"

"ABCDE—**A**irway, **b**reathing, **c**irculation, gross neurologic **d**isabilities, and body **e**xposure—all basic for any trauma victim. Because this person has a suspected head or neck injury, I'd also like to know more about the accident. From what height did he dive, how deep was the water, did he loose consciousness, was he moving his extremities at the scene? I'll look carefully for any facial injuries—anything that may acutely compromise his airway. Also, any abrasion or contusion will help me determine whether his neck was flexed or extended or just compressed when he hit. Of course, for all trauma patients we keep the cervical collar in place until a good physical examination and x-ray films tell us otherwise. So for him, without moving his head or neck, I'll feel for any swelling or tenderness around the collar if possible. In some cases it may have to be removed, so I'd have an assistant hold his head. Then, of course, I'd also do a thorough motor and sensory examination."

"How will you quantitate any muscle weakness?"

"Grading muscle strength on a five-point scale is standard. A score of 0 indicates no activity; 1 is palpable contraction without joint movement; 2 is joint movement with gravity neutralized; 3 is when the limb can be lifted against gravity; 4 is when movement against some resistance is possible; and of course 5 is normal strength."

"Good. The importance here of an extremely thorough neurologic examination cannot be overemphasized. You've got to start right up top with the cranial nerves. And at the other end of the spine, be sure to check for rectal tone and perianal sensation. In what seems like a complete spinal cord lesion, preservation of sensation in the sacral area carries a good prognosis for recovery because the cord may just be bruised and may resume conducting electricity after 1 to 2 days."

"So patients with complete motor and sensory losses can recover?"

"It's possible if it's just spinal shock. But after about 2 days, as spinal shock resolves, any fibers that were just bruised should be working. Whatever deficit is present at that time is permanent."

"How can you be sure spinal shock has resolved?"

"By testing for the return of a special spinal reflex—the bulbocavernosus reflex. Pressure on the glans penis or clitoris will normally cause tightening of the anal sphincter, but this reflex is absent during spinal shock."

"Now I remember. I've always wondered who discovered that one."

"Yeah, I guess it's not exactly one you'd want to attach your name to. But anyway, how about x-rays?"

"First, we have to get screening views without moving the neck, most importantly, a good cross-table lateral view that encompasses from C1 down to the C7-T1 interval. Almost 90% of unstable cervical spine injuries will be apparent on a good lateral x-ray. Of course, visualizing the complete C-spine can sometimes be tough in the trauma setting, so if this guy is headed for the CT scanner, I'd have the technician include fine cuts through the C-spine. The reformatted sagittal views would then give us a detailed look at the entire interval."

"What findings might suggest instability on this all-important screening lateral x-ray?"

"Well, first there are some clues to look for, aside from the appearance of the vertebrae themselves. Evidence of prevertebral soft tissue swelling—widening of the retropharyngeal space next to C2 or the retrotracheal space at C6—may indicate hematoma formation, suggesting a more severe injury than may be apparent on the single lateral view. In addition, the anterior and posterior surfaces of the vertebral bodies should normally follow nice smooth arcs, as do the posterior borders of the spinal canal at each level as well as the tips of the spinous processes. Disruptions or kinks in any of these lines require close attention, as does any widening of the normal space between vertebral bodies or spinous processes. Specifically, any translation of a vertebra more than 3 to 4 mm in front of or behind these lines, or any angulation more than about 15 degrees between adjacent vertebral endplates, likely represents an unstable injury."

"Great. The beauty of medicine is that it is not only interesting from an intellectual point of view, but it is also very practical. This must be our man now. Let's go to work."

PRINCIPLE: As exemplified by the C-spine lateral view, it is crucial to always look at x-ray films in a systematic and thorough manner to identify important findings beyond the appearance of the bones themselves.

A, Normal lateral cervical spine with smooth transitions of corresponding elements from one level to the next. **B,** Lateral x-ray from a patient with a fracture of the C2 vertebra. Note the disruption in the normal lordotic contour of the cervical spine.

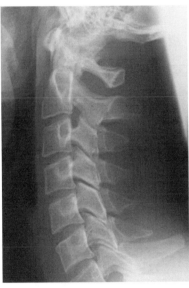

A

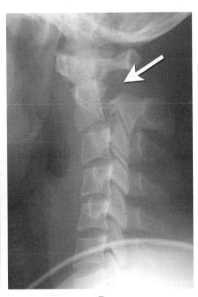

B

The doctors learn that this dive was part of a fraternity prank. The intoxicated young man never lost consciousness, and on arrival in the emergency room, he was mildly hypotensive and bradycardic. After initial stabilization, a detailed neurologic examination revealed full consciousness, normal function of cranial nerves I through XII, normal deltoid and biceps strength bilaterally, weak wrist extension bilaterally, and otherwise complete flaccid paralysis. Sensation was intact over only his shoulders and the lateral aspects of both upper limbs, including his thumbs. There was no perianal sensation to pinprick. The results of an additional test for sacral sparing—a gentle tug on the Foley catheter to see whether the patient had sensation at the bladder trigone—were also discouraging. A CT scan of his head revealed no acute hemorrhage.

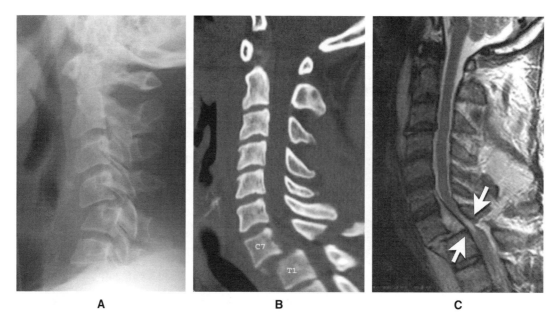

A **B** **C**

Examples of cervical spine injuries. **A,** Unilateral facet dislocation at C4-5. Note kyphotic deformity with anterior translation of C4 on C5 of approximately 25%. **B,** Sagittal CT showing bilateral facet dislocation at C7-T1 with greater than 50% anterior translation of C7. **C,** MRI scan demonstrating narrowing of the spinal canal with cord compression *(arrows)*.

"Dr. Jefferson, his physical findings and x-ray films are consistent with a complete spinal cord lesion at C6. It is not apparent whether he lost any blood, but he remains slightly hypotensive; yet he is bradycardic. I would expect him to be 'taching along' if he is hypovolemic."

"Your assumption is correct, but your premise is wrong. The injury has damaged not only his voluntary motor and sensory fibers but also the sympathetic fibers controlling vasomotor function and heart rate—neurogenic shock, not hypovolemic shock."

"Now I remember. That's why you gave him a vasopressor rather than fluid once you determined that he didn't have any source of occult bleeding. What are you going to do about his dislocation?"

"Well, that's where things get a little tricky. If he had an incomplete cord injury or evidence of worsening neurologic status, then I'd say we should emergently reduce his dislocation in order to relieve ongoing cord compression, either with skeletal traction or with open reduction in the operating room, followed by fusion of the unstable elements. With a complete neurologic injury, however, there is still debate regarding the optimal timing of surgery; in other words, urgent decompression versus an initial period of medical stabilization. But for right now, at least, we need to protect him against further neurologic damage, so we'll place him in skeletal traction with skull tongs. Then, when things stabilize, we'll give him the option of either surgical fusion of the unstable elements or a few months of immobilization in a halo vest external fixator. Both methods allow for early mobilization of the patient, which reduces the risks of pneumonia, bedsores, joint contractures, osteoporosis, thrombophlebitis, and so forth."

"You know, Dr. Jefferson, even though I know most of the facts about the emergency management of such a patient, I'm just beginning to comprehend. . . . This guy's washed up."

"Quite possibly, and if so, it will be at least a year before he can understand and cope with all the ramifications—physical, emotional, social. That's why the multidisciplinary care required is best provided in a regional spinal injury rehabilitation unit such as we have across town. Once he can sit up, it will be weeks before he can feed himself and months before he can transfer himself back and forth from his wheelchair to his bed. Eventually, most tetraplegic individuals with functioning C6 nerve roots can achieve a noninstitutional and at least semi-independent lifestyle."

"Why do you say C6?"

"Think about it. You noted on his examination that the deltoid, biceps, and a wrist extensor are working. With sufficient motivation and rehabilitation, that's enough to learn self-care activities. These will have to include intermittent self-catheterization for urine drainage and continuous weight shifting to avoid pressure sores over the insensate portions of his body. These functions can be enhanced by some carefully planned tendon transfers to provide some pinch function for manual dexterity and some elbow extension to assist with general mobility."

"Man, this guy needs all the help he can get. Let's do the tendon transfers tomorrow."

"Right and wrong. First off, he's still in spinal shock, so he's got a chance of at least a partial recovery. Second, these patients have much to learn about taking care of themselves both physically and mentally. They have to begin coping with the reality that they are severely disabled. They would be extremely disappointed with the results of the tendon transfers if done early. Once they've accepted their altered existence, they're grateful for anything we can do to increase their independence and overall quality of life."

"I see. What about injuries higher or lower in the neck?"

"Even at C5-6, which is the most common level for cervical spine injuries, the intercostal and abdominal muscles are paralyzed, so respiration depends mainly on the phrenic nerve coming from C3-5. Without a good cough potential, pneumonia is a constant threat. Moving up from C6, the complete absence of any upper limb function requires institutional care, and above C5 respiratory support becomes a necessity. Going the other way, injuries at C7 or C8 progressively spare more muscles in the forearm and hand, so more dexterity is preserved. For instance, patients with a functioning C7 nerve root will typically have good triceps strength. This aids significantly in transfer mobility. So even though these people are wheelchair bound, they are independent in most activities of daily living."

"How about thoracic and lumbar injuries?"

"Thoracic injuries aren't very common because of the extra stability provided by the ribs. Patients with complete lesions in the thoracic and upper lumbar spine can sometimes learn to walk using crutches and long-leg braces. It's strenuous though. Then those with lower lumbar injuries can walk with their ankles braced, assisted by canes if necessary. Injuries even as far distal as the sacrum still cause bowel and bladder impairment, so incontinence is a problem at all levels."

"How do you break the news of an injury like this to the patient? And his family?"

"We've got to be realistic, supportive, and available. We'll let their questions guide us about how much information they're ready to absorb. And remember, until the spinal shock wears off, there's hope that the deficits we see tonight might not be permanent. I see Dr. Chance. While you're writing your orders, I'll go say hi to my old friend.

"Hello, George. What brings you to the emergency room tonight?"

"I'm afraid it's the same fraternity party that brought you in, but the fellow in there jumped feet-first off the cabana roof. He initially hobbled away with just some heel pain, but then he called me about an hour ago because of numbness and weakness in his legs. I've known his family for years, so I came on over."

"Sounds like a lumbar vertebral burst fracture with some progressive instability."

"Right. I found no step-off or bulge by palpation of his spine at the area of tenderness, but the x-rays showed a compression-burst–type fracture at L2. Now he's having an MRI to ascertain the degree of spinal canal narrowing. At that level it's all nerve roots, no cord—just cauda equina."

"What's his neurologic examination like?"

"He's got some diffuse and patchy weakness and numbness in both lower limbs. It's gotten worse since I first examined him, so I expect some instability with retropulsion of a vertebral body segment into the canal at that level. Even though only a minority of lumbar fractures and fracture-dislocations cause neurologic injury, the presence of a deficit strongly suggests instability. This risks further damage if not carefully managed. Ah, here are his scans. Let's have a look."

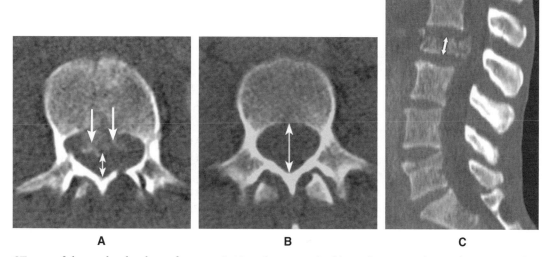

A	**B**	**C**

CT scan of thoracolumbar burst fracture. **A,** Note the retropulsed bony fragments *(arrows)* narrowing the canal space compared to, **B,** an unaffected level. **C,** Sagittal reconstructed view. Note the loss of vertebral height as well as canal compromise.

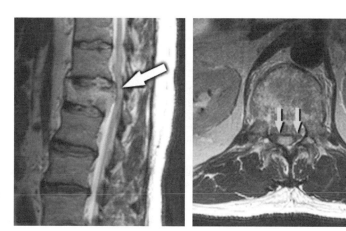

MRI of L2 burst fracture. Note the retropulsion of bony fragments into the canal *(arrows)*.

"Looks like there's definitely some canal compromise from the retropulsed bony fragments."

"Yeah, and in the face of his worsening neurologic picture, he needs to undergo decompression."

"So while you are there removing the bone fragments from the canal, will you go ahead and stabilize the spine with internal fixation?"

"Yes. You know, over the years I've had excellent results from postural reduction and several months of bed rest to allow for natural restoration of lumbar spinal stability. The newer methods of internal fixation, however, seem to reduce residual spinal deformity and pain, and they certainly allow for early mobilization and shorten the hospital stay."

"What did you tell him about his prognosis?"

"Well, assuming that strict spinal precautions are maintained until I get him decompressed and stabilized, I think it's pretty good. Maybe some residual weakness and numbness, but I suspect he'll be ambulatory—perhaps with some bracing and crutches. He may have to resort to a wheelchair to continue his marathoning interests. Bowel and bladder function? Sexual function? Time will tell."

"I can never get over the irony of these devastating injuries usually occurring in energetic, high-spirited young adults, instantly making them old and debilitated."

"That bothers me too. But it's heartening to see that these young bucks can redevelop a sense of self-worth and salvage productive, meaningful lives with a lot of multidisciplinary help."

"Yeah. S'pose so."

ADVANCED READING

Chance GQ. Note on type of flexion fracture of the spine. Br J Radiol 21:452-453, 1948.

Eismont FJ, Currier BL, McGuire RA Jr. Cervical spine and spinal cord injuries: Recognition and treatment. Instr Course Lect 53:341-358, 2004.

Kaiser JA, Holland BA. Imaging of the cervical spine. Spine 23:2701-2712, 1998.

Kirshblum S. New rehabilitation interventions in spinal cord injury. J Spinal Cord Med 27:342-350, 2004.

Levine AM, Eismont FJ, Garfin SR, et al. Spine Trauma. Philadelphia: WB Saunders, 1998.

McDonald JW, Sadowsky C. Spinal-cord injury. Lancet 359:417-425, 2002.

Patel RV, Delong W Jr, Vresilovic EJ. Evaluation and treatment of spinal injuries in the patient with polytrauma. Clin Orthop Relat Res 422:43-54, 2004.

Stiens SA, Kirshblum SC, Groah SL, et al. Spinal cord injury medicine. Optimal participation in life after spinal cord injury: Physical, psychosocial, and economic reintegration into the environment. Arch Phys Med Rehabil 83:S72-S81, S90-S98, 2002.

Vaccaro AR, Kim DH, Brodke DS, et al. Diagnosis and management of thoracolumbar spine fractures. Instr Course Lect 53:359-373, 2004.

21

Nadine

Russell Meldrum ✦ *Roy A. Meals*

A while back Dr. Eldridge, the pediatrician down the hall, asked me to see a 12-year-old girl. A school screening examination had identified a shoulder asymmetry, which was especially evident during forward bending.

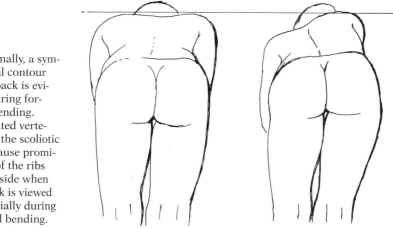

A, Normally, a symmetrical contour of the back is evident during forward bending.
B, Rotated vertebrae of the scoliotic spine cause prominence of the ribs on one side when the back is viewed tangentially during forward bending.

Her name was Linda, but she called herself Nadine, and even at her tender age, she had mastered the art of heavy makeup. Nadine lacked symptoms referable to her back, but she said that her dance instructor had been relentlessly trying to get her to stand up straight for at least a year. Dr. Eldridge had just finished a careful evaluation. She found no cardiovascular or pulmonary abnormalities and no pigmented patches of skin or subcutaneous masses. My findings showed a prominence of the right lower ribs and a slight elevation of the right shoulder when she was standing upright. Her iliac crests were level though. She had normal muscle strength in the trunk and limbs, and aside from her obvious disgust at being in my office, the results of her neurologic examination were normal.

What was going on here? Was this girl manifesting the slouch of teenage defiance? What should I have done?

✦ ✦ ✦

Defiant or not, the findings suggested scoliosis—a descriptive term for lateral curvature of the spine. This is, however, an over-simplification, as the disorder is really a complex three-dimensional deformity with angular and rotational components. At this point I didn't know whether the abnormality was structural in the spine or compensatory for a lower limb-length discrepancy. Measurement showed limb-length equivalence, and the asymmetry of her back did not disappear when she sat on a stool, which takes leg length out of the equation. From both assessments the abnormality appeared to be in the spine itself.

By far the most common type of scoliosis is the adolescent idiopathic type, but it is a diagnosis of exclusion. A careful physical examination is required to rule out causes such as neurofibromatosis, polio, syringomyelia, and other neurologic conditions. X-ray examination rules out congenital anomalies such as malformed vertebrae, absent discs, and fused or absent ribs. X-ray examination also assesses the secondary growth center of the iliac crest, the iliac apophysis, which helps indicate the time remaining to skeletal maturity. Although theories abound, the cause of idiopathic scoliosis remains, of course, unknown (otherwise it wouldn't be called idiopathic!), but there is familial predisposition and the common adolescent form affects girls far more often than boys.

What should I have recommended to this girl and her mother? Did she need any treatment at all? Nadine stressed the importance of a supple and sightly back for her intended dance career.

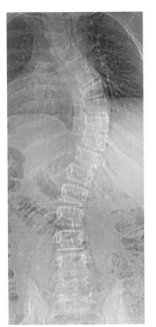

Thoracic curve of adolescent idiopathic scoliosis.

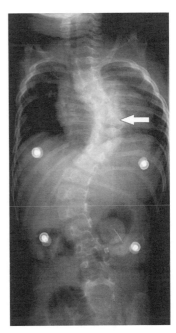

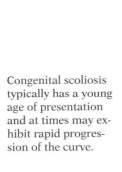

Congenital scoliosis typically has a young age of presentation and at times may exhibit rapid progression of the curve.

✦   ✦   ✦

Her spinal curve measured 27 degrees with the apex on the right side in the lower thoracic area. Compensatory curves had developed above and below the major curve to keep her head level and centered over her pelvis. The prominence of the ribs and scapula on the right was characteristic since a lateral bend imposed on the normal thoracic kyphosis and lumbar lordosis results in vertebral rotation. This rotation makes the posterior ribs more prominent on the convexity of the curve.

P R I N C I P L E :   Adolescent idiopathic scoliosis typically causes a right-sided thoracic curve (apex is on the right). A left-sided thoracic curve should raise suspicion for a primary neurologic or neuromuscular etiology.

Once the normal alignment of the spine is sufficiently disturbed, progressive deformity can be anticipated, particularly during periods of rapid growth. The rib hump associated with vertebral rotation becomes progressively more unsightly as the scoliosis increases. Untreated curves greater than 50 degrees will continue to progress even after skeletal maturity, and curves greater than 80 degrees pose a risk of cor pulmonale and untimely death. Back pain, however, is neither more common nor more severe in adults with untreated idiopathic scoliosis than in the general population. Early spinal fusion, of course, would halt the progression of the deformity, but it reduces the patient's ultimate height because of early epiphyseal closure. It also risks early degenerative arthritis at the ends of the rigidly fixed spine segments. Thus treatment must be carefully directed and timed to halt progression of the deformity in order to minimize disfigurement and interference with the patient's quality and length of life.

Treatment of adolescent idiopathic scoliosis is based on an estimation of the curve's risk of progression. This is dictated by both the magnitude of the curve and the patient's degree of skeletal maturity, as assessed by chronologic age, bone age, and menarchal status to name a few. In essence, large curves in immature patients tend to progress, whereas slight curves in more mature patients tend to remain stable. The worse the curve appears on initial evaluation and the longer the time to skeletal maturation, the greater the propensity for significant progression. In terms of curve magnitude, minor curves less than 25 degrees can be observed. Moderate curves between 25 and 45 degrees and minor curves showing progression require bracing until skeletal maturity is reached. Severe curves greater than 45 degrees and moderate curves showing rapid progression require surgical fusion of the affected spine segments.

Nadine was totally compliant with her exercise regimen to maintain spinal suppleness. She returned at 6-month intervals for follow-up. Although her initial x-rays showed a 27-degree curve, I didn't initiate bracing then because I didn't know whether the curve was progressing. A year later, the curve was 33 degrees. She had begun menstruating, and her iliac crests were now nearly capped, so skeletal maturity was approaching. Because the apex of her curve was well below T8, a custom-molded shell from under-arms to iliac crests provided the desired counterforce to prevent progression of the curve. By taking it off for a few hours per day, she could continue her dance lessons unimpeded. I last saw her when she was 16 years of age; the curve had stabilized at 35 degrees, and the truncal asymmetry was not obvious on casual observation. One change I did notice immediately, however, was the presence of a whimsical dragon tattooed over her lumbar paraspinal muscles. She asked me whether I thought it added to her image.

Several years later I was entertaining a British visitor, Dr. John Watson, at my favorite nightclub. Ironically, he asked me about recent advances in scoliosis surgery. He knew that placing stainless steel rods along the primary curve, jacking the spine as straight as possible, and fusing it there have comprised the standard treatment for years. I told him that curve corrections are thereby obtained with minimal risks of neurologic damage or pseudarthrosis and that newer means of spinal instrumentation allow additional straightening and derotation. Intraoperative monitoring of sensory evoked potentials from the feet into the cerebral cortex has reduced the concomitant risk of irreversible spinal cord injury. As I was sketching the new devices on a paper napkin, a smiling dragon gracing a dancer's bare flank distracted me. Nadine's rhythmic movements and lustrous, waist-length hair successfully camouflaged her deformities. After the performance, I whispered to Dr. Watson that Nadine had been a patient of mine and that she had scoliosis. With the widest of eyes, he said he hadn't noticed a bit.

ADVANCED READING

Bridwell KH. Surgical treatment of idiopathic adolescent scoliosis. Spine 24:2607-2616, 1999.

Lenke LG, Betz RR, Harms J. Adolescent idiopathic scoliosis: A new classification to determine extent of spinal arthrodesis. J Bone Joint Surg Am 83:1169-1181, 2001.

Reamy BV, Slakey JB. Adolescent idiopathic scoliosis: Review and current concepts. Am Fam Physician 64:111-116, 2001.

Roach JW. Adolescent idiopathic scoliosis. Orthop Clin North Am 39:353-365, 1999.

22

Hoop Fever

James E. Li ✦ *Roy A. Meals*

"John Hill! What's with the crutches?"

"Went up for a rebound yesterday and came down on one of those oaf's big feet. My foot turned in as I landed. Felt like something ripped. They called it an inversion injury in the emergency room last night after looking at the x-ray films. No fracture though. The ER doc told me to RICE my ankle until I could see you. I've been trying to put some weight on it, but it still hurts like hell."

"RICE it? What do you mean?"

"**R**est, in other words, crutches. **I**ce to reduce pain and swelling. **C**ompression wrapping with an elastic bandage. **E**levation to reduce swelling."

"Good, I agree with all that. I just hadn't heard that mnemonic used as a verb before. Let's have a look. Good pulses, skin is warm. Do you have good feeling everywhere?"

PRINCIPLE: Never forget to perform a careful neurovascular examination distal to any musculoskeletal injury.

"Yeah. Too good on the outside there."

"The swelling and bruising are localized around your lateral malleolus. I'm going to check for tenderness in two spots: just anterior and just distal to the lateral malleolus. Which spot hurts more?"

"Definitely anterior. Is that the ligament that runs anteriorly from the distal fibula to the talus?"

PRINCIPLE: A sound knowledge of musculoskeletal anatomy is the basis of a good limb examination.

"Right on. When the ankle is in its normal position, the anterior talofibular ligament, ATFL for short, is almost parallel to the axis of the foot. But with the foot in plantar flexion, the ligament becomes parallel to the axis of the leg. Then it functions as a collateral ligament, and because most ankle injuries occur in plantar flexion and inversion, this ligament takes the first hit. It's the most commonly damaged ligament in the body."

"I can believe it. I'm the third one on my intramural team this year, although Michi actually injured his for the first time while playing soccer."

"Yup. Running, basketball, soccer, any activity in which you unexpectedly come down on your foot when it's in plantar flexion during the swing phase of gait. It folds right under. The excess energy is absorbed by the weakest link in the system—in your case, the ligament—but sometimes the same injury mechanism results in a fracture. How well I remember my medical school injury. Took 2 years to get back my full basketball prowess."

"You also checked for tenderness just distal to the lateral malleolus. What's there?"

"The ligament that runs distally from the tip of the fibula to the calcaneus. Interestingly, this ligament becomes most taught with dorsiflexion and inversion of the ankle, as compared to the ATFL, which is more commonly injured by plantar flexion. Depending on the severity of the inversion force though, both can be torn, but isolated tears of the ATFL are at least three times as common as combined injuries."

"So other than tenderness, which seems rather nonspecific, how do you tell the two patterns apart?"

"Stress testing."

"Kind of like med school, eh?"

"Well then, this is just a quiz. Let me see your x-rays first. Don't want to be stressing a fracture."

"I brought 'em with me: anteroposterior, lateral, and mortise view, whatever that is."

"Mortise actually means square peg in a square hole. It's a carpentry term, but it describes nicely an almost anteroposterior view of the ankle but with the leg internally rotated about 15 degrees. See how the talus is not overlapped by either the fibula or the tibia, and see how the cartilage space is the same width medially, superiorly, and laterally.

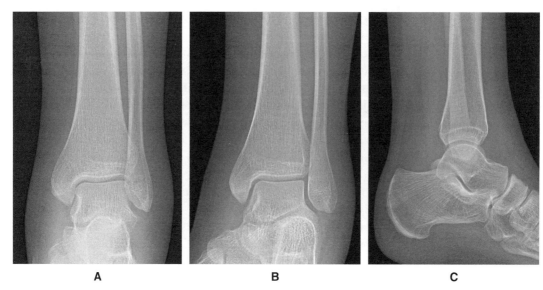

A, Anteroposterior view of the ankle. **B,** Fifteen-degree internal rotation view delineates the ankle mortise. **C,** Normal lateral view.

"Any shift or tilt of the talus in the mortise spells trouble. A shift of even a couple of millimeters can dramatically increase the stress on the articular cartilage with weight bearing. That can lead to early degenerative arthritis."

"The x-rays look fine to me. What's the point of stress testing?"

"We can't see torn ligaments on x-ray films, of course, so I'm going to gently stress those ligaments that attach your fibula to your tarsals. If they're completely torn, we'll see some abnormal motion. First, I stabilize your leg with one hand and gently invert your foot with steady pressure from the other hand."

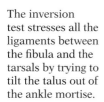

The inversion test stresses all the ligaments between the fibula and the tarsals by trying to tilt the talus out of the ankle mortise.

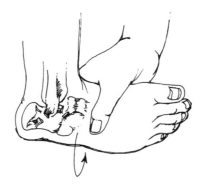

"If the degree of inversion is decidedly greater than on the uninjured side, or if the talus visibly tilts out of the mortise, then those ligaments are completely ripped. But your test looks OK."

"Good. Even though you were gentle, that's about my limit for pain."

"If stress testing is too painful, then some local anesthetic injected into the ankle can help."

"I'm a chicken for needles. Let's get on with it."

"OK. The inversion test I just attempted to tilt the talus out of the mortise sideways. The drawer test tries to pull it out anteriorly. Once again, I push steadily posterior on your leg with one hand and cup my other hand around your heel and try to draw the foot forward.

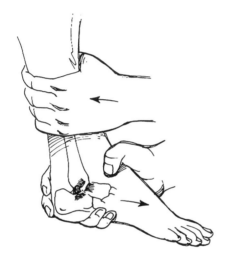

The drawer test stresses the anterior fibulotalar ligament by trying to pull the talus forward on the tibia and fibula.

"We do this with the ankle in plantar flexion and again in neutral. That seems all right too."

"What if it wasn't?"

"Then I'd put on a pair of lead gloves and repeat the stress tests under x-ray guidance so we could see precisely the degree of lateral tilt and anterior shift of the talus in the mortise compared to your nonstressed x-rays."

"So you're convinced I have a garden-variety ankle sprain?"

"Yup. X-rays are negative for ankle fracture as well as for any bony tarsal injuries. Sometimes peroneal tendon injury, synovitis, or some difficult-to-visualize fractures of the talus can mimic sprains, but your story and examination are pretty straightforward."

"So what do we do? My physical diagnosis course starts in 2 weeks; I'll be on my feet a lot."

"In the past there has been considerable controversy about the best method for treatment of ankle sprains, especially with complete ligament injuries in high-performance athletes."

"That's me of course."

"Roughly 85% of ankle sprains are going to do fine with conservative management. Even in those that don't, late surgical repair or reconstruction of the lateral ligaments gives a result equal to that achieved with early repair. Also, functional treatment is obviously cheaper and less risky than surgery."

"Functional treatment? What's that? Don't I need a cast?"

"Functional treatment includes early weight-bearing and only a brief period of taping or wrapping. Then range-of-motion and strengthening exercises provide the quickest return to full activity. Compared to casting or surgery, functional treatment is almost free from complications, yet it provides as good a result."

"What kind of complications are you talking about?"

"Wound breakdown, infection, muscle atrophy, deep venous thrombosis, sensitive scars."

"OK, OK; you've convinced me. When can I play ball again?"

"Well, when your swelling and tenderness have subsided in a week or so, I'll show you some strengthening exercises and gradually get you started on some running on the level. It'll probably be at least a month before you feel comfortable twisting, stopping suddenly, or hopping on that foot; and you may want to tape your ankle inside your high-top shoes for a while. It may even be several months before you are completely free of discomfort when you're playing ball. But I'll have you in peak condition for the student-faculty game. You'll need everything you have for that one."

ADVANCED READING

Frey C. Ankle sprains. Instr Course Lect 50:515-520, 2001.

Kannus P, Renstrom P. Current concepts review. Treatment for acute tears of the lateral ligaments of the ankle. J Bone Joint Surg Am 73:305-312, 1991.

Marder RA. Current methods for the evaluation of ankle ligament injuries. Instr Course Lect 44:349-357, 1995.

Quinn K, Parker P, de Bie R, et al. Interventions for preventing ankle ligament injuries. Cochrane Database Syst Rev 2:CD000018, 2000.

Wolfe MW, Uhl TL, Matacola CG, et al. Management of ankle sprains. Am Fam Physician 63:93-104, 2001.

23

Dr. Youngman

Raymond J. Chang ✦ *Roy A. Meals*

"Yes, I am Ruth Davis. You hardly look old enough to be a doctor, but neither do the others who have been in here already. Just like I told *them*, I'm 56 years old. When we were driving home from our ski trip last week, my right leg began to ache. We can normally make that drive in 12 hours, but the weather was so lousy it took more than twice that long. A day later my leg began to swell, first near my knee, then down toward my foot. Now it looks like this. I can't walk."

"Has this ever happened before, and have you had any fevers or chills?"

"No, no, and no. All you young doctors ask the same questions. No shortness of breath, chest pain, pounding heart, or coughing up blood either. Also, no tobacco, cancer, or birth control pills. What does all of this mean, anyway?"

"I'll tell you after I've had a look. Just like the student said, the swelling extends from the popliteal space to just above the ankle. It seems like most of your tenderness is posterior, and the leg is clearly red and warm compared with the left. I won't test for Homans' sign again; the medical student said you screamed when he tried to passively dorsiflex your ankle."

"I didn't mean to scare him, but that Homans sure must have been some kind of sadist. That really hurt. So do tell, what's wrong with me?"

"It seems like there's a blood clot in your leg. Venous sludging from prolonged inactivity like sitting for a long time is an obvious predisposing factor. We also see it after total hip and knee replacements, and during immobilization for lower extremity or pelvic fractures. Oral contraceptives, smoking, malignancies, and certain hematologic disorders are also implicated because they make the blood hypercoagulable. It's risky because once a clot forms, it can break loose and drift up to plug the arteries in your lungs."

"Can't you just give me those pills that thin the blood and let me go home?"

PRINCIPLE: Pulmonary embolus is the most common preventable cause of death in hospitalized patients. Aggressive prevention and treatment save lives.

"Well, not really. For two reasons. First, until we get your blood thinned, you are at risk for pulmonary embolus and possibly death, so we need to thin it relatively quickly. Warfarin, the pill you are referring to, has a pretty long delay from the time you start taking it until its therapeutic levels are reached. Heparin, given through your IV, works almost instantly, but of course you have to stay in the hospital for that. The second reason is a bit more complicated. As it turns out, warfarin acts on several factors involved in clotting and its regulation produced by your liver, some of which are actually anticoagulant factors. Ironically, these anticoagulant factors have the fastest turnover in your body, so they are the first to be affected by warfarin. This, in turn, causes a temporary, paradoxical prothrombotic state until the remaining clotting factors are affected. So that's why we like to have people take heparin when we start them on high doses of warfarin for a deep venous thrombosis. The good news about warfarin, though, is that you can take it by mouth at home, and because it has a long half-life, once-a-day dosing is routine. The bad news is that you will have to have your prothrombin time tested every few days because of warfarin's narrow therapeutic index.

"There are lots of new anticoagulant drugs out there that I haven't used much. Some, like the low-molecular-weight heparins and the synthetic factor X inhibitors, can be given as once-a-day injections to take the place of a continuous heparin drip. Direct thrombin inhibitors are also on the market that can be taken orally like warfarin but without the need to monitor prothrombin times. But no matter what the medication is, all of these anticoagulants have the propensity to cause bleeding complications, so we have to be vigilant even if frequent blood draws aren't needed."

NOTE: *Which procoagulant factors are affected by warfarin? Which anticoagulant factors are affected? What is another name for factor II?*

"One other thing, young man. My knee isn't what it used to be. I had a partial meniscectomy done arthroscopically several years ago. Dr. Honeychurch did it. I felt pretty good until I fell skiing last week; then it ached a little and would pop occasionally. I forgot to tell this to the medical student after he tried that Homans' test."

"That's very interesting and possibly very important. I'll see whether we can get an ultrasound of your leg right away, before we start the heparin. Let me make a phone call; then I'll come back and explain."

Later

"Hello, Dr. Honeychurch. Glad to see somebody closer to my vintage. These young doctors are nice, but I was admitted last night and they still haven't started the blood thinners."

"Well, they are actually doing a good job. I just saw the ultrasound results, and it looks like you probably have a Baker's cyst rather than thrombophlebitis. To make sure, we will get an MRI of your knee. If we're right, you won't need to take anticoagulants and you can avoid the attendant risk of bleeding complications."

"Now I'm really confused. What's a Baker's cyst? I haven't baked in years."

"No. It's named after the man who described the condition more than 100 years ago. He wasn't actually the first to describe it, but so it goes with eponyms."

"Just think, 'Honeychurch's cyst.' Sorry you missed out."

"Yeah. . . . Anyway, fluid buildup from some derangement, such as a torn meniscus, osteoarthritis, or rheumatoid arthritis, may form an outpocketing of the joint lining behind the knee. Repeated movements such as skiing, dancing, or jogging can pump the fluid out and expand the cyst. If its synovial lining becomes inflamed, the findings mimic thrombophlebitis, especially if the cyst extends for some distance down the calf as in your case. Just to confuse matters, a Baker's cyst can partially occlude the veins in the popliteal space, further mimicking or even contributing to the development of deep venous thrombosis."

"What about that damned Homans' sign, and what about the ultrasound?"

"Well, that's one of the problems with Homans' sign. First of all, not every deep venous thrombosis causes pain or inflammation in the popliteal space. On the flip side, passive dorsiflexion of the ankle stretches the calf muscles and will hurt whatever tissues in the area are inflamed. The test cannot distinguish between a deep venous thrombosis and an inflamed or ruptured synovial cyst, but an ultrasound usually can. It is a simple, noninvasive screening test. We can confirm a cyst with an MRI, which also happens to be quite good at finding out what type of intraarticular pathology might be causing the cyst in the first place. In the old days, we used to inject radiopaque dye along with some air into the knee joint itself. It would leak out into the cyst and show up on an x-ray. We don't do that too often anymore because it is relatively invasive and poses a risk of infection of both the cyst and the knee joint itself.

"Now, if the ultrasound had suggested a deep venous thrombosis, there are some different diagnostic tests we could use. Venography, injecting contrast medium downstream from an affected vein, is considered the "gold standard," but again it is not used much anymore. Actually, now that I think about it, with the advances in venous ultrasound imaging, that is probably all the confirmation we really need. An MRI venogram can sometimes be helpful in proximal or pelvic thrombosis where ultrasound doesn't work quite so well."

"So, say the MRI confirms a Baker's cyst; can I go home then?"

"Yes, but you will still need some bed rest, warm compresses, and antiinflammatory medication to manage the acute inflammation. Then, so the fluid buildup doesn't recur, we will need to deal with the underlying disease in your knee joint. If the cyst is as large as I suspect it is, from looking at your leg and at the ultrasound, I will also talk to you about resecting it to preclude further confusion with or contribution to thrombophlebitis."

"Oh, here's that nice doctor who admitted me last night. Good morning, young man."

"Good morning, Mrs. Davis. Hello, Dr. Honeychurch. I'm Steve Youngman, the new resident on your service."

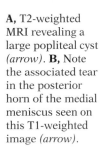

A, T2-weighted MRI revealing a large popliteal cyst *(arrow)*. **B,** Note the associated tear in the posterior horn of the medial meniscus seen on this T1-weighted image *(arrow)*.

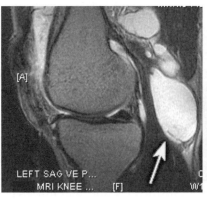

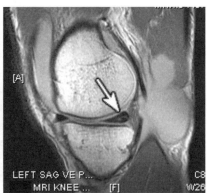

A   B

ADVANCED READING

Baker WM. The formation of abnormal synovial cysts in connection with the joints. St Bart's Hosp Rep 13:245-261, 1877.

Chaudhuri R, Salari R. Baker's cyst simulating deep vein thrombosis. Clin Radiol 41:400-404, 1990.

Handy JR. Popliteal cysts in adults: A review. Semin Arthritis Rheum 31:108-118, 2001.

Homans J. Thrombosis of the deep leg veins due to prolonged sitting. N Engl J Med 250:148-149, 1954.

McRae SL, Ginsberg JS. Initial treatment of venous thromboembolism. Circulation 110(9 Suppl):13-19, 2004.

Ramzi DW, Leeper DV. DVT and pulmonary embolism: Part I. Diagnosis; Part II. Treatment and prevention. Am Fam Physician 69:2829-2836; 2841-2848, 2004.

Sculco TP, Colwell CW, Pellegrini VD, et al. Prophylaxis against venous thromboembolic disease in patients having a total hip or knee arthroplasty. J Bone Joint Surg Am 84:466-477, 2002.

◆ *If your right hip is flexed 90 degrees and your left hip is abducted 10 degrees, flexed 100 degrees, externally rotated 90 degrees, and you then flex your left knee 100 degrees, where is your left lateral malleolus?*

24

Elbow Mac—A Detective Story

Yong Sung ✦ *Roy A. Meals* ✦ *Scott A. Mitchell*

It all started about 2 months ago, just after I returned from a trip to the mountains in pursuit of a fugitive. I had spent months tracking him—he had hijacked my Corvette and my favorite pair of skis after illicitly helping himself to the luxuries of my home. But again he eluded me. I'll have the best of him yet, though, as all this vigorous activity will increase his risk of needing revision surgery for his total hip arthroplasty. Of course, that may not be for another 10 to 15 years.

Having discovered my unique talent for sleuthing, I had recently offered my diagnostic services to our local orthopedic surgeon. I was waiting at the time in Dr. Goode's office late in the afternoon when I overheard a heated argument brewing in exam room 1. Suddenly there was a gasp and a thump, and the door flew open. A man with a wild eye and a scarred forearm stood there for an instant and then hobbled into the hallway. I rushed to the exam room. The doctor gasped, "I know that man," and then passed out, a stethoscope tied tightly around his neck. On the desk was what appeared to be the beginning of a medical history.

> Mac . . . [blood smudged the rest of the name]. A 37-year-old, left-handed stockbroker/taxi driver notes a 4-month progressive loss of manual dexterity and increasing numbness on the medial border of his right hand. Dorsal and palmar aspects are equally affected. Symptoms increase during busy days at the brokerage and during slow nights in the cab. No increase in symptoms with overhead activities. No recent injury. Elbow fracture as child. Medical history otherwise unremarkable. No history or symptoms suggestive of diabetes or other cause of peripheral neuropathy. Exam:

The doctor's note ended there. Not much to go on. I came to call this criminal "Elbow Mac." I queried the local brokerage firms and cab companies without success. I then went to the library to read about compression neuropathies. Pay dirt!

Elbow Mac's symptoms suggested ulnar nerve involvement. The most common site of compression is behind the medial epicondyle at the elbow, the so-called cubital tunnel. But it also can be compromised at the wrist. You can figure out the site of compression since the branch of the ulnar nerve supplying the dorsal medial aspect of the hand splits off in the forearm; an ulnar nerve compression at the wrist would affect only the palmar aspects of the hand and the ulnar two digits. A compression located more proximally at the elbow would affect both the dorsal and anterior aspects.

Ulnar nerve compression at the elbow affects sensation on both the dorsal and palmar aspects of the hand. Ulnar nerve compression at the wrist does not affect dorsal sensation.

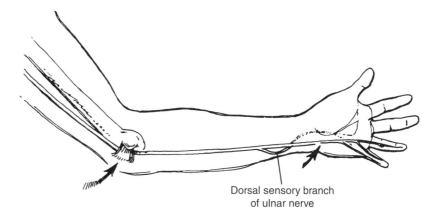

Dorsal sensory branch
of ulnar nerve

Likewise, the strength of the flexor carpi ulnaris and flexor digitorum profundus to the ring and little fingers might be affected by disease at the elbow but not by compression at the wrist. Long-standing ulnar nerve compression at either site would cause wasting of the ulnar-innervated muscles in the hand.

Long-standing, severe ulnar nerve palsy with marked wasting of the interosseous muscles and clawing of the ring and little fingers. Why are the index and middle fingers not clawed?

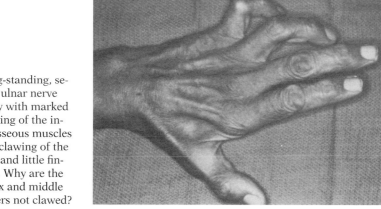

For further differentiation, the elbow acute flexion test will exacerbate symptoms within 1 minute if the nerve is rendered ischemic behind the medial epicondyle. Gentle tapping along the course of the nerve may also elicit paresthesias when the irritable area is struck. Unfortunately, the good doctor didn't record Elbow Mac's physical examination findings so I had only his history to go on, but it was a good start.

PRINCIPLE: Frequently a thorough history will be more helpful in making the diagnosis than results of either the physical examination or laboratory tests.

Cubital tunnel syndrome (known aliases: ulnar neuritis, tardy ulnar palsy) also may be mistaken for more proximal compressions such as thoracic outlet syndrome. Yet Elbow Mac didn't have increased symptoms with overhead activities, and it is well known that the shoulder positioned in abduction and external rotation aggravates the nerves passing through the thoracic outlet. Mac's numbness on both the dorsal and palmar surface of his hand suggested compression proximal to the wrist. Activities requiring prolonged elbow flexion (such as holding a telephone) and those causing direct pressure on the nerve (such as resting the elbow on an unpadded surface) are contributory. And sometimes an elbow injury, even one sustained many years previously, may lead to scarring and eventual nerve entrapment.

Although I knew it wouldn't help solve this crime, my curiosity compelled me to read about treatment. Avoidance of nerve irritation is the first line of defense—not resting the elbow on a hard surface while talking on the phone or studying, not sleeping with the elbow acutely flexed, and so forth. A night splint that holds the elbow in nearly full extension is often helpful for the latter. For patients with persistent symptoms, surgery is generally beneficial. Several procedures are available, and all have their proponents. Simple release of the fascial restraints over the nerve in the elbow area may be curative in early and mild cases. Transposition of the nerve anterior to the medial epicondyle certainly decompresses it. This also moves the nerve anterior to the center of rotation of the elbow, preventing stretching of the nerve that otherwise occurs with elbow flexion. The extensive mobilization required, however, at least temporarily interferes with the nerve's blood supply, potentially compounding the condition. Removal of the medial epicondyle decompresses the nerve and allows it to float anteriorly without the need for extensive mobilization. The forearm muscles originating from the medial epicondyle have plenty of remaining origin from surrounding fascia to prevent compromise, and although theoretically the ulnar nerve is more vulnerable to direct blows without the protective medial epicondyle, this is not a practical problem.

As I left the library armed with this information, I was convinced that this man had cubital tunnel syndrome. But maybe his stated occupations had been contrived, although those occupations could certainly predispose someone to cubital tunnel syndrome. The doctor's words came to mind: "I know this man." If Elbow Mac had been a former patient, I could search the office computer records by diagnosis to find him. Perhaps the elbow fracture in childhood was responsible for a case of tardy ulnar palsy. This possibility seemed sufficiently engaging.

It took some convincing for Dr. Goode's faithful staff to allow me access to his clinic charts—my not being a real detective or having any official position in the investigation. But they were kind enough to vacate the office overnight, leaving his charts guarded only by an easily picked padlock. Thoughtful of them, in my opinion. And as I painstakingly scanned through the files, I finally made my discovery. "Mackenzie Whitherspoon . . . Supracondylar humerus fracture age 8, complicated by compartment syndrome requiring emergent fasciotomy . . . Malpractice suit filed . . ." Elbow Mac, now with a compelling motive.

Before I could finish my search for more clues, however, I heard the main entrance door swing open. I quickly concealed my flashlight and peeked outside the records closet for a better look. I saw what appeared to be a maintenance worker headed straight for Dr. Goode's private office, where he produced a large ring of keys as he reached the door. As I watched the stranger fumble with his keys, I noticed something peculiar about his left hand. It appeared clumsy—he dropped the set twice before he found the one he was looking for. Then the small finger seemed to drift into abduction whenever he wasn't grasping something in the hand. A vague sense of familiarity began to wash over me. I intensified my scrutiny. The stranger had finally produced the requisite key, and now held it positioned between the pulp of his thumb and the radial aspect of his index middle phalanx—the common position we all use to turn a key. But what caught my eye was the interphalangeal joint of his thumb. He needed to flex this joint to produce enough strength to keep the key in place while he struggled to turn it in the lock. Most of us hold the interphalangeal thumb joint extended in this key-pinch position. He then hesitated, sensing my presence, and turned directly toward me. His eyes caught mine for but an instant, but that was enough. It was Elbow Mac.

In a siege of panic he bolted into the office, slamming it closed before I could reach him. But I couldn't let a shut door come between myself and this fugitive, so I did what any respectable detective would do and tried to ram it open with my shoulder. It didn't budge. After the stinging pain subsided, I realized that I hadn't actually checked whether or not it was still locked. A simple turn of the knob revealed a now-empty office. I searched diligently but could not produce the subject. My only clue was an open second-story window, although there was no fire escape in sight—only a broken row of concrete planters nearly 15 feet below that paralleled the sidewalk.

Somewhat disheartened, but nevertheless invigorated by my discovery, I returned to the library to confirm my observations. Sure enough, I had witnessed some of the more subtle, yet classic signs of ulnar neuropathy. Patients often describe clumsy or weak hands, even in the absence of atrophy or objective sensory changes. This occurs because the motor fascicles that supply the intrinsic muscles of the hand seem to be sensitive to early compression because of their superficial location within the ulnar nerve at the cubital tunnel. Clawing of the hand may occur in relatively severe cases due to significant intrinsic weakness, but some of the earlier manifestations include an abduction posture of the small finger as well as flexion of the interphalangeal joint of the thumb with attempted key pinch. The abduction deformity occurs as the weakened palmar interosseous muscle that normally adducts the small finger is overpowered by the oblique pull of the radially innervated extensor digiti minimi in the forearm. Thus the finger assumes an abducted position with attempted extension. Similarly, with attempted key pinch, the weakened adductor pollicis is unable to generate enough force to hold pressure in this position, so the patient learns to recruit the median-innervated flexor pollicis longus muscle (which flexes the distal phalanx of the thumb).

The next morning, quite proud of my newly discovered analytical skills but also growing fearful that our killer's trail would soon become cold, I headed straight for the local emergency room. I was quite confident that the assailant's fall the previous night would not have left him unscathed.

ADVANCED READING

Bozentka DJ. Cubital tunnel syndrome pathophysiology. Clin Orthop Relat Res 351:90-94, 1998.

Fujioka H, Nakabayashi Y, Hirata S, et al. Analysis of tardy ulnar nerve palsy associated with cubitus varus deformity after a supracondylar fracture of the humerus: A report of four cases. J Orthop Trauma 9:435-440, 1995.

Posner MA. Compressive ulnar neuropathies at the elbow: I. Etiology and diagnosis; II. Treatment. J Am Acad Orthop Surg 6:282-297, 1998.

Wartenberg R. Some useful neurological tests. JAMA 147:1645-1648, 1951.

◆ *If you ever awaken with your ulnar nerve asleep, try snapping your fingers to appreciate the devastation wrought by an ulnar nerve palsy.*

25

Frederick

Edward H. Parks ✦ *Scott A. Mitchell* ✦ *Roy A. Meals*

"I'm all over the keyboard. With laser beam precision, I shoot right pinky up to nail a 'p,' right ring taps the period key, then two quick thumb pumps on the space bar and we're tearing through the next sentence. It's poetry in motion. But it never fails; before I can finish a page, I wake up. That's when reality comes crashing in and the depression really hits the hardest. Then, after I'm soaked in the shower, hidden in a pair of socks, and finally jammed into a pair of smelly loafers, another boring day begins in the life of Fred. Fred the Foot. I suppose it could be worse, right? I could be stuck with a guy who stomps grapes or something." We both laugh.

Dr. Freiberg touches his pen to his lips and then points it at me. "That's the first real smile I've seen from you since we started these sessions, Frederick." He raises an eyebrow. "I honestly think we're making some progress here. I'd like to talk a bit more about these dreams, though. So tell me, how long have you had this subconscious desire to be a hand?"

"Well, to be honest, I guess it was sometime back in my early childhood," I explained. "You know, I used to *like* being a foot. Things were great in the beginning. Being a breech delivery, I led the way. The obstetrician held onto me for the first spanking. If I slipped then—bam, on the cold tile floor. I felt important. I had it good as an infant too—toes tickled, handmade booties. I was a star. But as I got older, I was forced to spend more and more of my time stuck in shoes, caged like an animal. Meanwhile, the hands are soaking up the glory: fancy rings, special 'hand' lotions, sexy leather driving gloves. I just don't get it. I mean, we're not *that* different looking. Why should hands be treated so much better than feet."

"Is there more, Fred?"

"Well, things were OK until the accident. That's when it became painfully obvious that if you want respect in this world, you have to be a hand. And hey, that really was an accident. I mean, I may have been depressed and all, but I never saw that bowling ball coming. I swear."

Dr. Freiberg sensed the nervousness in my voice. "That must have been very traumatic for you. But you know, all of us experience unpleasant events in our lives, Frederick. Take me, for instance. I had to have two operations on my hand—one for a spiral metacarpal fracture and the other for a completely torn thumb ligament." He held his hand down in front of me and wiggled his fingers, smiling. "As you can see, everything healed fine."

"Dr. Freiberg, this is exactly what I'm talking about. That bowling ball broke three of my toes and two of my metatarsals. But did I get an operation? Did I get plates and screws? Do I have macho scars to show off? No-o-o-o-o-o, not for Fred. I'm just a foot! I get a cheap plaster splint for a week and then some dorky cast. As if I didn't have enough trouble with odor to begin with. I've never felt so humiliated in my life!" I was trembling now and noticed a few beads of perspiration in my first web space. I curled my toes and continued, "It's one thing to be called names and made fun of, but getting gypped on health care, that's just too much. I lost my pride, my self-confidence. And that's when the dreams started."

Dr. Freiberg suddenly seemed alert and interested. "You mean to say that all your problems stem from this feeling of discrimination after the accident?"

"Hey, I'm not the only one. My lawyers think I've got a great case here."

"Fred, that's ridiculous," Dr. Freiberg responded, shaking his head. "The treatment you received was actually quite appropriate for your injuries. Hands may look like feet, but that's all. The treatment of hand and foot injuries is very different, mainly because of the difference in their functions. Hands are designed for fine manipulations, and this depends on the precise relationships between the bones, muscles, and other supporting tissues. And that bony anatomy needs to be maintained or restored, often surgically, when fractures are being treated. Feet are equally complex, but they provide the interface between our bodies and the earth's surfaces. Feet need to be strong, stable, and durable." He pulled a dusty anatomy text from the bookshelf. "Let's talk about metatarsal fractures. On the top of the foot, only a thin layer of skin and soft tissues covers the metatarsals. This makes them particularly vulnerable to injury when objects—bowling balls, for instance—are dropped. But on the other side, it is also important to consider that the metatarsals bear a considerable portion of body weight through the normal gait cycle, and they are exposed to even greater forces with many athletic activities. So even though direct trauma is the primary cause of metatarsal fractures, stress and insufficiency fractures are also common.

"Now the first metatarsal is shorter, wider, and stronger than the others, and as a result it's less often fractured; but of all the metatarsals, it withstands the most stress. The big toe, of course, also has the best motion and coordination."

"Coordination and motion?" I interrupted. "You just said that the hand reserves these features."

"Well, Fred, the big toe is a bit unusual in that regard. Although it can't really be compared to a thumb or finger, it's more like them than the other toes."

"Does that mean it's treated differently?"

"Exactly." Freiberg was getting excited. "You see, Fred, whenever function demands a wide motion arc, treatment has to accurately restore the original alignment and balance. Fractures of the first metatarsal that heal with bad angulation disturb the mechanics of the big toe. Because its mechanical demands are high, we have to ensure that the fracture heals in good alignment."

"So if that bowling ball had broken my first metatarsal, I would've gotten plates and screws?"

"Not necessarily. The first step would be to manually realign the fracture and then to apply a plaster splint. Most metatarsal fractures are stable once they are reduced."

"If they're stable, why the splint?"

"Well, they're not that stable. A cast would be preferable, for that matter, but casts don't allow for swelling. By stable, I mean the fracture fragments can maintain their position until they unite—usually within 4 to 6 weeks."

A, Multiple fractures involving the second metatarsal shaft, third and fourth metatarsal necks, and dislocation of the fourth and fifth metatarsophalangeal joints. **B,** Shown on the right is the post-reduction film. Even this complex injury is best managed nonoperatively.

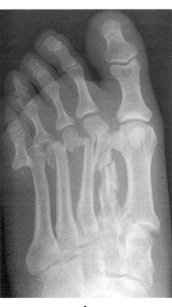

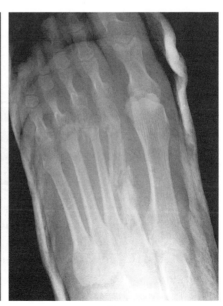

A   B

PRINCIPLE:	Do not place injured limbs in rigid circumferential casts until swelling has peaked.

"Wow! That's a long time to be hopping around on crutches, Doc."

"Crutches aren't needed the whole time, Fred. After 5 days or so, the swelling is down enough that the patient can have a short-leg walking cast."

"What if the reduction slips or cannot be secured in the first place?"

"Steel pins, screws, plates and screws. But remember, this is only if the alignment is unacceptable, which is unusual."

"So everything gets plaster?"

"Generally speaking, that's correct, Fred. Aside from the occasional unstable first metatarsal fracture, most metatarsal fractures are best managed with immobilization in a walking cast or hard-soled shoe. But there are some exceptions. As I was saying, the first metatarsophalangeal joint is a mobile, high-demand joint. If an intraarticular fracture there is displaced, the contour of the joint surface should be reestablished and held with pins or screws. Left untreated, arthritis would result. Fractures through the joints of the other toes are not as important because the demands on these joints are relatively low."

"Do they *ever* operate on fractures of the lesser metatarsals?"

"Rarely. If any broken bone is sticking through the skin, it needs to be thoroughly cleaned in the operating room, but that's a special situation. And there *are* a few oddball metatarsal fractures out there that don't play by the rules. Two famous troublemakers are march fractures and dancer's fractures. March fractures are fatigue fractures, also called stress fractures. They result from unaccustomed, repeated stress, like in military recruits. They are most common in the second and third metatarsals, as these are relatively immobile and bear significant stress with ambulation. However, especially in people who tend to oversupinate when they walk or run, the fifth metatarsal shaft may also be affected."

"I met a foot with that problem," I interjected. "She was no drill sergeant though, that's for sure. She was an aerobics instructor at the club. What a babe! She had the greatest set of malleoli on her. And a super-tight arch too. Anyway, she got this stress fracture and had to quit. She never really got better; she just got fat. She's like a triple E now. What a shame. . . . What about the dancer's fracture? Why is it rare? Was it named after an aerobics instructor?"

"Not quite. It's a spiral or oblique fracture through the distal aspect of the fifth metatarsal shaft, commonly seen in ballet dancers. These fractures can have significant rotational deformity and often require surgical fixation. Now there's a bit of confusion surrounding all of these eponyms given to fractures through different regions of the fifth metatarsal. The dancer's fracture is relatively distal, in the region of the metatarsal neck. Then moving more proximally into the diaphysis is the march or stress fracture, and then just a bit more proximal, right at the metaphyseal-diaphyseal junction, is a third important site. Sir Robert Jones was the father of British orthopedics in the early twentieth century. He sustained and named this fracture that occurs right at the metaphyseal-diaphyseal junction, a watershed region with a relatively poor blood supply. Because this region also experiences a large amount of stress during normal weight bearing, this fracture has a high incidence of nonunion."

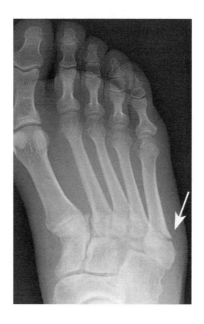

Considerable weight-bearing forces are transmitted across this fracture, and healing may be problematic.

"Now wait a minute, Dr. Freiberg. You just said that it is the first metatarsal that takes most of the heat during weight bearing. Looking at this picture in your book; the fifth metatarsal seems pretty wimpy to me. What makes you think it's under so much stress?"

"As a board-certified psychiatrist, I *know* it's under stress. . . ." We both laughed. "Seriously though, Fred, think of your footprints when you walk barefoot in the sand. The only part of the foot between the heel and the ball that touches the ground is the lateral edge, right where the fifth metatarsal is. In any event, this fracture should be treated carefully in a cast for the 6 to 8 weeks required for healing. If a nonunion occurs, this fracture will likely need bone grafting and internal fixation to heal. But be careful not to confuse Jones' fractures with the more common and slightly more proximal avulsion fracture of the fifth metatarsal base. Here an inversion injury tightens the peroneus brevis, avulsing its insertion. Avulsion fractures heal quickly in walking casts.

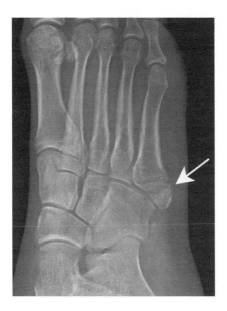

Weight bearing does not disturb this avulsion fracture, and healing is prompt.

"Here is another type of injury to the lesser metatarsals that doesn't quite fit the mold. It is named after one of the field surgeons in Napoleon's army who didn't actually describe the injury, but somehow the name stuck. Termed Lisfranc fracture/dislocations, these injuries encompass a spectrum of pathology around metatarsal bases at the junction of the rigid midfoot with the more supple forefoot. As I'm sure you are well aware, the second metatarsal is longer than the rest, and it fits in a recess proximally at the tarsometatarsal joint. The Lisfranc ligament itself originates from the lateral aspects of the medial cuneiform and attaches to the medial aspect of the second metatarsal base. This strong plantar ligament provides the only soft tissue link between the medial ray and the lesser metatarsals (there are no ligamentous connections between the first and second metatarsals). Injury to this joint complex, either from dislocation of the tarsal-metatarsal joints or, more commonly, a fracture through the second metatarsal base, can result in a chronically painful and functionally unstable foot with weight bearing. If any displacement is apparent on x-rays, these fractures/dislocations need to be reduced and operatively stabilized to minimize the risk of ending with this debilitating outcome."

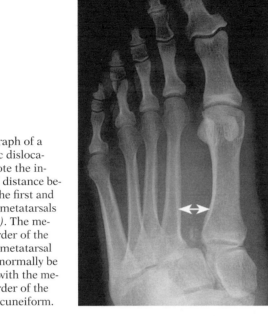

Radiograph of a Lisfranc dislocation. Note the increased distance between the first and second metatarsals *(arrows)*. The medial border of the second metatarsal should normally be in line with the medial border of the middle cuneiform.

"I'm impressed; who knew I was so intricate? What about toe fractures? Do they ever need surgery?"

"Only very rarely, again because toes have such limited function. The exception would be a widely displaced, intraarticular fracture of the big toe. For the other 99% of toe fractures, satisfactory healing occurs regardless of treatment. Pain relief during healing can be aided by taping the injured toe to an adjacent toe or, better yet, by wearing a wooden-soled sandal so that the toes remain motionless during ambulation."

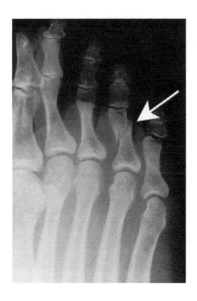

Typically, a person sustains this injury by stubbing his or her toes.

"You know, Dr. Freiberg, I'm glad we had this talk. I feel much better now that I understand why I was treated the way I was. I'm glad I'm not some temperamental, prima donna, sissy-like appendage that has to be wheeled off to the operating room when things get rough. Strength and stability—that's me all the way. Besides, how many of your patients tell you they have a *hand* fetish?

ADVANCED READING

Buzzard BM, Briggs PJ. Surgical management of acute tarsometatarsal fracture dislocation in the adult. Clin Orthop Relat Res 353:125-133, 1998.

DeLee JC. Fractures and dislocations of the foot. In Mann RA, ed. Surgery of the Foot, 7th ed. St Louis: CV Mosby, 1999.

Jones R. Fracture of the base of the fifth metatarsal by indirect violence. Ann Surg 35:697-700, 1902.

Lawrence SJ, Botte MJ. Jones' fractures and related fractures of the proximal fifth metatarsal. Foot Ankle 14:358-365, 1993.

LeVay D. The History of Orthopaedics. Carnforth, United Kingdom: Parthenon, 1990.

Philbin T, Rosenberg G, Sferra JJ. Complications of missed or untreated Lisfranc injuries. Foot Ankle Clin 8:61-71, 2003.

Rosenberg GA, Sferra JJ. Treatment strategies for acute fractures and nonunions of the proximal fifth metatarsal. J Am Acad Orthop Surg 8:332-338, 2000.

Wilson IN. Fractures of the metatarsals and phalanges. In Helal B, Wilson D, eds. The Foot. Edinburgh: Churchill Livingstone, 1988.

◆ *From an orthopedic perspective, what was wrong with the Hunchback of Notre Dame?*

26

Separation Anxiety

Scott A. Mitchell

It had already been a long night. What had begun as a gentle beating had turned into a frank blowout. The teammates' heads hung lower with each possession, too disheartened to even look at the scoreboard any longer. John Hill had been their downfall, seemingly unstoppable on both ends of the court. The rumored ankle injury hadn't slowed him down a bit.

But then a spark, a momentary triumph, as Arthur managed to pick the pocket of the opposing forward as he blazed toward the rim preparing for yet another uncontested layup. A quick spin, then the outlet pass up to midcourt, then another, leading the break. Then, in slow motion it seemed, the image of Ty leaping in stride over the ducking defender, hanging in midair for just an instant longer than seemed possible, then finishing with a two-handed dunk. Redemption.

Unfortunately, what the scene revealed next was the formerly frozen defender pivoting backward in an attempt to avert the shame of being dunked on. With this ducking maneuver, he managed to knock Ty's legs out from under him as he hung gloating from the rim. Then, as he spun nearly 180 degrees while falling from the rim, arms flailing and unable to catch himself, Ty sustained a direct blow to his right shoulder as he struck the ground. His temporary glory somewhat shaken by this tumble, he attempted to rise but was quickly halted by the pain. It was his teammates who first noted that the skin over his distal clavicle appeared tinted.

"I may be just a simple man," claimed Dave, "but that just don't look right. I think you may be done for the day."

"But you guys saw that, right?" Ty pleaded with an insuppressible grin."

"Yeah, yeah, too bad you blew it with that fall."

"How 'bout some props for my steal," Arthur interjected. "You never would have been that open on the break if it weren't for my lightning quick hands."

"Sure thing, fat boy . . ."

Several hours after the incident, the teammates stood in a cramped ER examining room surrounding a somewhat intimidated medical student. But despite his hesitancy, he performed a thorough physical examination. He localized the tenderness to the acromioclavicular joint and noted the superior displacement of the distal clavicle relative to the acromion. Although the overlying skin remained tinted and contused, no lacerations were apparent. Fortunately, the distal neurovascular status of the right arm was also intact. As the medical student pointed out, traction injuries to the underlying brachial plexus are not uncommon with injuries about the clavicle. The remainder of Ty's musculoskeletal examination was normal. Shortly after the medical student politely excused himself from the examining room, Ty was taken by wheelchair, much to the amusement of his audience, for x-ray examination of his shoulder and clavicle.

"But you can't kick me out of here!" a distant voice pleaded, "Do you realize what I've been through?" His tone escalated. "No, I'm not a patient. As I told that security guard, I'm trying to find . . . No, I don't know if he's a patient or not. That's the whole point . . . You're not listening. My name is Quentin B . . ."

The closing of the door to the examining room door silenced the gentleman's rising voice.

"Funny to see you guys here," Dr. Michael remarked with feigned surprise as he stepped into the room. "What, you don't get enough of this place with your day jobs, eh?" His fellow teammates returned his sarcasm with shaking heads.

"You have got to be kidding me," Ty pleaded, "Don't they give you any time off?"

"Sure, just long enough for the game and then right back into the trenches. Thought I told you guys I was on call tonight."

"We thought you were just making excuses for your lousy jump shot. What happened out there? You used to at least *look* like you knew what you were doing. The price you pay for being an orthopedic resident, huh?"

"Yeah, yeah, I guess my game has suffered just a bit. At least I can still outjump Arthur." Dr. Michael then paused, cleared his throat, and in his best attempt at a New York accent began one of his favorite impersonations. "Hey Art, you fallin' asleep on me back there. Name the three muscles that insert on the clavicle."

"Uh, uh, the deltoid?"

"No, I said, insert not arise. Pay attention. You're killin' me." He began stomping about the small examining room. "Don't you ever read nothin'? That's it, you're out. How 'bout you, next to him. Yeah, you. I'll switch it up for ya. You've already got one, so tell me the other two muscles that *arise* from the clavicle."

"You're getting that impression down," Ty interrupted. "Still got a few more years to work on it I'm sure. So why don't you tell me what happened to my shoulder."

"Alright, alright. All kidding aside, our fine student, Dr. Kim, has filled me in on the details of your medical history and physical examination. And I pretty much saw, firsthand, the debacle that led to this injury, as impressive as the effort was. So that just leaves your x-rays for us to review.

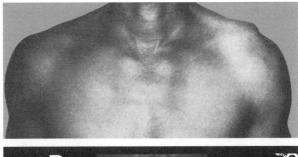
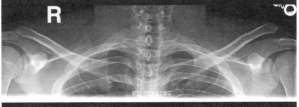

Example of complete acromioclavicular separation.

"Looks like you sustained a dislocation of the acromioclavicular joint—a separated shoulder as it is commonly referred to. Not to burden you with details, but there are a few points that are worth mentioning. Acromioclavicular joint injuries are most often caused by a direct blow to the tip of the shoulder, usually with the arm adducted, essentially driving the acromion inferiorly. Less commonly, injury may result from an indirect force transmitted through the arm as a result of a fall on an outstretched hand. As our teammates kindly pointed out earlier, simple inspection is often sufficient for a presumptive diagnosis. A prominent distal clavicle with a step-off down to the sagging acromion is highly suggestive. X-rays, of course, are confirmatory and are needed to distinguish this injury from a very distal clavicle fracture. If there is uncertainty regarding the degree of ligamentous injury, having the patient hold a 10- or 15-pound weight while x-rays are being taken will typically accentuate any ligamentous incompetence."

Ty cringed, "Uh, wouldn't that kind of hurt."

"Well sure; but we can't let that get between us and a diagnosis now, can we?" replied Arthur. "If you guys had just listened to me back when . . ."

"Remind me not to bring you guys along for the show next time."

Dr. Michael, amused by the friends' playful insults, continued, "Now there are two important ligamentous complexes that stabilize the acromioclavicular joint—the only bony link between the axial skeleton and the upper extremity, I might add. The first group consists of the ligaments and capsule of the acromioclavicular joint itself. Obviously, from the displacement apparent on your x-rays, you have sufficiently disrupted those. Some people, however, sustain isolated minor sprains of just these ligaments, in which case only minimal displacement of the distal clavicle is evident. Such injuries are nicely treated with a 1- to 2-week period of sling immobilization followed by range-of-motion exercises. Recovery is usually quite rapid. Now, the second group of ligaments—arguably the most important vertical stabilizers of the distal clavicle—are the coracoclavicular ligaments. With sufficient downward force directed against the acromion, as in your case, these ligaments too will rupture, producing the superior displacement of the distal clavicle we see on your x-ray films. This, however, is a bit misleading, as it is really a downward displacement of the acromion and scapula from the weight of the arm due to the loss of these supporting links to the clavicle."

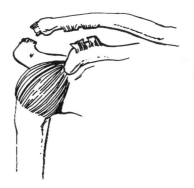 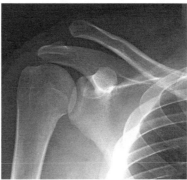

Both the coracoclavicular and acromioclavicular ligaments are torn in a complete acromioclavicular separation.

Modified from the American Orthopaedic Association. Manual of Orthopaedic Surgery, 6th ed. Chicago: American Orthopaedic Association, 1985, p 131.

"That's mighty interesting and all, but what does all that mean for me? I've got my basketball career to think about you know? How are we going to deal with this?"

"Dude, what are you thinking? You're a neurology resident," Dave ever so kindly pointed out. "What kind of basketball career are you referring to? I don't think the scouts really come to watch pickup games with you playing in scrubs."

"Yeah, looks like you'll have to save it for next year, lefty . . ." Arthur chimed in.

"Actually, he does sort of have a valid point," Dr. Michael continued. "First off, there does not appear to be any posterior displacement, button-holing of the distal clavicle through the trapezius or deltoid, severe elevation, or open injury, any of which might otherwise have pushed us toward early surgical management. So this leaves you with a bit of a treatment dilemma. Obviously this injury leaves you with a bit of a cosmetic deformity about your right shoulder."

"I think he needs all the help he can get in that department," Dave interrupted. "You have got to give the man a break."

"Uh, as I was saying, with proper nonoperative management we can expect some soft tissue healing and remodeling. This, along with some exercises to strengthen your deltoid and periscapular musculature, should allow you to return to normal activities without significant disability, although the separation will likely persist. In most people, particularly sedentary or elderly people, or neurology residents, for that matter, this approach can be expected to achieve excellent functional results. Treatment of this type of acromioclavicular injury still remains controversial, however, despite the frequent success of nonoperative management. The argument *for* surgery is that with this degree of displacement, muscle fatigue, discomfort, and difficulty with overhead loads may result. But it is really only in manual laborers, who must do repetitive overhead lifting, or in select high-level athletes, that these types of problems typically arise. For most patients, the results after operative and conservative management are equivalent. The decision essentially becomes a tradeoff between a bump and a scar over the distal clavicle. There are some additional disadvantages of surgery that I should point out, including the possibility of skin breakdown or infection as well as the risk of painful acromioclavicular arthritis down the road. I think that for these reasons most orthopedists now prefer nonoperative treatment initially, with the option of delayed surgical reconstruction should pain or instability persist."

"So how long do you think I'm going to be out if we decide to treat this with just a sling?"

"Well, it varies somewhat but my guess is your pain will subside in about 2 weeks, at which point we will get you out of the sling and start some range-of-motion exercises to keep the shoulder loose. But it will really be at least 6 weeks until we can really get you back to strength training and the sort."

"I don't get why it's going to take so long. It's not like there are any broken bones."

"Ah, glad you mentioned it. Actually, depending on the position of the arm, the location of contact, and the direction of the offending force, these types of falls can produce a fracture of the clavicle rather than acromioclavicular separation. Despite its relatively linear appearance on chest x-rays, the clavicle is actually an S-shaped bone. This may be best viewed by tilting the x-ray beam in the cephalic direction to approximate an orthogonal view to the standard anteroposterior view. Fractures of the clavicle most commonly occur through an area of relative weakness in the middle third as its contour moves from convex to concave. Fractures in this location typically cause the sternocleidomastoid to pull the proximal fragment upward while the weight of the limb pulls the distal fragment downward. The pectoralis major and latissimus also pull the shoulder toward the midline, causing the fracture ends to override and producing the characteristic subcutaneous bone spike palpable at the fracture site. Fractures of the distal third, on the other hand, though less common, can disrupt the insertions of the coracoacromial ligaments, creating a functional shoulder separation as well. Injury to these ligaments in the context of a distal clavicle fracture allows increased fracture displacement, which may interfere with healing.

"Treatment of clavicle fractures is also predominantly nonoperative, at least initially. Of course in open fractures, associated neurovascular injury, severe displacement with skin tenting and impending breakdown, significant shortening, or posterior displacement risking vital neurovascular and intrathoracic structures, operative fixation is indicated. But in most cases, a simple sling for comfort, or a figure-of-eight brace that keeps the shoulders in a retracted position to help reduce the fracture fragments is sufficient until the pain resolves in a few weeks. If displacement is significant, however, there is a considerable risk of nonunion, and some prefer plate fixation. The other exceptions to this are distal third clavicle fractures involving the coracoacromial ligaments. Injury through these stabilizing structures allows increased fracture displacement, so the incidence of nonunion is quite high. Although still somewhat controversial, many surgeons prefer operative fixation of the clavicle in this subtype of fracture.

"Just in case there are any budding orthopods in our midst, I brought along some x-rays to show you."

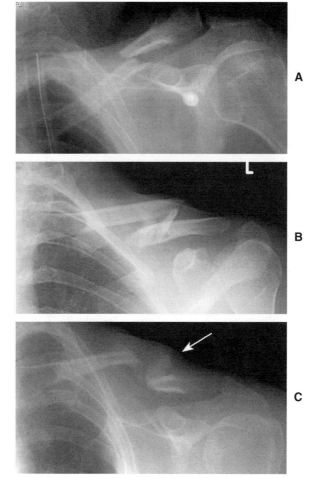

A, Distal third clavicle fracture. **B,** Displaced fracture of the middle third of the clavicle. **C,** Same fracture as in *B,* now a nonunion. Note the abundant callus formation and overlying soft tissue prominence *(arrow)* from the nonunion.

"Thanks for the lecture and all, Doc," Ty interrupted, "but you forget we all went to medical school together. We already did the Google search for acromioclavicular joint and clavicle injuries on my PDA while we were sitting in the waiting room."

"That would have been nice to know. So, was I at least convincing?"

"Don't worry; you did alright. Sounded like you may actually know what you're talking about. Good thing too, after your field-goal percentage on the court earlier. Now if you will be so kind, I think there may be a sling somewhere around here with my name on it."

ADVANCED READING

Anderson K. Evaluation and treatment of distal clavicle fractures. Clin Sports Med 22:319-326, 2003.

Bradley JP, Elkousy H. Decision making: Operative versus nonoperative treatment of acromioclavicular joint injuries. Clin Sports Med 22:277-290, 2003.

Clarke HD, McCann PD. Acromioclavicular joint injuries. Orthop Clin North Am 31:177-187, 2000.

Guttman D, Paksima NE, Zuckerman JD. Complications of treatment of complete acromioclavicular joint dislocations. Instr Course Lect 49:407-413, 2000.

Nuber GW, Bowen MK. Acromioclavicular joint injuries and distal clavicle fractures. J Am Acad Orthop Surg 5:11-18, 1997.

Rockwood CA Jr, Green DP, Bucholz RW, et al. Fractures in Adults, 4th ed. Philadelphia: Lippincott-Raven, 1996.

27

The Oral Exam

Roy A. Meals ✦ *Scott A. Mitchell*

"So Nick, I'm Dr. Jeffrey. I hope you're not frightened by my reputation for being a tough examiner. You guys have it easy these days. Back in my time, they wouldn't lay off during these sessions until you were nothing but a heap of babbling nonsense. Where's your shirt and tie, by the way? You better not be seeing patients in those scrubs."

"No sir. They just called me out of the operating room to come see you right away."

"Fine. So tell me, where did you do your surgery clerkship?"

"Six weeks at the VA and 6 weeks here at University Hospital."

"You've probably never had an oral examination before, but you'll have some others later; so this is a good place to start. Did you rotate on orthopedics?"

"Yes, sir."

"Well then, let me present you first with a 30-year-old patient just brought to the emergency room by ambulance. He was riding his bicycle and was struck by a car. Now he's complaining of pain in his left thigh. He is alert. Vital signs are stable. Tell me how you would manage him."

"Those could be fairly high-energy impact injuries, both when the car struck him and when he struck the ground. Most anything is possible—head, spine, chest, abdomen, pelvis, or limb injuries. It's a trauma setting, so I would start with the basics—the "ABCs." Even though you've told me he is alert, I would still quickly assess his airway, make sure he is able to talk without difficulty, and doesn't have any evidence of facial or neck trauma that could cause airway obstruction. Breathing is next, so I would look for how fast his respirations are and whether his chest is rising symmetrically. I would also look for any evidence of rib fractures and listen to his lungs to make sure he doesn't have a pneumothorax. Then circulation, so I would get him on a monitor to measure his heart rate and blood pressure, check his extremities for distal perfusion—pulses, warmth, and capillary refill. To protect against the possibility of occult blood loss somewhere, I would get the nurse to start a large-bore IV and draw some blood to check the hematocrit and collect a sample for the blood bank. Finally, I would do a quick neurologic check to make sure the patient is able to move and feel all of his extremities.

"Assuming all these basics check out, I would move on to a bit more in-depth secondary survey. I would get a brief history, ask him about the accident and where he's having pain. Make sure he doesn't have any medical problems. Medications and allergies, of course. Also, when his last meal was, just in case he needs to go to the operating room right away. While talking to him, I would do a brief head-to-toe physical examination. His clothes are already off, I presume, so I won't miss any contusions or other evidence of injury. I would carefully move all of his joints and palpate the pelvis, long bones, and spine for any tenderness. Got to be careful in these trauma patients, because the presence of one injury can distract from other injuries that you wouldn't want to miss."

"Fine. The only sore area you find is his left thigh, with a superficial abrasion and deep ecchymosis on its lateral aspect. Everything else checks out."

"OK, so for the moment I'm going to focus on the leg. I need to check and document the distal neurovascular status more carefully than during the initial survey. It is very important not to overlook an associated nerve or arterial injury."

"Let's say his pedal pulses aren't palpable on the injured side."

"Then I have a couple of options. First, I would continue his fluid resuscitation and make sure that he wasn't just hypotensive. Then, assuming he has a fracture that you haven't told me about, I would reduce any gross deformity and put him in a long splint to make sure that the vessels weren't kinked near the fracture site. I would also check the temperature, color, and capillary refill in the foot. I'd want to know if he still had perfusion through collateral vessels or if the leg was completely ischemic. A warm, pink foot, even without a palpable pulse, is a bit different from a cold, white foot. I would also recheck the pulses with a Doppler. The presence of a Doppler signal can be misleading, however, because a greatly reduced arterial pressure can still produce an audible signal. Ideally, I would use the Doppler signal along with a blood pressure cuff on the calf to find out exactly what the pressures were in the distal leg. If the pressures aren't bilaterally equal, he probably should be referred for a vascular surgery consultation."

"OK, OK, OK. Let's say his Doppler pressures are equal. What next?"

"Well, sounds like he may have a femur fracture, so I would ever so gently feel clear around the thigh, checking for breaks in the skin posteriorly. I would try palpating the greater trochanter and condyles of the femur to check for alignment, and I'd compare this to the other side. Then, of course, we would need to get some x-rays."

"Good. Here is a film, but while you are in radiology, the nurse tells you that his blood pressure has dropped to 105/55 and his pulse is up to 110."

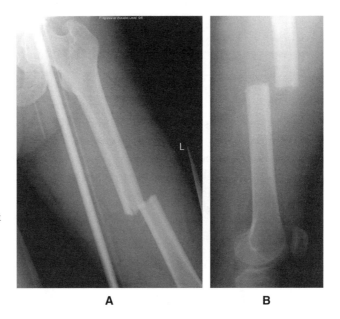

A, Noncomminuted transverse midshaft femur fracture with lateral displacement and apex medial angulation. B, Lateral view showing posterior displacement.

A   **B**

"In this setting it sounds like hypovolemic shock. His x-rays confirm a displaced transverse femoral shaft fracture. You didn't mention any external bleeding, so he is likely bleeding into his thigh from this fracture. One can lose a liter or more into the thigh without much visible evidence of it. The pelvis is the other place for major occult blood loss, although the results of that examination were negative. I would ask the general surgeons whether they wanted to get a CT scan of the abdomen to look for bleeding or even do a peritoneal lavage if he is unstable. For now I would give him a bolus of IV fluids. That brings me to another point; we have gotten x-rays of the femur, but we haven't gotten all of the films we need yet. Every trauma patient should have at the very least three x-rays while in the trauma bay—lateral cervical spine, anteroposterior chest, and anteroposterior pelvis. The latter would give us a good idea about whether to suspect blood loss from a pelvic fracture, which can at times be massive."

"OK, so the CT scan of his belly is negative, there is no pelvic fracture, and the cervical spine is clear. Any more studies you want?"

"Well, the x-ray you gave me didn't show his hip as well as I would have liked. There might be an associated femoral neck fracture. It only happens in about 3% of femur fractures, but when it does it can easily be missed. Any patient with a femur fracture needs a dedicated x-ray of the hip."

"Very well. How do you want to treat the fracture and when do you want to do it?"

"In the past, fractures like this were treated first for about 6 weeks of skeletal traction to maintain the length and some semblance of alignment; then a spica cast was used for another 6 weeks. Not only is that length of time in the hospital exorbitantly expensive these days, it is not physiologic to be on your back that long—pneumonia, pressure sores, osteoporosis, muscle atrophy, and so forth. Surgical options include opening and plating the fracture or slipping a rod down the intramedullary canal. Doesn't sound like there is a need for an external fixator here, although if he was hemodynamically unstable or if this was an open fracture with severe soft tissue injury, I would consider it. Right now this is not a life-threatening emergency that requires getting him to the operating room immediately, but the sooner the fracture is stabilized, the sooner he can sit up and get up. This reduces the risk of pulmonary complications and various metabolic derangements."

"Excellent. Would you expose the fracture site to put the rod in?"

"Only as a last resort. Bone has both a periosteal and an endosteal blood supply. We can assume that because of the fracture the endosteal blood supply has been at least partially disrupted. Opening the fracture and exposing the bone ends would further strip away the periosteum, rendering the fracture ends quite avascular. Then osteomyelitis and nonunion become greater risks. I think this fracture should get an intramedullary nail placed through an entry site next to the greater trochanter."

"What if the x-ray showed several large, loose fragments at the fracture site? With that degree of comminution, would you still use a rod? Wouldn't the femur just shorten up and possibly rotate on the rod when the patient contracted his quadriceps or put any weight on it?"

"Right. Intramedullary nailing used to be just for noncomminuted transverse fractures and short oblique fractures, for the reasons you mention. But rods can now be locked with screws that are placed transversely through the bone and through the rod using small stab incisions under image-intensifying fluoroscopy. The locking screws prevent shortening and rotation, and they have basically eliminated the need for opening and plating a femur fracture. The patient is up on crutches with toe-touch weight bearing and out of the hospital in just a few days, other injuries permitting. Much less chance for the knee to get stiff too, as there is less trauma to the thigh musculature than with a formal open reduction and plating. Also, compared to a plate, the rod is less likely to break and is easier and safer to remove after healing is complete."

"Quite impressive. So let's say he gets a rod and the next day the nurse calls you to say the patient seems disoriented and restless."

"First things first; what are his vital signs?"

"Blood pressure 120/80; pulse 120; respirations 30 per minute."

"Pulmonary embolus is always a possibility, but in this setting I would give serious consideration to fat embolism. It occurs 1 to 3 days after injury in patients with long-bone fractures; the more fractures, the greater the likelihood. Opinions vary as to whether it is actually small fat globules from the bone marrow at the fracture site that enter the circulation or primarily an inflammatory or metabolic derangement. Either way, it's bad news for the lungs, so I'd draw a blood gas and order a chest x-ray. While I was waiting, I would look for the characteristic petechiae on the conjunctiva, buccal membranes, and chest wall. I'd spin a urine sample to look for fat."

"What would you expect from the x-ray and blood gases?"

"With fat embolus, the x-ray would show bilateral patchy infiltrates, exactly like adult respiratory distress syndrome. The hypoxemia would cause a low oxygen pressure, and the resultant tachypnea would cause a low carbon dioxide pressure as well. If he's not intubated, he needs to be. He also needs positive end expiratory pressure to hold the alveoli open throughout the respiratory cycle. I am actually a little surprised that he is developing fat emboli. That is one reason to fix his fracture as soon as possible, because fat embolism can be fatal in 10% to 15% of cases. Although early fracture stabilization reduces its incidence, it does not eliminate the risk entirely."

"Extraordinary. Let's say that the patient does well. How about his 9-year-old son, who was struck by the same car and also sustained a midshaft femur fracture? Somebody didn't know what else to do, so they put him in skeletal traction. It's now 2 weeks later. Here is his x-ray. Can you get the other doctor out of this mess?"

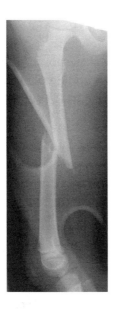

Femur fracture with significant fragment overriding in a 9-year-old boy.

"I guess by 'mess' you mean that the fracture ends are overriding, and there is complete anterior displacement of the distal fragment with some apex posterior angulation. Actually, for a kid this position will probably be fine, providing the rotational alignment is OK. That cannot be determined very easily from the x-ray films, so I would have to see the boy and make sure that while he is supine his anterior iliac spine, kneecap, and second toe are all pointing straight up. If his patella and toe are pointing out, for instance, he has a rotational malalignment of his fracture."

P R I N C I P L E :   Anteroposterior and lateral x-rays give an incomplete view of the three-dimensional world. Only a clinical examination will identify subtle rotational fracture malalignment.

"So we'll say that the rotation is OK. What about the overriding? Do you want him to end up with a short limb?"

"Of course not, but neither do I want him to end up with the limb longer than the opposite one. In kids a femur fracture produces a regional hyperemia that lasts for more than a year—well after the fracture has healed. This increased blood flow to the area stimulates the epiphyses, so the bone overgrows relative to the uninjured side. In fact, it is not uncommon for the fractured side to end up 1 to 1.5 cm too long."

"So what do you propose?"

"Well, I think we have a couple of options. In any child with a femur fracture, a spica cast is always an option. Some people put them on right away, and others use a period of traction beforehand to help maintain length and wait until the ends of the bone get sticky from early callus formation. However, spica casts have some practical downsides that limit their utility in older children. First, older kids simply do not tolerate the amount of immobilization imparted by a spica cast as well as younger ones. Also, you have to consider the size of the patient. The parents must be able to lift and reposition the child every couple of hours while he is in the cast, which may be as long as 6 weeks. For these reasons, spica casts seem to work best for children less than 6 years old. Another option, and in my opinion the best option for a patient over 6, is fixing the fracture with several percutaneously placed flexible nails. A bit different from the intramuscular rods we used in his dad though. Usually requires at least two of these thin, flexible nails placed in the medullary canal to maintain alignment and length. Not as strong as the adult intramuscular rods either, but these flexible nails preclude the child spending several weeks immobilized in a hip spica."

"So why not just use a standard intramedullary nail? You just told me they work great for adult femur fractures."

"Well, because as pediatricians like to say, children aren't just miniature adults. Let's not forget about the growth plates. There are three of them, after all, in the immature femur—two proximally in the femoral head and greater trochanter, and one distally. To put an adult nail in would require disruption of the trochanteric apophysis and possibly the distal femoral physis, the site of almost 75% of the longitudinal growth of the femur. With the flexible nails, you can make a small cortical hole in the distal femoral metaphysis and slip the nails up without damaging any of these physes. Also, the vascular anatomy of the proximal femur in children seems to be a bit more temperamental than in adults. The risk of avascular necrosis of the femoral head from a proximal entry point is higher and best avoided."

"OK, so you've given me a lot of information, but you have not yet answered my original question. What do you want to do with this kid's femur."

"Sorry, sir. Given that it's been 2 weeks since the fracture occurred, there is probably a good bit of healing already, so I don't think we need to take this patient to the operating room and struggle to realign the fracture enough to slide flexible nails in. Nor do we really need to worry about the reduction, so long as the rotational alignment is acceptable. So in this case I'd suggest leaving him in the hip spica cast and sending him home, providing there is someone at home strong enough to turn him every couple of hours to prevent pressure sores."

"Why not just a long-leg cast? And what about the angulation?"

"A long-leg cast leaves the hip free. This would allow motion at the fracture site—not beneficial for either comfort or prompt fracture healing. That extra angulation in the femur will remodel with growth over the next several *years,* especially since it is in the plane of knee motion. Medial-lateral angular deformities don't remodel so well, and rotational deformities don't remodel at all."

PRINCIPLE:	**Compensate for the age-related growth and remodeling potential of the patient's bones when planning treatment.**

"Why, that's what I was going to show you. Here are four x-rays of another 9-year-old who had an oblique fracture of the femur."

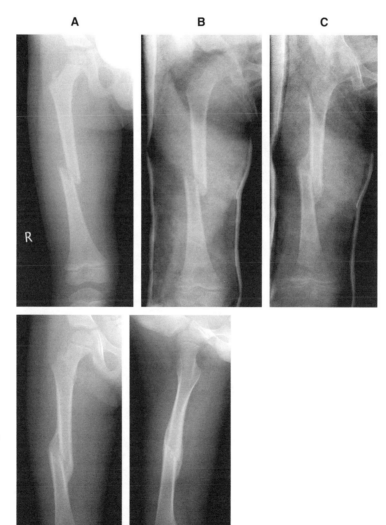

A, Oblique femur fracture in a skeletally immature patient. **B,** Radiograph after spica cast placement. Is this degree of displacement acceptable? **C,** One month after injury. Note the abundant callus formation that has bridged across the fracture site. **D,** Two months after injury. Note the callus maturation and bony remodeling that have already begun.

"Nick, you've been most impressive with your answers. More like an orthopedist prepared for the board examination rather than a third-year medical student on your first clinical rotation. You are quite knowledgeable."

"Thank you. Maybe you missed my full name. I'm Nicholas Andry, XIII. My namesake, Nicholas Andry, was interested in skeletal deformities. In 1741, at age 83, he coined the word 'L'Orthopédie' from the words for 'straight' and 'child' to describe the art of straightening deformities by mechanical aids and improved posture. He likened it to tying a crooked tree to a stake to straighten it out. All Andrys since then have been interested in musculoskeletal disorders."

"Well, that is very interesting. Holding back on me are ya? I wish I'd known. Maybe I can still tie you to a stake. Let's talk about a 50-year-old woman with long-standing melorheostosis who has just been discovered to have alkaptonuria. . . ."

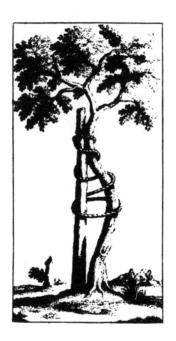

Illustration from Nicholas Andry's book published in 1742.

ADVANCED READING

Andry N. L'Orthopédie ou L'art de Prévenir Dans les Enfans, les Diffonnités du Corps, vol 1 and 2. Paris: 1742.

Bliss B, Bradley JWP, Fairgrieve J, et al. Vascular injuries. J Bone Joint Surg Br 71:738, 1989.

Gardner MJ, Lawrence BD, Griffith MH. Surgical treatment of pediatric femoral shaft fractures. Curr Opin Pediatr 16:51-57, 2004.

Jaarsma RL, van Kampen A. Rotational malalignment after fractures of the femur. J Bone Joint Surg Br 86:1100-1104, 2004.

Pryor JP, Reilly PM. Initial care of the patient with blunt polytrauma. Clin Orthop 422:30-36, 2004.

Sponseller PD. Surgical management of pediatric femoral fractures. Instr Course Lect 51:361-365, 2002.

Winkelaar GB, Taylor DC. Vascular trauma associated with fractures and dislocations. Semin Vasc Surg 11:261-273, 1998.

Wolinsky P, Tejwani N, Richmond JH, et al. Controversies in intramedullary nailing of femoral shaft fractures. Instr Course Lect 51:291-303, 2002.

✦ *What should you assume when a patient has a scapula fracture or first and second rib fractures?*

28

Joe's Bugaboo

Joe Katz lays tile. He's been doing it since the oil fields dried up, and he's quite good at it. From crawling around all day, the skin on his knees is even tougher than the skin on his feet. He didn't used to wear knee pads. That's how his bursitis first developed.

An enlarged bursa will develop in the area between the skin and the patellar tendon in anyone who is on their knees a lot. Bursa means purse or sac, which develops in areas of direct pressure or friction. Think of it as a synovial-lined pouch; the synovial fluid lets the tissues glide friction-free over one another, as in joints and around tendons. With repeated, forceful pressure, such as Joe on his knees, the bursal sac thickens and fluid accumulates, causing a puffy, possibly tender swelling over the lower part of the kneecap. In this location bursitis is called housemaid's knee, but can you remember the last time somebody scrubbed a floor on their knees? Plumbers, tile setters, carpet layers, and roofers are more likely contemporary candidates. Unfortunately while the fluid accumulation may be adaptive to repetitive pressure, the synovial fluid itself is a great culture medium for bacteria. A puncture wound or indirect spread of bacteria from an infected sore on the leg can infect the bursa.

Joe crawled onto a nail and broke the skin; 2 days later he was in his doctor's office with a red, painful swelling on the front of his knee and an unwillingness to flex the joint. He thought his knee joint was infected, but the signs of inflammation were isolated to the prepatellar area. Dr. Honeychurch explained that the pain with knee flexion was related to further stretching of the inflamed prepatellar bursa and not from inflammation within the joint. He then confirmed the diagnosis by aspirating pus from the bursa, and the next morning he opened and drained the infected bursa in the operating room. Joe wore knee pads after that.

Joe also likes to fish on the weekends, far more than he likes to maintain his dinky outboard motor. Consequently, it doesn't start too easily sometimes. Joe wonders whether the bursitis at his elbow came from repetitively yanking on the starter cord or from striking his olecranon sharply against the gunwale. Here is the photograph Dr. Honeychurch took that following Monday.

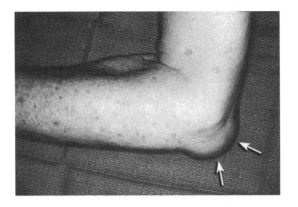

Swelling and thickening of the olecranon bursa over the extensor surface of the elbow.

His diagnosis was olecranon bursitis, also known as "student's elbow." He drained the serosanguineous fluid with a needle and syringe, and Joe wore an elastic compression bandage for a week or so. Then after three more attacks, Joe finally got his motor tuned. But the bursa persisted, and Dr. Honeychurch excised it. Since then, Joe hasn't had any more trouble with his elbow or his boat motor.

Patients with rheumatoid arthritis are also susceptible to olecranon bursitis. The intraarticular disease stimulates production of synovial fluid, which leaks into the bursa. If this type of bursa becomes infected, the joint is also at immediate risk, obviously with much more serious consequences.

Several years after his elbow problem (and this time for no good reason), Joe got trochanteric bursitis—between the bony prominence of his greater trochanter and the overlying gluteus maximus tendon and iliotibial band. Joe thought he had arthritis. Every time he flexed his hip, one of these tendons would snap sharply over the bone. When Dr. Honeychurch passively put the hip through the same motions, the snapping was absent because the muscles were relaxed. Joe's pain was localized to the lateral aspect of his hip over the greater trochanter, and he was quite tender to palpation in this area. Pain from arthritis in the hip joint is usually described as groin pain, which is more medial than trochanteric bursitis pain. Patients do not usually have any local tenderness to palpation on examination, but passive internal rotation of the hip will typically reproduce their arthritic pain. So Dr. Honeychurch was fairly confident after his clinical examination that Joe's pain was bursitis rather than the more ominous hip arthritis. After an x-ray ruled out hip joint disease, Dr. Honeychurch infiltrated the tender area with long-acting cortisone, which took care of the problem.

PRINCIPLE: When symptoms arise from a discrete, identifiable area, cortisone injection frequently has a higher benefit-risk ratio than oral nonsteroidal antiinflammatory medication.

In how many other areas can Joe potentially develop bursitis? More than 150 bursas have been identified in the human body, but commonly just several more are problematic.

There are two bursas just superior to the Achilles tendon insertion at the back of the heel—the subcutaneous calcaneal bursa (also called the Achilles bursa), located superficially between the skin and tendon, and the retrocalcaneal bursa, located deeper between the calcaneus and tendon. Inflammation of either of these bursas caused by repetitive trauma or overuse can cause pain at the posterior heel. Pressure from the back of a tight-fitting shoe can also irritate the superficial bursa—therefore its name, 'pump bump.' The overlying skin is inflamed and reddened, and walking barefoot characteristically relieves the pain. If the deeper, retrocalcaneal bursa becomes inflamed, symptoms are similar but the pain is localized just anterior to the Achilles tendon and signs of skin inflammation may be absent. A lateral x-ray may show an enlarged upper posterior corner of the calcaneal tuberosity, which may contribute to impingement between this prominence and the Achilles tendon. Protecting the inflamed bursa with adhesive tape or foam rubber and changing shoe styles are usually curative. Sometimes the bursa must be excised, and to prevent recurrence the offending prominence on the calcaneus can be trimmed.

The anserine bursa lies on the medial side of the knee beneath the conjoined tendinous insertion of the sartorius, gracilis, and semitendinosis muscles, termed the pes anserinus (literally translated 'goose's foot,' presumably likening the common tendinous insertion to its webbed appearance). Anserine bursitis is an overuse syndrome commonly seen in athletes and long-distance runners, particularly those who run on uneven terrain. It is thought to arise, in part, from tight medial hamstrings, which are also common in runners. Pain typically radiates along the medial joint line at the extremes of knee flexion and extension, and is characteristically bothersome when climbing stairs. This malady must be differentiated from medial joint pathology (meniscal tear, osteoarthritis) or strain of the medial collateral ligament. Hamstring stretching and activity modification are typically curative.

Joe doesn't know it yet, but he is also due for a bout of subacromial bursitis. Down at the lake, he holds his arms overhead to trim the trees around the cabin; then he plays volleyball until it is too dark to see.

The rotator cuff tendons cross over the head of the humerus en route to their insertions on the greater tuberosity. The overlying acromial arch prevents the shoulder from dislocating superiorly, but it also creates friction as the rotator cuff rubs against its undersurface with shoulder abduction. Does this sound like a likely place for a bursa?

When Joe's subacromial bursa becomes inflamed, pinching it between the humeral head and the acromion with abduction or external rotation maneuvers will cause pain. After his weekend of vigorous overhead activities, he'll notice pain when trying to push up a sticky window, for instance. A cortisone injection or two usually suffices. Subacromial bursitis is part of the impingement syndrome, in which not only the bursa but also the rotator cuff itself gets pinched between the acromion and the humerus. Then tendinitis, sometimes with a calcific deposit seen on the x-ray film, is noted.

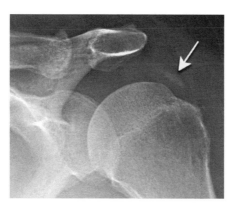

Calcific deposits in the supraspinatus tendon *(arrow)*.

Surgical decompression of the rotator cuff by partial acromion excision may be required to avoid an attritional tendon rupture. But you will hear about Johnny Mann later. So you see, although bursas have been Joe's bugaboo, at least he is active. Imagine getting ischial tuberosity bursitis from sitting too much.

ADVANCED READING

Butcher JD, Salzman KL, Lillegard WA. Lower extremity bursitis. Am Fam Physician 53:2317-2324, 1996.

Morrison DS, Greenbaum BS, Einhorn A. Shoulder impingement. Orthop Clin North Am 31:285-293, 2000.

Myerson MS, McGarvey W. Disorders of the Achilles tendon insertion and Achilles tendonitis. Instr Course Lect 48:211-218, 1999.

Reveille JD. Soft-tissue rheumatism: Diagnosis and treatment. Am J Med 102:23S-29S, 1997.

Salzman KL, Lillegard WA. Upper extremity bursitis. Am Fam Physician 56: 1797-1806, 1997.

◆ *Has anyone with only one hand ever played major league baseball?*

29

The Legal Secretary

A 62-year-old secretary to the busiest medical liability plaintiff's attorney in the state has been awakened at night over the past 6 months by tingling and numbness in the fingers of her dominant left hand. More recently, similar symptoms have appeared on the right. She also notes symptoms when driving for more than 20 minutes, such as when she visits her new grandson. She is uncertain which digits are involved but thinks the index and middle fingers are the worst. She denies having paresthesias in her feet and other symptoms suggestive of peripheral neuropathy. Symptoms characteristic of thyroid disease are absent. Personal and family histories for diabetes are negative. Examination shows normal light touch and two-point discrimination in all fingertips. The muscles in the hand, the intrinsic muscles, are all of normal bulk and strength. Thumb opposition is full. Tenosynovial thickening is not evident in the palm or distal forearm. Gentle tapping over the palmaris longus tendon at both wrists elicits paresthesias in the index fingers.

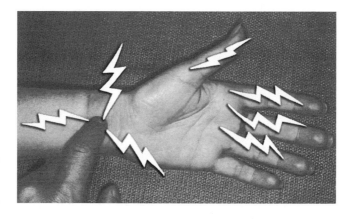

Gentle tapping at a site of nerve irritability will cause depolarization. The patient will have paresthesia in the nerve's distribution.

Letting the wrists flop into flexion and leaving them there for 30 seconds reproduces the severe paresthesias the patient experiences at night.

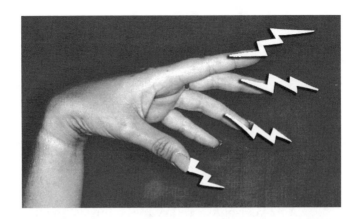

Wrist flexion further insults an ischemic median nerve and will thereby produce symptoms within 1 minute.

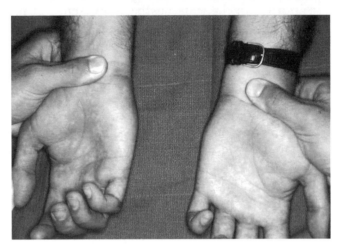

Another simple maneuver that is perhaps the most sensitive and specific test for carpal tunnel syndrome involves applying pressure with the examiner's thumb directly over the carpal tunnel. This test is positive if the patient's symptoms are reproduced by this compression within 30 seconds.

The ulnar, median, and radial nerves are not irritable around the elbow. Testing for thoracic outlet syndrome by having the patient hold her shoulders in abduction and external rotation does not reproduce the symptoms. The neck exhibits full range of motion without any paraspinal tenderness. Axial compression of the cervical spine does not cause pain. Nerve conduction velocities are as follows:

	Right	Left	Normal
Sensory latency across wrist	3.6	3.7	≤3.5 msec
Motor latency across wrist	4.4	4.5	≤4.5 msec

What's your diagnosis? What's in your differential diagnosis? Do you want any other diagnostic tests? What treatment do you recommend?

Median nerve compression within the carpal canal is known as carpal tunnel syndrome. Nine digital flexor tendons and the median nerve pass through the unyielding bony and ligamentous canal, and any tenosynovial thickening or other local enlargement causes increased pressure on the nerve and thereby decreases capillary perfusion. The ischemic nerve is easily depolarized when mechanically stimulated by direct tapping. With wrist flexion or direct pressure from the examiner's thumb, the nerve is further compressed causing depolarization and tingling. This is the basis for the wrist flexion test and possibly the cause for the nearly pathognomonic symptom of night waking with paresthesias.

PRINCIPLE: Nerve tissue is very sensitive to ischemia. Neurons are among the few cell types in the body that are exclusively dependent on a continuous supply of glucose to meet energy requirements, which is thought to account for their susceptibility to ischemia. What other tissues share this characteristic?

Compression of the median nerve at the wrist results in local ischemia and impaired axonal transport. This initially causes a neurapraxia, a situation in which the nerve is in full anatomic continuity but not functioning normally. Typically this is associated with a conduction block caused by focal demyelination of axons within the carpal tunnel. Prolonged, unrelenting pressure, however, will cause disruption of the axon within its connective tissue sheath—axontomesis. In this situation, progressive axonal loss leads to thenar muscle wasting and impaired opposition. Two-point discrimination, a function of innervation density, is relatively spared in early carpal tunnel syndrome when axons remain in continuity. However, with axonal loss from long-standing carpal tunnel syndrome, impaired two-point discrimination develops.

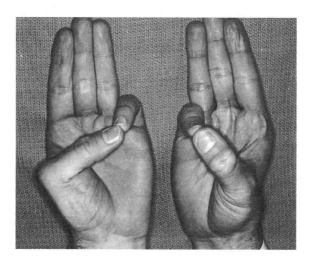

In long-standing, severe carpal tunnel syndrome, the median innervated thenar muscles weaken and atrophy, causing incomplete opposition, as seen on the left.

The etiology of carpal tunnel syndrome involves both local and systemic factors. Local causes of elevated carpal tunnel pressures can include tumors, osteophytes, fractures, anomalous muscles, infection, and other inflammatory conditions. Work-induced carpal tunnel syndrome results from proliferation of the tenosynovium related to repetitive wrist and finger motions in occupations such as word processing, meat packing, and grocery checking. Prolonged extremes of wrist flexion and extension also elevate pressure within the carpal canal and may also play a role. There are several systemic disorders associated with carpal tunnel syndrome. These include obesity; rheumatoid arthritis; endocrine abnormalities such as diabetes, hypothyroidism, and acromegaly; and amyloidosis. Also, a nerve may be compressed at more than one site, a condition known as double-crush syndrome. For instance, pressure on the nerve in the neck, at the thoracic outlet, or at the elbow will make it more susceptible to even mild pressure in the carpal canal. Likewise, nerves compromised by diabetes or chronic alcoholism are also more sensitive to compression. Most commonly, however, carpal tunnel syndrome is "idiopathic" (medical obfuscation for "the doctors don't know") and tends to affect middle-aged and older women.

Nerves elsewhere in the body can be entrapped similar to the median nerve at the wrist. Common sites include nerve roots in the cervical and lumbar areas and the ulnar nerve at the elbow. If the doctor knows the motor and sensory distribution of the region's nerves, a careful history and physical examination can usually pinpoint the site of compression.

P R I N C I P L E :   Knowledge of anatomy and diagnostic acumen go hand in hand.

N O T E :   *The ulnar nerve passes through a lesser-known osteoligamentous canal in the wrist adjacent to the carpal canal where it also is prone to compression. How would signs and symptoms of ulnar nerve compression at the wrist differ from carpal tunnel syndrome? Which muscles in the hand are innervated by the median versus the ulnar nerve?*

Treatment is directed at relieving pressure on the nerve. In patients with neurapraxia of only a few months' duration, protecting the wrist from prolonged flexion and extension by use of a splint and injecting a long-acting cortisone preparation into the canal to reduce tenosynovial thickening are frequently curative. In patients with symptoms of longer duration, which may be associated with axontomesis, surgical release of the transverse carpal ligament may be required. Although this procedure is straightforward and generally successful in relieving symptoms, a return to the work activities that initially incited symptoms may promote a recurrence. Thus work-induced carpal tunnel syndrome needs to be prevented by introducing improved work habits, wrist postures, and tool designs.

Follow-up Note 1: The nerve conduction velocities confirmed the history and physical examination by identifying slowing of median nerve conduction across the wrist. In confusing situations, electrical studies also may help identify more proximal sites of compression or evidence of generalized peripheral neuropathy. With one steroid injection, night splinting, and pacing her word-processing responsibilities at work, the secretary has been completely relieved of symptoms. Her boss is 'eternally grateful' to you for getting her valued employee back to work.

Follow-up Note 2: Nine months later, the legal secretary returns to your office, this time accompanied by her boss. Her symptoms have returned and worsened over the past 3 months. While her boss is taking notes, your patient demands to know why your treatment has failed.

In your typical thorough and patient manner, you explain that while relief provided by splinting and steroid injection is often successful initially, symptoms may recur as the antiinflammatory effects of the injection wear off. You inquire about her work habits. She quietly relates that she is now doing double-duty word processing since the other secretary has been on maternity leave. Her keyboard is awkwardly placed causing her to type with her wrists in constant flexion. Her boss's glare does not diminish your calm demeanor.

Follow-up Note 3: The patient's symptoms did improve after a temp assumed the overflow word processing and after the secretary's work station was rearranged such that her keyboard was directly in front of her and at a height that allowed her to position her forearms parallel with the floor while her wrists were straight. She appreciates that she was previously abusing her median nerve and asks if there are any secretarial openings in your office.

ADVANCED READING

Durkan JA. A new diagnostic test for carpal tunnel syndrome. J Bone Joint Surg Am 73:535-538, 1991.

Gellman H, Gelberman RH, Tan AM, et al. Carpal tunnel syndrome. An evaluation of the provocative diagnostic tests. J Bone Joint Surg Am 68:735-737, 1986.

Katz JN, Simmons BP. Clinical practice: Carpal tunnel syndrome. N Engl J Med 346:1807-1812, 2002.

Michelsen H, Posner MA. Medical history of carpal tunnel syndrome. Hand Clin 18:257-268, 2002.

Osterman AL, Whitman M, Porta LD. Nonoperative carpal tunnel syndrome treatment. Hand Clin 18:279-287, 2002.

Phalen G. The carpal tunnel syndrome. Seventeen years' experience in diagnosis and treatment of 654 hands. J Bone Joint Surg Am 48:211-228, 1966.

Steinberg DR. Surgical release of the carpal tunnel. Hand Clin 18:291-298, 2002.

Tinel J. Nerve Wounds. London: Bailliére, 1917, p 34.

◆ *To heighten appreciation for the sensibility on your fingertips, cover the pulps of three or four digits with Band-Aids for a day.*

30

The Morning After

Roy A. Meals ✦ *Scott A. Mitchell*

"Why is everybody checking my back? I tell you it's fine. It's my foot that's killing me. Don't you guys have any morphine or heroin or something?"

"Well, when somebody jumps or falls and lands on their feet hard enough to break their heel bone like you have, there are often additional injuries that we have to look for. The lower back, for instance. One or more of the vertebrae can collapse from the compressive load absorbed at impact. This would certainly be enough to cause a howling backache on its own, but with enough energy, portions of the vertebra can literally explode back into the spinal canal, putting pressure on the cord and nerve roots. But fortunately, the results of your back and neurologic examinations seem OK. So tell me, how far did you fall?"

PRINCIPLE: An estimate of the energy absorbed at impact will suggest the likelihood of otherwise unsuspected regional injuries.

Calcaneal fractures are commonly associated with other axial loading injuries, including compression/burst fractures of the vertebral bodies and fractures of the proximal femur. Be alert for these injuries as the discomfort from the calcaneus fracture may distract both patient and physician alike.

"Fall? Hell, I jumped. Right out of the window. I've done it before but not from the third story. Good thing I did, too, since . . . ouch! What are you doing now?"

"Checking the pulses in your feet. You see how swollen your foot is already, and over the next 2 or 3 days it's going to get worse: black and blue, for sure; big blisters sometimes. It'll hurt even more if it's lower than your heart. The good news is you've got normal sensation on the sole of your foot. That rules out nerve impingement from a calcaneal fracture fragment."

"Hey Doc, Is this one going to mess me up? I broke my elbow as a kid. Fell out of a tree. Other than the ugly scar from the skin graft, it hadn't bothered me too much until lately. Been getting

189

some pain and tingling feelings from my elbow down to my little finger for a few months, and my hand has been a bit clumsy. Saw the doc about it, but that didn't seem to work out so well."

"I noticed those skin grafts on your arm. No muscle wasting in your hands as best I can tell. Sounds like you may have a case of tardy ulnar nerve palsy. That reminds me, any other medical problems, allergies, or medications we should know about? You don't smoke, do you?"

"Naw, I'm a pretty healthy guy, aside from getting my elbow jacked up. They had to take me to surgery twice on the same day 'cause it hurt so much. Got myself a nice little settlement for that debacle."

"Well, you landed on a concrete planter this time. Wanna see your x-rays?"

"Sure. Since I'm going to be here watching TV through my toes, might as well learn what I can."

"This is a view of your calcaneus or heel bone. It sits off a little to the outside of the bone above it, the talus.

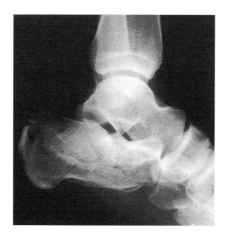

A severely comminuted calcaneal fracture with distortion of the articular surface contacting the talus.

"When you bash them together, the calcaneus splits apart and sometimes even shatters into multiple fragments. The joint between these two tarsal bones is the talocalcaneal joint, though it's usually called the subtalar joint. It allows you to turn your foot in and out, inversion and eversion as we say, so you can plant it securely even on irregular ground."

NOTE: *The axes of rotation of the tibiotalar and subtalar joint complex are nearly perpendicular to each other, quite similar to the design of the universal joint used in auto mechanics. By coordinating ankle flexion-extension and subtalar inversion/eversion, this unique configuration creates an almost hemispherical range of motion (rather than the uniplanar motion afforded by each joint independently). This allows the foot to be placed in nearly any position within this range, creating a mobile base for weight bearing even while moving on uneven terrain.*

"Think you lost me on that one, Doc. So where's the break?"

"Good point. This is a view of your uninjured heel. We took it for comparison. Here you can see the normal height and angle of the calcaneus on the lateral view."

Opposite, uninjured side for comparison. Normally the angle drawn above ranges from 25 to 40 degrees, but in fractures it decreases and may even become negative. Try drawing similar lines across the calcaneus on this patient's injury film. Loss of this angle indicates significant impaction of the calcaneus as well as disruption of the subtalar joint.

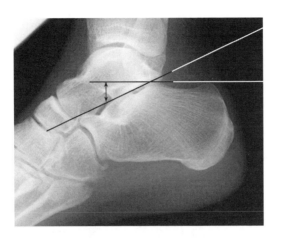

PRINCIPLE: To analyze a complicated fracture problem, compare the x-ray findings with those on the unaffected side.

"Hey, man, get on with it. You said you'd show me the break."

"Actually, I did, but you've got a point. Fractures of the calcaneus don't appear as impressive on x-rays as your elbow. In fact, they are sometimes quite difficult to see on x-rays because the breaks don't line up with the x-ray beam. That's why we use the calcaneal height and that angle to alert us to the presence and severity of fractures. You can see how the shape of the bone on the injured side is different and how the subtalar joint looks scrunched. Here's another view for you, this time looking from the top down onto the back of your heel."

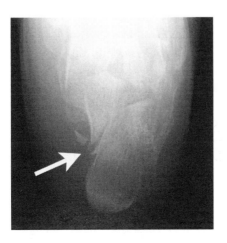

Axial view of the heel showing a comminuted calcaneus fracture.

"Looks bad, even to Superman."

"Sure does. When someone sustains a high-energy axial loading injury from a fall or from a motor vehicle accident with the foot planted against the floorboard, the soft cancellous bone of the calcaneus is forced apart by the talus. This creates complex patterns of impaction and comminution of the calcaneus. So in the end, you are left with a crushed calcaneus, an incongruent subtalar joint, and a short, wide heel."

Examples of calcaneal fracture patterns. **A,** Low-energy fractures tend to produce a sagittal split through the length of the calcaneus. This fracture is difficult to visualize on standard radiographs. **B,** High-energy mechanisms result in impaction of the talus into the calcaneal body with comminution.

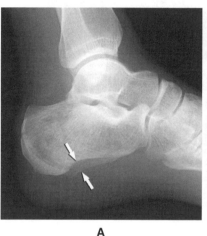
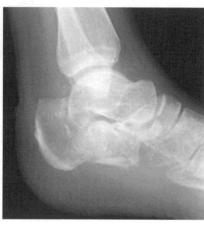

A   B

"So what can you do about it?"

"In the past, not much. Just wait for the swelling to go down and then put a cast on for protection and let you gradually start walking on it. Pretty sore for a year or so, and even then not much inversion or eversion, hard to walk on the beach or on rough ground. If it stays really painful, then we can go in surgically and fuse the two bones together or maybe even do a triple arthrodesis."

"Triple what? I know about triple plays, triple crowns, and triple threats, but Triple Arthur Deesus? Who's he?"

"Sometimes the pain is really bad and all the bones in the area have to be stabilized. So these joints here, the talonavicular and calcaneocuboid, as well as the subtalar joints are fused."

"So you said, 'in the past.' What's new?"

"I've scheduled you tomorrow for a CT scan, which shows the fracture pattern much better than regular x-rays. If the configuration looks promising, we can try to surgically realign the subtalar joint and hold the major fragments together with screws. This reduces the chances of arthritis down the road and the need for an eventual fusion. I'll be back after your CT scan tomorrow to check on things."

NOTE:	*Open reduction and internal fixation improve the overall shape and contour of the calcaneus. This allows for more comfortable shoe wear and may reduce malalignment of the subtalar joint. Any residual incongruity or damage to the cartilage from the injury itself, however, commonly results in arthritis. Patients should be warned that this outcome is possible even with internal fixation.*

"Sounds great. On the way down the hall, tell that nurse to bring me another morphine. The pain's a bitch."

PRINCIPLE:	Intraarticular fractures in weight-bearing joints of the lower extremity benefit from perfect anatomic reduction.

Follow-up Note: The next morning the CT technician and the police came looking for the patient at about the same time. Then we all looked. His phone number and home address were bogus. Eventually he might show up in a shoe store that sells split sizes because his injured heel is definitely going to require a wider shoe than before. And he is likely going to want a shoe with a nicely cushioned heal to alleviate pain from subtalar incongruity. But I didn't mention this long shot to the police.

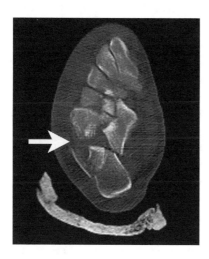

CT scan showing in greater detail the degree of fracture displacement. What is the white curved line?

ADVANCED READING

Buckley RE, Tough S. Displaced intra-articular calcaneal fractures. J Am Acad Orthop Surg 12:172-178, 2004.

Lim EV, Leung JP. Complications of intra-articular calcaneal fractures. Clin Orthop Relat Res 391:7-16, 2001.

Rammelt S, Zwipp H. Calcaneus fractures: Facts, controversies, and recent developments. Injury 35:443-461, 2004.

Thermann H, Krettek C, Hufner T, et al. Management of calcaneal fractures in adults. Conservative versus operative treatment. Clin Orthop Relat Res 353:107-124, 1998.

31

Preparation for Conference

Roy A. Meals ✦ *Scott A. Mitchell*

"Were you moving when you got hit, Leanne?"

"No, I'd just pulled up to the red light, and wham, out of nowhere one of those monster SUVs slammed into the back of me, smashing me right up into the next car. These darn LA drivers. Think they own the road. I had my seat belt on, of course, but the airbag did a number on me when it deployed. And I guess in retrospect, my headrest probably wasn't as high as it should have been; but all things considered those things probably saved me from a stint in the neuro-ICU."

"Did your neck start hurting right away?"

"Actually, no. I thought I was fine while the officer was writing up his report, and by bedtime it was only aching a little; I took some aspirin and fell asleep. But when I tried to lift my head in the morning, I could barely move it at all. The hot shower helped some, and I took some more aspirin. I asked my husband to drop me off here on his way to work. I thought about ordering x-rays on myself, but I wasn't sure what views you'd want."

"That's good. You shouldn't try to be your own doctor, not much objectivity. Any pain, numbness, paresthesia, or weakness in your limbs?"

"I thought about that, and, fortunately, no. Would you believe that I'm presenting at Spine Conference next week? The topic is neck pain. I was going to start my preparation today."

"I think you already have. I'll make a point to be at the conference; I'm certain your presentation will be quite authoritative. Let's have a look. Your natural cervical lordosis, where the spine is concave posteriorly, is preserved. How far can you move it, just gently? Flexion? Extension? Now try turning your head to the right, the left. OK, how about lateral bending? Can you put your ear on your shoulder? Your neck muscles are really tight and tender, although I

don't find any point tenderness. For completeness, I'll check the reflexes, sensation, and strength in your limbs and then get some
x-rays."

Later

"You're back already; that didn't take any time at all."

"Well, being a radiology resident has its perks. What do you
think? The films look fine to me."

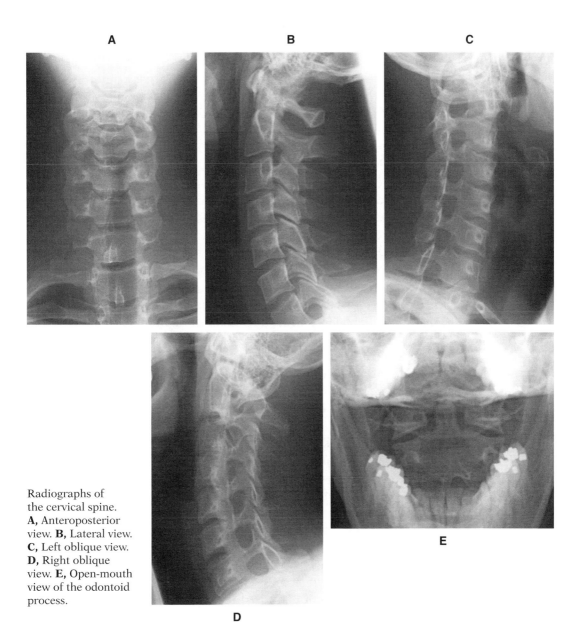

Radiographs of
the cervical spine.
A, Anteroposterior
view. **B,** Lateral view.
C, Left oblique view.
D, Right oblique
view. **E,** Open-mouth
view of the odontoid
process.

"The anteroposterior view shows straight alignment. The lateral view confirms the normal lordotic curve without any step-offs. As I'm sure you know, reversal of that normal lordotic curve can suggest a major injury such as a ligamentous tear, subtle fracture, or facet joint problem even if you can't see the injury directly. And see how you can follow the smooth lines created by the anterior and posterior margins of the vertebral bodies? That tells me that there is no subluxation of the vertebrae. All of the disc spaces are of approximately equal height, and there is no abnormal separation of the spinous processes in the back that would suggest ligamentous injury. Soft tissue shadows look fine—that can also be an important clue if you see significant soft tissue swelling, even in the absence of obvious bony problems. The lateral view, by the way, is probably the most important, at least in the trauma setting. The oblique films show wide-open neural foramina, and the open-mouth anteroposterior x-ray gives me a clear view of your odontoid process."

"So what's wrong? It hurts like hell."

"Ironically, this is an important part of your preparation for the conference. The neurosurgeons and orthopedic surgeons will want to hear why those soft tissues, which don't x-ray well, make your neck hurt. Basically, that sudden, totally unanticipated acceleration-deceleration type of injury acutely stretches the neck muscles, and a strong stretch reflex with forceful muscle contraction ensues. The injury is at a cellular level, so there is rarely obvious hemorrhage or edema. And because major nerves aren't affected, there are no sensory or motor changes or immediate pain. If the muscles get stretched beyond their physiologic limits, then tearing occurs in the spinous ligaments and joint capsules. We don't see these severe injuries so often since the advent of headrests in cars, but you were right, the support has to come up at least to your occiput for it to prevent a severe cervical hyperextension injury.

"As far as your diagnosis goes, many would call this 'whiplash,' but I think that's kind of a wastebasket term. It evokes strong imagery, but 'cervical strain' for muscle stretch and 'cervical sprain' for involvement of the ligamentous and capsular supports are the preferred terms. Some have proposed 'cervical acceleration-deceleration injury' or 'cervical hyperextension injury' for their more descriptive nature. Unfortunately, these types of soft tissue injuries are among the most common and yet least understood disorders of the spine. The severity of the trauma does not seem to be correlated with the degree of clinical problems, and unfortunately complaints of chronic pain and disability following these injuries are among the most common subjects of litigation."

"So what's going to happen? Am I going to be able to present next week?"

"I'm certain of it. I'll write prescriptions for some nonsteroidal antiinflammatory pills and a muscle relaxant. I'll give you a soft cervical collar and a copy of my file on neck pain that you can read at home for a couple of days. While your acute spasm is subsiding, we'll start you on some gentle range-of-motion exercises to do while you are in the shower. The sooner the better, really. We don't want those injured neck muscles to get deconditioned from wearing that collar for too long. Although in the past we typically recommended wearing the collar for several weeks, it now seems that early active rehabilitation helps to prevent chronic pain and disability. You may still have some aching for several months, but most people improve considerably within the first 8 weeks or so. I don't anticipate any long-term problems."

PRINCIPLE: When the inflammation is diffuse, use systemic medication rather than local injection for antiinflammatory treatment.

"Sounds good. Thanks. Before I go, can I show you this x-ray that I found in the teaching file? When my neck hurts as much as it does with normal films, a guy with this much degenerative change must have excruciating pain."

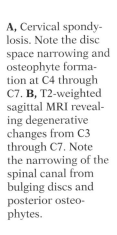

A, Cervical spondylosis. Note the disc space narrowing and osteophyte formation at C4 through C7. **B,** T2-weighted sagittal MRI revealing degenerative changes from C3 through C7. Note the narrowing of the spinal canal from bulging discs and posterior osteophytes.

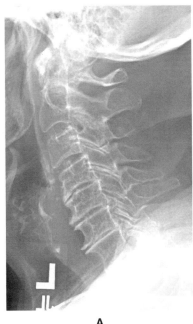

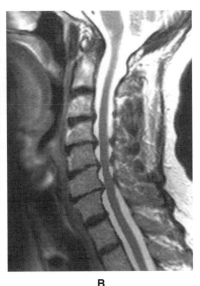

A

B

"Let me have a close look . . . very interesting. You can see disc space narrowing and osteophytic lipping at C5-6 and C6-7 but you know, that's actually my film from 2 years ago, and I'm fine. Cervical spondylosis is like that. Even without injury, the discs gradually narrow with age, and everybody over 50 is going to show some arthritic changes on their neck films. As the vertebral bodies settle closer together, their facet joint alignment is altered, and osteoarthritic spurs form. The associated soft tissue inflammation waxes and wanes, just like osteoarthritis elsewhere in the body. I was having neck and shoulder pain when I had these x-rays taken, and although several foramina were markedly narrowed on the oblique views, I have never had any symptoms of nerve root impingement. In general, motor and sensory changes are unusual except perhaps a diminished deep tendon reflex. That's certainly not always the case though, and cervical spondylosis can present in a variety of ways. Most commonly, it's like me with intermittent bouts of neck pain and radicular symptoms. Unfortunately, however, the osteoarthritis spurs from the vertebral bodies and facet joints, along with posterior bulging of the discs as the vertebrae settle, can also cause compression of the spinal cord—cervical myelopathy it's called. Patients may develop problems with balance, incoordination in the hands, and even bowel or bladder dysfunction. Neck pain may be minimal or even absent in these cases.

"Fortunately, with some conservative treatment like I've just outlined for your strain, my symptoms subsided. My motion is fine except I have a hard time looking over my shoulder to back up my car. And you can hear the crepitation if I go to the limit. My point is simply that there is poor correlation between neck pain and the x-ray changes, so it's important to consider the whole picture—history, neurologic examination, and imaging studies—together. And again, in most cases conservative treatment is the best first line. Now when a patient has evidence of cord compression, best confirmed by MRI, I might add, then it's a bit of a different story and early surgery can often prevent further deterioration."

"That's fascinating. I'd like to show your x-rays at the conference. This MRI of a prolapsed cervical disc isn't yours too, is it?"

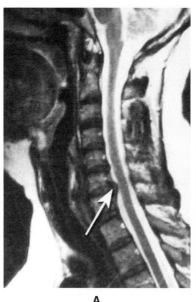 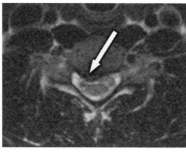

Sagittal **(A)** and axial **(B)** MRI views of an intervertebral disc herniation at the C6-7 level. Based on these images, what signs and symptoms would you predict?

A   **B**

"No, but I'm surprised you found an example of a cervical disc protrusion; they're much less common in the neck than in the low back. What do you know about the patient?"

"From the chart, a slip and a twist at work. No big deal for a couple of days. Then fairly severe pain and stiffness in the neck followed by pain radiating as far distally as the right hand and paresthesias in the thumb and index finger. Questionable biceps weakness and a definitely diminished biceps reflex on that side. X-rays are normal."

"Sounds like a C5-6 disc herniation with pressure on the C6 root, a common level for both disc disease and spondylosis. With disc prolapse, part of the gelatinous nucleus pulposus pushes through a weak area in the anulus fibrosus posterolaterally and stretches the well-innervated posterior longitudinal ligament—hence the neck pain. When the protrusion is large enough, it herniates through the ligament and impinges on the nerve root leaving the spinal canal at that level—hence, the radiating pain and any motor or sensory changes. Actually, here's a good pimping question for you to practice with. Both cervical and lumbar disc herniations usually cause symptoms in the distribution of the caudal-level nerve root. So a C6-7 herniation would cause symptoms in the C7 nerve root, right? But the anatomic reason for this is different in the cervical spine compared to the lumbar spine. Can you explain that?"

"That's a good one. Let's see if I can get this straight. So in the cervical spine, each nerve root is numbered according to the vertebra below the foramen through which it exits. I just remember that the C1 root exits between the occiput and C1, and that C8 exits between C7 and T1. Disc herniations in the cervical levels typically occur laterally, compressing the nerve root as it is entering the neural foramen. So for instance, a herniated C5-6 disc will compress the exiting C6 nerve root, producing symptoms of biceps weakness and pain/paresthesias in the thumb and index finger. In the lumbar spine, however, the numbering system is different. Nerve roots are numbered based on the vertebrae above the foramen through which they exit (L1 root exits between the L1 and L2 vertebral bodies). However, in the lumbar spine, disc protrusions most often occur more posteriorly than in the cervical spine—typically called posterolateral herniations. This spares the exiting nerve root (it passes lateral to the herniation as it exits); rather it compresses the traversing nerve root that will actually exit at the next level below. Thus a L5-S1 herniation will miss the L5 nerve root that actually exits at this level but compress the traversing S1 nerve root, producing gastrocnemius weakness and sensory symptoms in the sole of the foot."

"Excellent. That's an important concept that I think is often overlooked. Now for another curve ball. With advancing age, x-rays may show even severe arthritic changes, but the arthritis may be entirely asymptomatic and only coincidental to the disc prolapse. The clinical picture of the two conditions—cervical spondylosis and disc herniation—can be similar, although the latter does typically affect somewhat younger patients. And since the nerve root pressure is typically more acute in disc prolapse, the radicular pain is often worse and there are more clearly defined findings in the limb. Now for the good news. Although the diagnoses may overlap, the treatment for the two conditions is similar. You know, immobilization, rest, antiinflammatory medication. Intermittent cervical traction tends to relieve nerve root compression as well. As the inflammation around the nerve root subsides with these measures, symptoms usually resolve. Sometimes the body can even resorb the extruded disc material. So what happened to this patient?"

"Just like you said. With conservative treatment the symptoms gradually resolved. So tell me, do you ever have to operate for neck pain?"

"Only rarely. If symptoms correlate to one or possibly two levels, and if conservative measures fail to relieve pain, particularly if there is corresponding motor weakness, then removal of the discs and fusion of the involved vertebrae can often help. Surprising as it may seem, such procedures can be performed through an anterior approach—drawing the esophagus aside and gaining access to the offending discs and vertebral bodies. As in the lumbar spine, though, surgery seems to work much better for radicular pain in the arms than it does for neck pain alone."

"But doesn't a fusion leave the neck permanently stiff even if it relieves pain?"

"That's a good question. Roughly half of neck flexion and extension occurs between the occiput and the first vertebra, and roughly half of rotation occurs between C1 and C2. The remaining motion occurs rather evenly throughout the rest of the cervical spine. So fusing one level anywhere below C2 is not going to cause much restriction; and if it relieves pain and muscle guarding, motion at other levels may return to normal, actually increasing overall range of motion."

"Thanks for all your help. Presenting this conference topic is not going to be such a pain in the neck after all. I hope to have time to sketch my mechanism of injury."

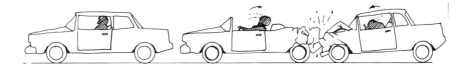

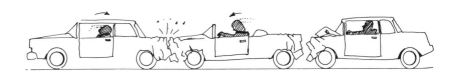

Common mechanism of cervical sprains.

ADVANCED READING

Boyce RH, Wang JC. Evaluation of neck pain, radiculopathy, and myelopathy: Imaging, conservative treatment, and surgical indications. Instr Course Lect 52:489-495, 2003.

Eck JC, Hodges SD, Humphreys SC. Whiplash: A review of a commonly misunderstood injury. Am J Med 110:651-656, 2001.

Gunzburg R, Szpalski M, eds. Whiplash Injuries. Current Concepts in Prevention, Diagnosis, and Treatment of the Cervical Whiplash Syndrome. Philadelphia: Lippincott-Raven, 1998.

Lawrence JS. Disc degeneration: Its frequency and relation to symptoms. Ann Rheum Dis 28:121-138, 1969.

Lovell ME, Galasko CS. Whiplash disorders—a review. Injury 33:97-101, 2002.

Rao R. Neck pain, cervical radiculopathy, and cervical myelopathy: Pathophysiology, natural history, and clinical evaluation. J Bone Joint Surg Am 84:1872-1881, 2002.

Riew KD, McCullock JA, Delamarter RB, et al. Microsurgery for degenerative conditions of the cervical spine. Instr Course Lect 52:497-508, 2003.

Scholten-Peeters GG, Bekkering GE, Verhangen AP. Clinical practice guideline for the physiotherapy of patients with whiplash-associated disorders. Spine 27:412-422, 2002.

◆ *Which portions of the spine are normally lordotic? Which portions are normally kyphotic?*

32

San Vicente

Eugene DellaMaggiore ✦ *Roy A. Meals*

I remember how San Vicente Boulevard used to look in late June. To the motorists it was just a tree-lined parkway, but to me it was freedom—freedom after a month in the library studying for the National Boards. I was in such poor shape that all I wanted to do was run. I even bought new running shoes to mark my return to the world of fitness.

I started with a gentle stride and pace. But the gunner medical student instinct along with the hip-hop beats pounding through my iPod drove me ever faster and longer. I soon began to notice a nagging, dull ache in my right shin during and after my runs, but I pressed on, trying to ignore it.

I trained religiously, but the pain worsened. I thought that as I got into better shape and my muscles got used to the activity, the discomfort would work itself out. But it sure didn't. Originally it only hurt when I ran, but by the Fourth of July the pain lasted all day. I remember watching the fireworks that night and feeling the tender, swollen area on my shin.

The next morning I broke down and went to Student Health. The x-ray examination was negative, and the doctor told me I had shin splints. He gave me some antiinflammatory medication and told me to lay off running for a week or two. I guess I should have taken his advice, but San Vicente beckoned.

Despite cutting my workouts to alternate days, the pain worsened. I returned to Student Health and saw Dr. Godot, the orthopod. She listened to my story and then examined my leg, localizing the problem to the anterior proximal aspect of my tibia. She asked whether I had experienced any acute trauma to the area, and I replied "no." Although my problem could be shin splints, she said it seemed more consistent with a stress fracture.

> PRINCIPLE: In any patient with a history of new or intensified athletic training, always think about possible stress fractures.

As I looked at her in disbelief, all I could picture in my mind was San Vicente and its cool breeze as one approaches the Pacific. I refocused my thoughts on matters at hand and asked what the difference between shin splints and stress fractures was. She explained that "shin splints" is often used as somewhat of a "garbage can" term for chronically painful leg conditions. Like a stress fracture, it usually occurs after a bout of unusually strenuous activity. The pain of shin splints, however, is musculotendinous in origin and usually is localized to the medial border of the tibia, where the tibialis posterior muscle originates.

Dr. Godot was good at weaving together basic science facts with clinical findings. She started by describing the difference between insufficiency fractures—fractures that occur when normal activity or stresses are placed on abnormal bone, such as that seen in patients with osteoporosis—and stress or fatigue fractures. A stress fracture, she explained, is a gradually enlarging crack that develops in an otherwise normal bone because of repeated, unaccustomed impact loading. Bone is an active, dynamic tissue that responds to applied forces by constantly remodeling through the concerted action of osteoblasts and osteoclasts. Bone resorption can occur more rapidly than deposition, however, leading to a temporary weakening of the bone. With repetitive loading during this period, a fatigue fracture can occur. Beginning as a small cortical crack, it can progress to involve the entire circumference with possible bone displacement. Although new or intensified training is commonly cited as the primary etiologic factor, there does appear to be a complex interplay with other factors such as bone density, nutrition, endocrine disturbances, and fitness level that may predispose certain patients to the development of stress fractures.

> PRINCIPLE: Bone remodels to resist applied stresses but breaks if the stress is too sudden or forceful.

Stress fractures in the second, third, or fourth metatarsals are also known as march fractures because they commonly occur in military recruits unprepared for the rigors of boot camp. Even unaccustomed walking, particularly in persons with osteoporosis, can produce march fractures.

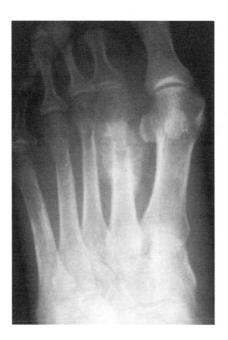

Healing stress fracture of the second metatarsal.

Heavy, repetitive loading of the femur risks femoral neck and shaft stress fractures, which are also seen in military recruits. Stress fractures of the femoral neck, particularly in thin adolescent females, should also alert the physician to the possibility of osteopenia secondary to estrogen deficiency.

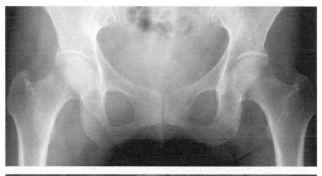

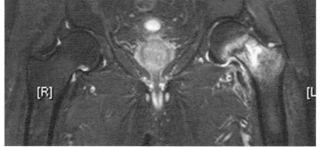

Which femoral neck has a fatigue fracture?

Dr. Godot also explained that runners get stress fractures in the proximal tibia as well as in the distal fibula, tarsals, and metatarsals. Gymnasts, javelin throwers, and paraplegics are among those at risk for similar fatigue fractures in their upper limbs. Even chronic, strenuous coughing can stress ribs to the breaking point. Stress fractures in the interfacet region of a lumbar vertebra cause an unlinking of normal spinal stability, a condition known as spondylolisthesis.

By then repeat x-rays had been processed, and the bone looked fine. "Great! No fracture," I thought, "but something is definitely wrong."

Dr. Godot said that the differential diagnosis included infection and neoplasm as well as other overuse syndromes, but based on my story, she was almost certain I had a fatigue fracture. To prove it she ordered a technetium bone scan.

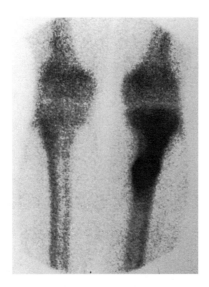

Technetium bone scan shows increased uptake in the proximal tibia.

Radioactive technetium is tagged to a phosphorus analog. The analog accumulates in areas of high blood flow and high osteoblastic activity, which in turn displays increased activity on the scan. To my surprise, there was a hot spot right in the area where my pain was. I've since learned that theoretically a scan can be positive even before the onset of pain because rapid remodeling precedes the fracture and the associated symptoms. MRI is another useful modality to detect stress fractures, often showing marrow edema in the affected region before either x-rays or bone scans become positive. It also can be a useful tool to visualize soft tissue pathology if a diagnosis of stress fracture is uncertain.

I remember checking my watch and telling Dr. Godot it was time for my run. It was only a joke, but she didn't think it was funny. She stated emphatically that I must stop running and even use crutches if walking perpetuated the symptoms. Otherwise she would put me in a cast to minimize the risk of fracture displacement. I complied.

P R I N C I P L E :   Most stress fractures can be managed conservatively by stopping the offending activities. An important exception is the tension-side femoral neck stress fracture, which often requires internal fixation to prevent displacement and the attendant risk of avascular necrosis. Which side of the femoral neck, the top or the bottom, is under compression with normal weight bearing and which side is under tension?

Ten days later there was much less pain, and an x-ray finally showed the damage.

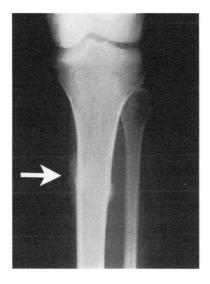

X-ray shows subperiosteal callus formation *(arrow)* around an otherwise invisible stress fracture.

She let me begin running again when the pain and tenderness were completely gone and the x-ray showed further healing. My osteoblasts were keeping up with their destructive associates, but by then I was immersed in my clinical clerkships. My exercise was restricted to taking the hospital's steps two at a time—decent exercise, but unfortunately without San Vicente's soothing influence.

ADVANCED READING

Kaeding CC, Spindler KP, Amendola A. Management of troublesome stress fractures. Instr Course Lect 53:455-469, 2004.

Pell RF IV, Khanuja HS, Cooley GR. Leg pain in the running athlete. J Am Acad Orthop Surg 12:396-404, 2004.

Tuan K, Wu S, Sennett B. Stress fractures in athletes: Risk factors, diagnosis, and management. Orthopaedics 27:583-591, 2004.

Wilder RP, Sethi S. Overuse injuries: Tendinopathies, stress fractures, compartment syndrome, and shin splints. Clin Sports Med 23:55-81, 2004.

◆ *What is the only solid tissue in the body that heals without scar formation?*

33

Overheard at the Tavern

"Hook, you rabid seadog. I haven't seen you in years."

"Silver? Johnny Silver? You crusted barnacle, is that you?"

"Aye, Captain. And I must say, the years have treated you well. The gray beard becomes you, and what's this? No hook! You've grown a hand!"

"Pipe down, Johnny boy, it's a new prosthesis. Slide on in here and share a pint or two. We've got some catching up to do since our swashbuckling days. I must be growing deaf though, as well as gray. I didn't hear that peg of yours on the floor. Remember how you tried to surprise me in Santo Domingo, but your wooden leg gave you away? I jumped overboard and swam ashore. No easy feat with an above-elbow amputation and a hook."

"Well, if you think swimming is tough without a hand, try walking around most of your life on an above-knee amputation stump. Not to mention trying to stay balanced during a swell with that blasted peg for a foot. At least I don't get so winded now with my new prosthesis; it's far more efficient . . . and quiet too—heh heh."

"You know, I never heard how you lost your leg. Cannon fire or cutlass wound?"

"A musket ball shattered my tibia, but it was the infection that finally did me in. That on top of the diabetes and clogged arteries— a dreadful combination I daresay. Nowadays, infections can be controlled much better with those new antibiotics, so there's only an occasional amputation from gangrene. Given the same fracture today, the medics probably could save my leg. But when the nerves and arteries ain't workin,' amputation is still probably the best bet, even in healthy folk."

PRINCIPLE: Limb salvage following high-energy fractures in the lower extremity at times becomes a quite lengthy process, involving multiple surgeries and months of rehabilitation. Amputation performed shortly after such severe injuries, however, can allow patients to be up and around on their new prosthesis in relatively short course. Thus, although amputations are sometimes viewed as salvage procedures, in many ways they are reconstructive surgeries that enable patients to regain function expediently.

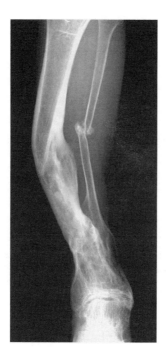

Radiograph obtained following multiple surgical procedures and prolonged antibiotic treatment for severe soft tissue and bony trauma. Would an early amputation have better served this patient?

"Wait a minute now, are you telling me that you had diabetes all those years on the bounding main? Just imagine if your crew had known . . . 'Ol' Long John's down below shootin' insulin. Let's cut off his supply and mutiny!'"

"Shut up you old albatross. Only my surgeon knew, and I disposed of him in about 60 seconds after my stump finally healed. Got his reward alright. At first he amputated through my shin, said I'd be more functional with my knee intact. Used a bit of the rum I was drinkin' to keep things clean. Cut through my leg with one fell swoop of that guillotine blade he had, then cauterized the bleeders with a red-hot poker. Said that was worlds better than the boiling oil they used to use. 'Course I still got most of the common complications: blood accumulatin' in the stump, skin splittin' open, pus drainin,' and agonizing pain in my missin' foot. Things got so bad I had to go back for another round. He moved above the knee the next time and tried things a bit different. Tied off the vessels with a thread from my britches; plus he whacked the nerves sharply, one at a time, and let the ends retract. Then that stump healed right up.

"I understand that now they've got drugs that work a bit better than my trusted spiced rum for pain control. That and a wrap to keep things bloodless give modern medics time for careful cuttin' —that lets things heal up darn quick. And helps keep the stump from hurtin' all the time. Times do change. My surgeon took about 30 seconds on me each time. Guess he and I are about even now.

By the way, how'd you come by your hook, Captain? I heard that croc story was just for kids and that you actually gnawed your own arm off to avoid . . . "

PRINCIPLE: In amputation surgery, preserve all possible length consistent with good surgical judgment.

"Truth be told I was actually born this way, but through the years I've certainly concocted a few accounts as the need suited me. No better way to gain respect from the crew than to tell 'em a gruesome tale or two. And of course I could always work some sympathy from the ladies with a finely crafted yarn. Although I was born with my hand missin,' most folk these days lose theirs from major injuries or nasty growths.

"Done wonders with the field of replacement parts too, they have. Only one I ever had was that rusty meat hook that everyone talks about. Now they start babies out at about 6 months with a sort of learning tool—a limb extender with a mitt on the end. Let 'em start crawling around at a spry young age. After their first birthday, they get a spring-loaded pincher. And by age 2, they're using a body-powered cable so they can latch onto things all on their own. Just look at these newfangled electric contraptions they've got now.

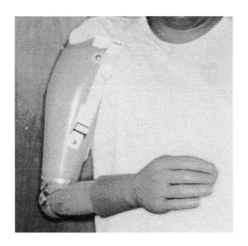

Myoelectric prostheses use electrical impulses generated by the residual muscle bellies in a stump to signal motion at the terminal device. The battery, motor, and electronic circuitry are all concealed within the prosthesis itself, and an aesthetic, flexible glove covers the mechanical digits.

"It's a trade-off between function and appearance, however. When I'm digging up doubloons that I put away for retirement, I use my hook—a bit unsightly but quite rugged and functional for hard work. When I'm out for a night of carousing in town, I wear my myoelectric unit. Gretchen, the barmaid over there, wears highly aesthetic artificial fingers—no motion or sensation, but they mask the memories of misfortune."

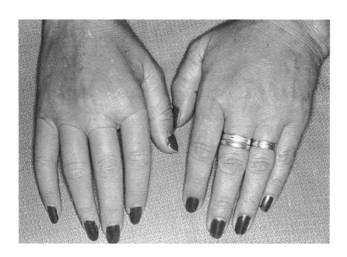

Cosmetic prostheses on the amputation stumps of the right index, middle, ring, and little fingers.

"Let's see. Gretchen! More grog! Ah, still a fine lass. And what pretty hands. Hah. Stomping on toes is no way to turn my tide, you wench, at least not on that foot. Ouch! Hey, those are real. Hook, make her stop."

"Be nice, Gretchen, or you'll feel the power of my pinch. Now hurry with the grog. Tell me, Silver, how does your new above-knee prosthesis mask your infirmity so well from my ear and Gretchen's eye?"

"Ship carpenters never dreamed of a bucket and peg so comfortable, lightweight, and functional. With the total contact socket the weight's evenly distributed over all my thigh rather than just on the end like before—no more skin breakdown or sensitive scars from poorly padded bone. And with the suction fit I tossed overboard that bothersome waistband and shoulder harness I had to wear to keep that infernal bucket from flying off every time I took a step. With my new hinged knee and flexible ankle, I can even dance a bit of the hornpipe.

"I'm told that now even limbs with clogged arteries and diabetes can often be saved at the ankle or at least below the knee. And keeping the knee is important for rehab—lets patients get around without wasting all the energy it takes me with my above-knee amputation.

| NOTE: | *Prediction of tissue healing capacity is critical in planning an appropriate amputation level. Doppler waveform analysis, transcutaneous oxygen pressures, dermofluorometry, and thallium scanning are helpful in assessing local tissue perfusion.* |

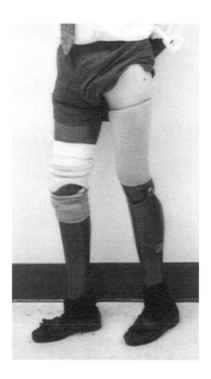

Examples of lower limb prostheses: above-knee amputation on patient's left, below-knee amputation on patient's right.

"But enough about our ailments, Captain. I want to ask you about that time in Port-de-Paix when . . ."

ADVANCED READING

Krebs DE, Edelstein JE, Thornby MA. Prosthetic management of children with limb deficiencies. Phys Ther 71:920-934, 1991.

Letts RM, Lyttle D, eds. Amputations and artificial limbs. Clin Orthop Relat Res 256:1-86, 1990.

Moshirfar A, Showers D, Logan P, et al. Prosthetic options for below knee amputations after osteomyelitis and nonunion of the tibial. Clin Orthop Relat Res 360:110-121, 1999.

Rosenberg GA, Patterson BM. Limb salvage versus amputation for severe open fractures of the tibia. Orthopedics 21:343-349, 1998.

Stevenson RL. Treasure Island. London: Cassell, 1883.

Thorwald J. The Century of the Surgeon. New York: Pantheon, 1957.

Tooms RE. General principles of amputations. In Crenshaw AH, ed. Campbell's Operative Orthopaedics, 7th ed. St Louis: CV Mosby, 1987, pp 597-606.

Uellendahl JE. Upper extremity myoelectric prosthetics. Phys Med Rehabil Clin N Am 11:639-652, 2000.

34

Checkmate?

The parents of 12-year-old Trevor bring him to your office because they have noticed him limping. They had initially attributed this to merely a defiant swagger as he entered his teenage years, although Trevor insists that it is his normal stride. He denies having any pain, and he has been quite healthy except for several previous injuries. At age 9 he was struck by a car and had a right femoral shaft fracture treated by traction and casting. Then a year ago he had a distal epiphyseal fracture of the left femur when he was tackled from the side by his oldest brother.

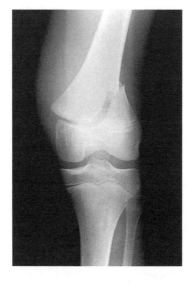

A distal femur fracture passes through the open epiphyseal plate and includes a fragment of the metaphysis. Future longitudinal bone growth from this injured epiphysis is uncertain.

As you watch him walk down the hall, his trunk seems to rise during stance phase on the right and then drop during heel strike and stance on the left, somewhat similar to wearing a high-heeled shoe just on the right foot. On examination, the ranges of motion in his back and lower limb joints are full, and no tenderness is elicited in his back or lower extremities. Strength, reflexes, sensation, and pulses are normal. As he starts to put his shirt back on, you (1) notice a lumbar scoliosis, (2) order x-rays of his spine, and (3) hurry on to the next patient. A bit later your assistant tells you that the family walked out before having the x-rays taken. They told her that Trevor's problem was in his legs and that they were going back to the doctor who treated his fractures.

PRINCIPLE: Hastily ordered tests cannot substitute for a careful history and physical examination.

What else could you have done during the examination to localize the source of his limp? What area would have been more appropriate for x-ray examination?

COMMON CAUSES OF PEDIATRIC LIMP:

Always Consider	Age <3 Years	Age 4-10 Years	Age 10-16 Years
Trauma	Developmental hip	Transient synovitis of	Slipped capital femoral
Septic arthritis	dysplasia	the hip	epiphysis
Osteomyelitis	Toddler's fracture	Developmental dysplasia	Perthes' disease
Malignancy	Tibial stress fracture	of the hip	Limb-length discrepancy
	Foreign body in foot	Perthes' disease	Stress fracture
	Cerebral palsy/neuro-		Tarsal coalition
	muscular disease		Juvenile rheumatoid
			arthritis
			Osteochondritis dissecans
			(knee)
			Gonococcal septic arthritis

Modified from Phillips WA. The child with a limp. Orthop Clin North Am 18:489-501, 1987.

Determining the cause of a limp can be a difficult diagnostic challenge. It is helpful to be aware of the common disorders in children of different age groups that may present with limping. As with most orthopedic disorders, however, a systematic clinical evaluation is essential. The history here gave some clues, but a more thorough physical examination could have clinched the diagnosis. For instance, as the previous doctor had noted, the scoliosis disappears when the patient is bending forward as well as when he is sitting, indicating that it is postural rather than structural. And with the boy standing, the pelvic rim is higher on the right than on the left. Placing a stack of magazines underneath the left foot in the standing position levels his pelvis and also straightens his spine. Obviously he has a discrepancy in the length of his lower limbs equal to the thickness of the magazine stack. With a few more simple examination maneuvers, the discrepancy can be further localized.

Lower limb-length discrepancies of 1 cm or less are common among adults and cause no difficulty whatsoever; in fact, most often people are completely unaware of them. With greater discrepancies, however, an asymmetrical gait is noted and, more important, a compensatory postural scoliosis develops to keep the shoulders and eyes level. Backache may follow. The most common cause of limb-length inequality is skeletal injury and subsequent growth disturbance, but various hip disorders, congenital malformations, and tumors of bones, muscles, or blood vessels also should be considered.

When Trevor broke his right femur at age 9, the bone ends were intentionally overlapped approximately 1 cm in anticipation of a similar amount of overgrowth from regional hyperemia. For reasons that are poorly understood, however, some femurs overgrow more, some less, although the usual overgrowth is between 1 and 1.5 cm. For equally obscure reasons, overgrowth seems to be less prominent in surgically treated femur fractures using intramedullary rods. We don't know whether Trevor's limb lengths actually equilibrated after his first injury. There is some confounding information in this case because his more recent left distal femoral fracture may have injured the growth plate. Although the femur and tibia have epiphyses at both ends, 70% of the femur's growth comes from the distal growth plate, and 60% of the tibia's growth comes from its proximal one. Thus physeal fractures around the knee can have devastating effects on limb length. The growth arrest that occasionally follows these fractures may involve only part of the physis, producing an angular deformity caused by continued growth of the unaffected side; or it may involve the entire physis, producing a limb-length discrepancy, as may be Trevor's case.

By examining the patient supine with hips and knees bent, the relative location of the knees will reveal whether the majority of a length discrepancy is in the femur or tibia.

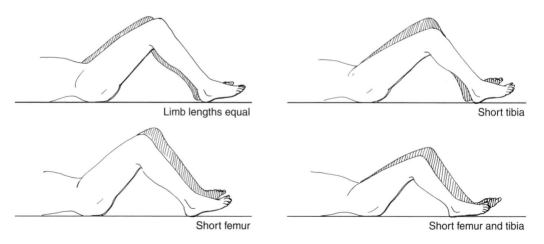

A gross length discrepancy in the femur, tibia, or both can be localized with the patient supine having the knees flexed.

In terms of treatment planning, however, a more accurate determination is usually required. Having the patient stand with one foot on progressively thicker wooden blocks until the pelvis becomes level can quantify the total clinical limb-length discrepancy. Precise localization of where the difference comes from—the hip, femur, tibia, or a combination thereof—requires special scanograms incorporating a metal ruler, or CT scans of the hips, knees, and ankles.

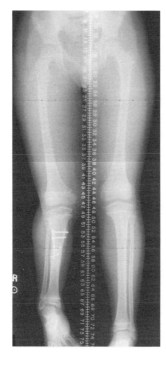

A scanogram takes perpendicularly oriented radiographs sequentially through the hips, knees, and ankles without moving a central metal ruler. The precise lengths of the femurs and tibias can then be calculated. Here the right tibia is 6 cm shorter than the left and the right femur is 1.5 cm shorter than the left.

At this point, planning the type and timing of treatment becomes somewhat of a chess game. The goal, of course, is to have the patient's lower limbs of equal or nearly equal lengths at skeletal maturity. This requires knowing not only the precise location and amount of shortening, but also the patient's age to provide an estimation of the amount of growth remaining. Because adolescents mature at different times and rates, this is best accomplished by measuring bone age. Comparing landmarks on an x-ray of the hand and wrist against standardized norms for boys or girls of various bone ages can help determine how close a patient is to skeletal maturity. Specialized graphs and charts are available that use past and current limb-length discrepancies along with the patient's bone age to project the ultimate discrepancy once maturity is reached.

If the projected difference is less than 2 cm, a shoe lift may be required, but such differences are usually well tolerated. For discrepancies greater than 2 to 2.5 cm, some type of surgical intervention is appropriate. The decision then becomes whether to shorten the long limb or lengthen the short one. Shortening, either by surgical destruction of one or more normal physes or by midshaft segmental osteotomy and internal fixation, is technically easier and generally preferred. Shortening, of course, leaves the total height shorter than otherwise and is generally reserved for projected discrepancies between 2 and 6 cm. Tall stature is esteemed, so if the patient is already shorter than his or her peers, lengthening has an appeal. Gradual distraction with an external fixator over several months can gain as much as 10 cm without permanent damage to nerves, vessels, or muscles. Complications abound, however, and include infection, nerve palsy, joint stiffness and subluxation, compartment syndrome, and psychological disturbances.

Follow-up Note 1:   The family returns. You hadn't given them a chance to say that Trevor had already had spine and lower limb x-rays taken. They went to pick them up. You lucked out this time. Trevor's scanogram shows a femoral difference of 2.7 cm and tibial equality. The left femoral distal epiphysis is narrow, and the right is wide open. Comparing landmarks on his hand x-ray against standardized norms for boys indicates that Trevor's bone age closely approximates his chronologic age. After a thorough discussion, this time regarding the causes of Trevor's limp, you arrange to see the family back in your office at 4- to 6-month intervals to track the discrepancy. You predict that Trevor will likely require shortening of his right leg, so the more information the better when it comes to timing this surgical intervention.

Follow-up Note 2:   Trevor is now 13 and already taller than his parents. You have obtained serial scanograms at 6-month intervals. The femoral discrepancy has increased to 3 cm, and his left distal femoral epiphysis is closed. The charts predict an additional 3 cm of growth from his right femur. After another detailed discussion with Trevor and his parents, they agree that a right-sided epiphysiodesis (surgical fusion) of the distal femoral and proximal tibial growth plates is best. You won't know whether this accomplishes your goal for several more years.

A D V A N C E D   R E A D I N G

Birch JG, Samchukov ML. Use of the Ilizarov method to correct lower limb deformities in children and adolescents. J Am Acad Orthop Surg 12:1441-1454, 2004.

Dahl MT. Limb length discrepancy. Pediatr Clin North Am 43:849-865, 1996.

Green SA. Patient management during limb lengthening. Instr Course Lect 46:547-554, 1997.

35

Zeke's Kin

It was Zeke's grandmother who first came to see me shortly after I treated her grandson for a septic hip. At the time I had taken care of her for carpal tunnel syndrome. She is currently 66 and in good health, but she has been bothered for a few months by a painful catching in her dominant left ring finger, worst in the morning. When I ask her what she thinks is going wrong, she says she is worried about arthritis. Her proximal interphalangeal joint suddenly snaps from a fully extended position to a fully flexed position when she makes a fist. Then she has to use her other hand to gingerly straighten out the digit.

PRINCIPLE: Ask your patients about their assessment of their problems. You will be surprised by their otherwise unvoiced concerns.

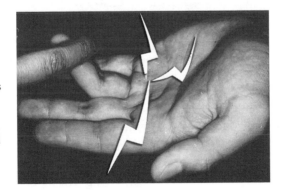

Pain and tenderness in the distal palm with the digit snapping back and forth between flexion and extension are characteristic of trigger finger.

The only positive finding during examination is a tender nodule in the palm over the head of the fourth metacarpal that moves with both active and passive flexion and extension of the digit. There are no Heberden's or Bouchard's nodes suggestive of osteoarthritis.

NOTE: *Osteoarthritis of the hand preferentially involves the distal interphalangeal joints, and to a lesser extent the posterior interphalangeal joints of the fingers. The trapeziometacarpal joint at the base of the thumb is another common site. Heberden's nodes refer to the fusiform swelling of the arthritic distal interphalangeal joint formed by growth of marginal osteophytes. Similarly, bony enlargements of the posterior interphalangeal joints are referred to as Bouchard's nodes.*

Next, Zeke's mother, Mary, comes in. She is 34 years old and in good health except for painful thickenings over both radial styloids and restricted, painful thumb motions. The symptoms started when Zeke was about 2 months old, got somewhat better when Zeke was in the hospital 4 months later, but are now getting worse again. The firm, visible thickenings on the radial styloids are tender. Resisted thumb extension is painful as is simultaneous thumb flexion and wrist ulnar deviation.

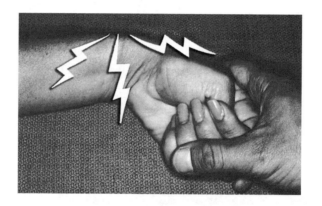

Forcibly drawing the inflamed tendons into the narrowed first dorsal tendon compartment increases the pain of de Quervain's disease.

Slightly distal to the radial styloid, the scaphoid is nontender, and just beyond that, the trapeziometacarpal joint is also asymptomatic.

Several days later, Zeke's Uncle Isaac limps into the office. Thirty-nine years old and a tree trimmer by trade, he also plays in two basketball leagues. He has been having pain in his right elbow and right heel. He, like his relatives, recalls no acute injury. Neither area hurts at rest, but forceful gripping such as when using his pruning shears or lifting a full pan off the stove causes pain on the lateral side of his elbow. Activities such as standing on a ladder or jumping for a rebound cause pain in his heel.

There is a tender area just distal to his lateral epicondyle. Elbow, forearm, wrist, and finger motions are full, but resisted wrist extension causes pain at the elbow.

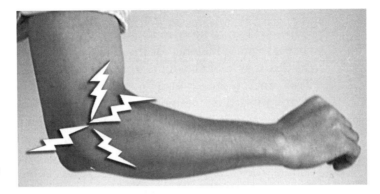

Forceful wrist extension tugs on the origin of the extensor carpi radialis brevis at the lateral epicondyle and reproduces the symptoms of tennis elbow.

There is also tenderness along his right heel cord near its insertion onto the calcaneus.

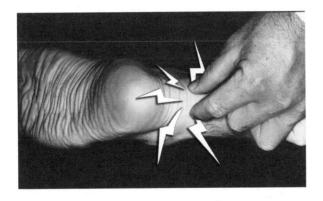

Pinching an inflamed heel cord causes pain.

Zeke's kin all share a frequent malady of active adults, commonly referred to as tendinitis. Although *-itis* means "inflammation," it's not actually the tendon that becomes inflamed but its bony attachments or the enveloping synovium or paratenon in sites where the tendon is mechanically constrained. Isaac, for instance, has tendinitis of his Achilles tendon near its insertion on the calcaneus. Here the paratenon surrounding and nourishing the tendon becomes inflamed, usually related to a sudden or substantial increase in running distance. This is frequently accompanied by inflammation in one or both of the bursa located immediately anterior and posterior to the tendon as it inserts onto the calcaneus. Another common malady of runners, shin splints, is thought to arise from tendinitis of the origin of the tibialis posterior muscle from the deep surface of the tibia.

Zeke's mother and grandmother do not have tendinitis at the motor units' origins or insertions but rather where the tendons are tightly constrained as they cross joints. If there were no retinacular ligaments in such locations, the tendons would "bowstring" directly from origin to insertion across the flexed joint, limiting the compactness and efficiency of the limb. Within restraining tunnels on the flexor side of the digits, on the flexor and extensor sides of the wrist, and on the extensor side of the ankle, synovial fluid nourishes and lubricates the tendons. Repetitive gliding of the tendon under the restraining sheath may exceed the lubricating capacity of the synovial fluid. The resulting friction generates inflammation, which results in thickening of the tendon or the sheath, or both. Of course, the thickening then further restricts tendon gliding, which generates more friction, and so forth. When the thickened sheath is in a subcutaneous location such as the first dorsal wrist compartment, a firm mass is visible. When a flexor tendon thickens at the base of the digit, the thickened portion may pop in and out of the sheath with active excursion, akin to pulling a knotted rope through a narrow piece of pipe.

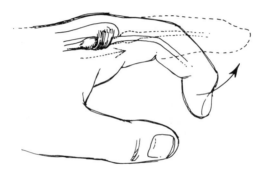

A thickened area of tendon glides fitfully beneath the restraining ligament to cause the snapping that is characteristic of trigger finger.

The mother's type of tendinitis was first described by Fritz de Quervain, a nineteenth-century Swiss surgeon who reported first dorsal compartment tendinitis in a washerwoman. By wringing wet clothes by hand all day, the woman was chronically irritating her abductor pollicis longus and extensor pollicis brevis tendons. Repetitive lifting of an infant child is a far more likely cause these days.

The grandmother's tendinitis is named for the observed phenomenon of the proximal interphalangeal joint snapping suddenly from one extreme to the other as the thickened tendon pops in and out of the retinacular sheath. Some macho poet named it "trigger finger" because of the appearance of the flexed digit being pulled into extension by a finger on the other hand. It is most common in the middle and ring fingers and the thumb, and it usually occurs in middle-aged and older individuals. Infants occasionally get fixed contractures of the thumb interphalangeal joint from trigger finger nodules on the flexor pollicis longus tendon.

✧ *How many other common sites of tendinitis can you think of?*

Although the traditional thinking has been that tendons become inflamed and hurt where they attach to bone or run through tunnels, the role of inflammation in this heterogeneous group of disorders has recently been called into question. It appears that the pathology in certain conditions results from chronic tendon degeneration with a notable absence of inflammation. It remains unclear whether the initial insult is secondary to mechanical strain, ischemia, or inflammatory mediators, but the end result is an inability of residing tenocytes to maintain structural integrity of the tendon. Put in another way, it represents an imbalance between synthesis and breakdown of the intratendinous matrix. Although a healing response ensues, it may be disrupted by even trivial stresses from repetitive use. This cycle of injury and disorganized healing ultimately progresses to further tendon degeneration.

Isaac has chronic pain around the origin of his wrist and finger extensor muscles from the lateral epicondyle, commonly known as *lateral epicondylitis* or "tennis elbow." From repetitive use/overuse, portions of these tendon-bone attachments have separated slightly, with attendant inflammation during acute flare-ups. Chronic symptoms, however, are typically marked by degeneration of the tendon substance at this insertion. Other common sites for this type of tendinitis (more appropriately referred to as *tendinosis* or *tendinopathy* to distinguish it from the *-itis* of an acute inflammatory process) include the rotator cuff tendons at their insertions onto the greater tuberosity of the humerus; the knee extensor mechanism immediately proximal and distal to the patella, known as "jumper's knee"; and the flexor/pronator origin from the medial epicondyle of the elbow, known as "golfer's elbow."

Treatment for any type of tendinitis focuses on relieving inflammation and preventing repetitive injury. Discontinuance of all aggravating activities is easily prescribed, but compliance is quite difficult. Once an area becomes aggravated, even minor activity provokes further irritation. Therefore complete rest is best; but most mothers, for instance, are not willing to have their thumbs and wrists cast or to quit picking up their babies. Likewise, most people with Achilles tendinitis still have to climb some steps, even if they quit playing sports. Therefore injection of a long-acting cortisone preparation into the sheath or next to the bony attachment may break the vicious cycle and allow healing. Multiple injections of cortisone, however, can lead to tendon atrophy and rupture. This risk is minimized by limiting the number of injections and spacing them apart by several months. Nonsteroidal antiinflammatory drugs (NSAIDs) also are useful, particularly when a site is diffusely involved or when multiple sites are involved. NSAIDs, however, are not without their own side effects, so they must be prescribed with some degree of circumspection. Application of local heat also may hasten healing by stimulating vasodilation and thereby enhancing nourishment of the affected areas. For tendon entrapments resistant to these measures, release of the constricting sheath should be curative, although care must be taken to preserve sufficient retinaculum to prevent bowstringing.

P R I N C I P L E :   Medicine can make a patient worse.

Follow-up Note: Zeke's mother responded well to cortisone injections into her first dorsal compartments. Several months later, she felt "80% better." Zeke started walking, and she was carrying him less. Her de Quervain's disease resolved completely after a second injection.

Isaac, with much regret, quit his basketball leagues and took NSAIDs for 2 months while he continued to work. Not surprising to me, he wasn't entirely symptom free until about 6 months later. That seemed like an eternity to him. He grudgingly accepted the reality of impending middle age and played in only one basketball league the following winter.

Zeke's grandmother had always refused to have anything to do with guns and would not let me call her condition "trigger finger." She didn't like "stenosing tenovaginitis" much better, however, so we settled on simply "tendosynovitis." A long-acting cortisone injection cured the condition in the left ring finger, but several months later the right middle finger and thumb were affected. She could not easily accept that she was one of those unfortunate persons who seems predisposed to various nerve and tendon entrapments sooner or later. Two injections into the symptomatic sheaths in the right hand did not give her lasting relief. Therefore I released the proximal portion of her offending tendon sheaths using local anesthesia. Relief thereafter was permanent in those digits.

ADVANCED READING

Almekinders LC. Tendinitis and other chronic tendinopathies. J Am Acad Orthop Surg 6:157-164, 1998.

de Quervain F. Ueber eine form von chronischer tendovaginitis. Korresp Schweiz Arz 25:389-394, 1895.

Fulcher SM, Keifhaber TR, Stern PJ. Upper-extremity tendinitis and overuse syndromes in the athlete. Clin Sports Med 17:433-448, 1998.

Khan KM, Cook JL, Bonar F, et al. Histopathology of common tendinopathies. Update and implications for clinical management. Sports Med 27: 393-408, 1999.

Paavola M, Kannus P, Jarvinen TA, et al. Achilles tendinopathy. J Bone Joint Surg Am 84:2062-2076, 2002.

Retting AC. Wrist and hand overuse syndromes. Clin Sports Med 20:591-611, 2001.

Sharma P, Maffulli N. Tendon injury and tendinopathy: Healing and repair. J Bone Joint Surg Am 87:187-202, 2005.

Walker L, Meals R. Tendinitis: A practical approach to diagnosis and management. J Musculoskeletal Med 6:244-254, 1989.

◆ *Can you reach your feet with your elbow fully flexed? Can you reach your face with your elbow fully extended? If you had to have your elbow fused, what position would be best?*

36

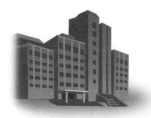

CASE RECORDS
OF THE
ELSA WARE GENERAL HOSPITAL

Weekly Clinicopathologic Exercises

FOUNDED BY OTTO NOSISTUF, SR.

DAVID J. HAK, MD, *Editor*

ROY A. MEALS, MD, *Associate Editor*

CASE 23-2005

PRESENTATION OF CASE

A 32-year-old woman was admitted to the hospital with a fracture of the right proximal tibia. The patient was well until 1 year before admission when she noted the onset of pain in her right knee. She related this to a twisting injury on the tennis court and a flare-up of an old medial-collateral ligament sprain sustained some years previously during a karate tournament.

She stopped playing tennis but was seen by her family doctor 4 months later because of persistent pain that awakened her at night. The pain was dull, intermittent, and unrelieved by aspirin. Examination showed no knee effusion, joint-line tenderness, or ligament instability. Knee motion was full. Back and hip examinations elicited normal findings. An elastic bandage and a course of nonsteroidal antiinflammatory medication were prescribed.

The patient next came to the hospital's ambulatory clinic 1 week before admission with increasing knee pain and localized swelling. Knee joint aspiration and fluid analysis showed straw-colored fluid of normal viscosity with normal protein and glucose content and only an occasional white cell. X-rays did not show any joint space narrowing irregularity. She was given crutches and an appointment at the sports medicine clinic.

On the morning of admission, she slipped in the shower, striking her right leg forcibly against the wall. The previously noted area of swelling was enlarged, and weight bearing caused severe pain.

Three additional items are of note in this patient's medical history. She grew up on a sheep ranch in South America and later spent 2 years as a missionary in a jungle village in Southeast Asia. Four years before admission, she underwent an extensive endocrine workup for possible hyperparathyroidism. She consumes little alcohol, takes no medications, and does not smoke. Her weight has been stable. A review of systems, social history, and family history indicate that they are noncontributory. The details are recorded in the electronic case records accessible online.

On the physical examination the patient was thin, well nourished, and healthy except for obvious swelling in the proximal portion of the leg. Vital signs were normal. The complete physical examination record is available online. Abnormal findings were restricted to her right lower extremity. Swelling, tenderness, and patchy ecchymosis without generalized erythema were present over the subcutaneous portion of the right proximal tibia. The knee joint itself appeared to be uninvolved, but motion was restricted because of pain. The distal neurovascular system was intact.

Urinalysis, routine blood chemistry, and complete blood count showed normal values. The erythrocyte sedimentation rate was 10 mm/hr.

X-rays of the right knee were obtained. A diagnostic procedure was performed.

DIFFERENTIAL DIAGNOSIS

DR. ADMIR L. JEFFREY*: May we review the radiologic findings?

DR. LEANNE RAY: The x-rays (Figs. 1 and 2) and CT scan (Fig. 3) of the right knee obtained at the time of admission show an expansive lytic lesion of the proximal tibial metaphysis. The lesion extends to the articular surface. The borders are well marginated, but there is minimal surrounding sclerosis. There appears to be a minimally displaced pathologic fracture extending transversely through the lesion. The lesion is more clearly defined in the lateral view. Soft tissue swelling is apparent. I am unable to rule out extraosseous extension of the tumor given the presence of the pathologic fracture.

DR. JEFFREY: This patient's history of chronic knee pain and the probable pathologic fracture suggests many diagnostic possibilities. On rare occasions, hyperparathyroidism may produce marked focal changes known as a brown tumor. This may easily be identified by serum studies for parathyroid function, which were normal for this patient 4 years ago, but hyperparathyroidism may have developed more recently. Histologically, a brown tumor appears identical to a giant cell tumor of bone. The patient's residence in Southeast Asia raises the possibility of tuberculosis. Hematogenous spread of the mycobacterial "red snapper" can produce a chronic granulomatous infection in bone, even without pulmonary involvement. As my predecessor Dr. Potts noted, tuberculous osteomyelitis most commonly affects the spine, but long-bone involvement is possible.

Hydatid cyst disease, caused by the *Echinococcus* tapeworm, also must be considered because of the patient's history of exposure on a South American sheep ranch. The parasite normally cycles between dogs and sheep, but humans can be an intermediate host with cystic infestations occurring in the liver, lungs,

*Director of Orthopedic Oncology, Elsa Ware General Hospital; Professor of Orthopedic Surgery, Elsa Ware Medical School.

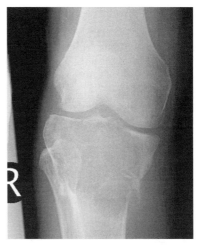
Fig. 1. Lytic lesion of the proximal tibia.

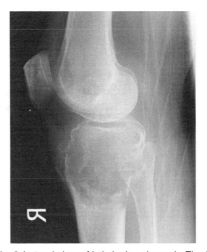
Fig. 2. Lateral view of lytic lesion shown in Fig. 1.

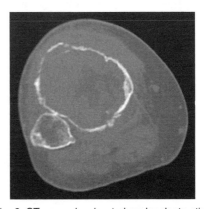
Fig. 3. CT scan showing trabecular destruction and cortical thinning.

bones, brain, and so forth. When the organism implants in bone, it usually occurs in the epiphyseal region, causing trabecular destruction and cortical erosion with a potential for pathologic fracture.

Neoplastic processes also must be considered: benign tumors such as a giant cell tumor of bone and chondroblastoma, and malignancies such as osteosarcoma, fibrosarcoma, and malignant fibrous histiocytoma.

Dr. David J. Hak: Dr. Carlson, will you give us your impressions before the diagnostic procedure?

Dr. Nicholas E. Carlson: I believe that a tumor is first on the differential diagnosis for a 32-year-old, otherwise healthy woman who presents with a possible pathologic fracture after several months of pain. I do not believe we have heard any evidence indicating that an infectious cause is anything other than an extremely remote possibility. Likewise, findings from a previous endocrine workup were negative. My differential diagnosis based on her age and location of the lesion would include a giant cell tumor, chondroblastoma, osteosarcoma, aneurysmal bone cyst, and metastatic disease. The x-ray examination, although showing a fair amount of expansion, does not show the degree of cortical destruction typical of a malignant process. Before the diagnostic procedure, I thought the most likely diagnosis was a chondroblastoma.

Dr. Hak: Dr. Hyzer, may we have the medical students' diagnosis?

Dr. Sheri Hyzer: The medical students considered the causes of a painful, lytic bone lesion of the proximal tibia in an otherwise apparently normal young adult. Their differential diagnosis included infectious causes, neoplastic causes, metabolic causes, and posttraumatic degenerative causes. Despite considerations in the patient's history suggestive of tuberculosis, parasite infestation, or endocrine abnormality, they believe that the most likely cause based on the patient's age, tumor location, and x-ray appearance was a giant cell tumor of bone.

CLINICAL DIAGNOSIS

Giant cell tumor of bone.

DR. ADMIR L. JEFFREY'S DIAGNOSIS

Tuberculosis complicating hydatid cyst disease.

DISCUSSION OF PATHOLOGY

Dr. Hak: An open biopsy was performed. Cortical and cancellous bone samples and adjacent soft tissue samples were submitted for pathologic review. The histology showed numerous multinucleated giant cells amidst a stroma of monotonous mononuclear cells with nuclei that appeared similar to those in the giant cells. Mitotic figures were abundant. Occasionally osteoid matrix was seen in small foci. The histologic findings are consistent with a giant cell tumor of bone.

A giant cell tumor of bone is a benign neoplasm with a unique histologic, radiographic, and epidemiologic presentation. It is often locally aggressive with a high incidence of recurrence following treatment. A giant cell tumor, unlike most bone tumors, is slightly more common in women than men. The peak incidence occurs in the third decade of life.

The clinical presentation is nonspecific and similar to that of other bone neoplasms. Most patients present with pain of varying severity. Some have localized swelling. A pathologic fracture may occur through the area of bone weakened by the tumor.

Giant cell tumors are located at the ends of long bones. The most common sites are the distal femur, the proximal tibia, and the distal radius. They typically appear near the epiphyseal-metaphyseal junction, but often extend into the epiphysis to form juxtaarticular lesions. Their location in the subchondral bone adjacent to joints is an important clue in the differential diagnosis, as relatively few tumors preferentially involve the epiphysis. Chondroblastomas occur here, but only in skeletally immature individuals. Conversely, giant cell tumors almost never occur in skeletally immature persons.

Although giant cell tumors are usually benign, occasionally a tumor will metastasize to the lung. These benign pulmonary metastases are treated by excision and do not show the same tendency to recur as do primary tumors. A separate classification of malignant giant cell tumors is reserved for rare cases in which the patient presents with a frankly malignant histology and clinical course. Most of these cases occur in patients who have previously undergone radiation treatment for a benign giant cell tumor. Therefore radiation should be used only if the tumor is surgically inaccessible.

Will you tell us about the subsequent course of the patient, Dr. Carlson?

DR. CARLSON: Following the open biopsy and a definitive diagnosis, the lesion was curetted and the resultant cavity was packed with bone cement. Traditionally, giant cell tumors have been treated by curetting the tumor and strengthening the remaining bone with an autologous bone graft. Microscopic nests of tumor cells are probably left behind, which helps account for local recurrence rates of nearly 50% with this treatment alone. Various forms of chemical and thermal adjuncts have been used to achieve additional tumor cell killing and reduce recurrence rates. Rinsing the cavity with phenol or freezing it with liquid nitrogen are two examples. In this patient the cavity was packed with polymethylmethacrylate bone cement, which solidifies with an exothermic reaction. The heat kills adjacent tissue for small distances and theoretically may destroy any remaining neoplastic cells. The recurrence rate with this method is about 10%.

Currently the patient is 1 year postoperative and ambulates normally without assistance. She has not shown any evidence of recurrence, but annual follow-up examinations will be required for life.

DR. JEFFREY: Argh! My favorite tumor and I blew it. I sure went down the tubes on this one. The last time you invited me here to discuss a case, I discounted an esoteric diagnosis and was wrong. This time I went for the most obscure possibility I could think of, and I was wrong again.

PRINCIPLE:
When you hear hoofbeats, it's more likely a horse than a zebra.

ANATOMIC DIAGNOSIS

Giant cell tumor of bone.

ADVANCED READING

Aboulafia AJ, Temple HT, Scully SP. Surgical treatment of benign bone tumors. Instr Course Lect 51:441-450, 2002.

Eckardt JJ, Grogan TJ. Giant cell tumor of bone. Clin Orthop Relat Res 204:45-58, 1986.

Szendroi M. Giant-cell tumour of bone. J Bone Joint Surg Br 86:5-12, 2004.

Temple HT, Scully SP, Aboulafia AJ. Benign bone tumors. Instr Course Lect 51:429-439, 2002.

✦ *Why would a knee fusion be more suitable for someone 66 inches tall than for someone 76 inches tall?*

37

The Vermin

Lawrence Shin

Once upon a midnight dreary, while I pondered weak and weary,
Suddenly I heard them chewing, gnawing through the hardwood floor.
Climbing up onto my bed, they covered me from toe to head,
Biting through my skin and swimming, through my veins into my core.
Thus began my living horror.

Nodules formed beneath my skin. Their young gestating deep within,
Hatching with an appetite, to digest joints, to maim and gore.
Tendons ruptured. Fingers twisted. Despite drugs the pain persisted.
Swollen joints choked with pannus, filled with rheumatoid factor.
Rheumatoid forevermore.

Next they did digest and wreck, the transverse ligament in my neck.
Nothing left to keep my odontoid from slipping posterior.
With a craniocervical junction that threatened my spinal function,
One false nod or sneeze would snap my neck—then adios, señor.
Noggin rolling 'cross the floor.

Shooting pains from neck to arm. Incontinence, to my alarm.
Hands so weak and numb and clumsy, felt like boxing gloves I wore.
Hoffmann's sign and ankle clonus. Vertigo an extra bonus.
Spastic legs that carried me plodding, like through deep sand on shore.
Myelopathy forevermore.

Head held tightly 'tween my hands, I ran to see the ortho man,
Schooled in bones and joints and spines by wizards from the days of yore.
Looking at my MRI, he sternly gave me his reply,
"Stability of your floppy neck is what we must restore."
To him for help I did implore.

"Kill the pain with anesthesia, and of course postop amnesia,"
Was my simple plea for mercy that the surgeon did ignore.
Wakened from my gloomy dream, with tube in throat I could not scream.
Heavy straps on arms and legs kept me from running out the door.
Awake I lay in the OR.

Scalpel sharp midline incision. Blunt dissection for division
Of the paraspinal muscles off the neck posterior.
Bone from hip placed as strut to fuse, from occiput through C2.
Held in place by twisted wires salvaged from a harpsichord,
To fuse my neck stiff as a board.

Lastly in this ritual, four screws were twisted in my skull,
Fastened to a ring with bars constructed of titanium ore.
Frames placed on my back and chest, I stood up in my halo vest.
'Til the day my fusion healed, this torturous vise I wore.
Neck unstable nevermore.

Numbness better. Pain is gone. My muscles reclaiming their brawn.
All my bowel and bladder functions did the surgery restore.
After weeks of countless number, finally now at night I slumber,
Dreaming of atlantoaxial subluxation nevermore.
Subluxation nevermore.

✦   ✦   ✦

Cervical spine involvement in patients with rheumatoid arthritis is common. Attenuation or destruction of the cervical joints and ligamentous connections from inflammatory arthritis may lead to instability and compression of neurovascular structures.

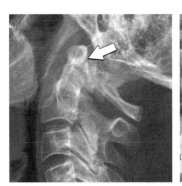 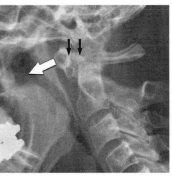 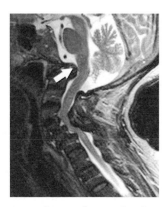

A	B

A, Normal atlantoaxial relationship when neck is extended. The odontoid process of C2 rests against the anterior portion of the C1 ring *(arrow)*, leaving ample posterior room within the C1 ring for the spinal cord. Normally, a transverse ligament maintains this relationship even with cervical flexion. **B,** When the transverse ligament is weak, the head and C1 slip forward on C2 during flexion (area between *black arrows*), narrowing the spinal canal and causing life-threatening neurologic symptoms.

Sagittal MRI of severe basilar invagination. Note the superior migration of the odontoid process *(arrow)* and the resulting deformation of the brainstem.

Among the most common manifestations of cervical spine involvement in patients with rheumatoid arthritis is atlantoaxial instability. Erosive synovitis leads to destruction of the ligaments stabilizing C1 and C2, allowing anterior translation of the atlas (C1) with neck flexion. This results in an increased distance between the odontoid process of the axis (C2) and the anterior aspect of the C1 ring seen on x-rays, and, more importantly, narrows the posterior space available for the cord. When severe, this subluxation may compress the spinal cord when the neck is flexed. Additionally, rheumatoid pannus, a proliferating mass of inflammatory cells and granulation tissue within the synovium, may lead to external compression of the spinal cord even without x-ray evidence of instability. Finally, bony erosion from synovitis in the occipitoatlantal and atlantoaxial joints may lead to the cranium settling onto the cervical vertebrae, with superior migration of the odontoid process into the foramen magnum. Referred to as *cranial settling* or *basilar invagination,* this process may lead to rapid neurologic deficits caused by compression of the brainstem and upper spinal cord.

Neck pain is typically the earliest symptom. The pain may radiate into the head, back, or limbs. Compression of the vertebral arteries may lead to transient episodes of dizziness, nystagmus, or sudden postural collapse without unconsciousness. Progressive spinal cord compression may lead to cervical myelopathy. Patients complain of vague, generalized weakness and clumsiness, worst in the upper extremities. They have trouble with fine motor tasks such as writing or buttoning a shirt. Difficulty with balance leads to a wide-based, ataxic gait. Loss of voluntary bladder or bowel control may follow. The cause of these symptoms may be attributed erroneously to peripheral neuropathy, severe joint deformity, or generalized weakness from chronic disease—all of which are common in rheumatoid arthritis. Myelopathy may be detected from a careful physical examination, giving particular attention to the presence of long-tract signs: hyperactive deep tendon reflexes, ankle clonus, Babinski's sign, and Hoffmann's sign (involuntary flexion of the thumb when the nail of the middle finger is stimulated).

Significant atlantoaxial instability may exist without clinical findings. The process is potentially life threatening, and sudden death may occur if the head is suddenly jarred or forcibly moved. If the anesthesiologist is aware of cervical instability, special steps for endotracheal intubation can be taken to avoid such an injury during surgery.

PRINCIPLE: Obtain preoperative lateral cervical spine flexion and extension x-rays for patients with rheumatoid arthritis.

Progressive neurologic deterioration, progressive instability, and intractable pain are indications for surgical stabilization. Surgically fusing the unstable bony elements to one another is usually sufficient without formal decompression of the spinal cord.

✧ *What is lost by fusing to the occiput? In other words, what is the predominant motion that normally occurs between the occiput and C1?*

What is the downside of sparing the occiput-C1 level from fusion in a patient with rheumatoid arthritis? Think about another cervical spine disorder common in patients with rheumatoid arthritis that is sometimes associated with atlantoaxial instability.

Damage to the spinal cord is a potential intraoperative complication. In days of yore, patients were wakened from anesthesia intraoperatively to verify that they could still move their hands and feet. This so-called 'wake-up test' has been replaced with intraoperative monitoring of somatosensory evoked potentials. Electrodes are placed on the feet to stimulate sensory nerves while the electroencephalogram is continuously monitored. Any change in the EEG alerts the surgeon to potential spinal cord damage.

Postoperatively, the neck requires immobilization until the fusion mass has solidified. This is most commonly achieved with a halo jacket consisting of pins screwed into the outer table of the skull and attached to a halo ring, which connects by vertical rods to a semirigid vest. In the past, fusion was typically carried to the occiput, but newer internal fixation devices allow isolated C1 and C2 fusion. This preserves flexion-extension at the occiput-C1 level and may obviate the need for postoperative halo immobilization.

ADVANCED READING

Bohlman HH, Emery SE. The pathophysiology of cervical spondylosis and myelopathy. Spine 13:843-846, 1988.

Boyce RH, Wang JC. Evaluation of neck pain, radiculopathy, and myelopathy: Imaging, conservative treatment, and surgical indications. Instr Course Lect 52:489-495, 2003.

Dreyer SJ, Boden SD. Natural history of rheumatoid arthritis of the cervical spine. Clin Orthop Relat Res 366:98-106, 1999.

Lipson SJ. Cervical myelopathy and posterior atlanto-axial subluxation in patients with rheumatoid arthritis. J Bone Joint Surg Am 67:593-597, 1985.

Lipson SJ. Rheumatoid arthritis in the cervical spine. Clin Orthop Relat Res 239:121-127, 1989.

Rao R. Neck pain, cervical radiculopathy, and cervical myelopathy: Pathophysiology, natural history, and clinical evaluation. J Bone Joint Surg Am 84:1872-1881, 2002.

38

Weekend Warrior

Last Saturday Sidney Freiberg, a 37-year-old right-handed psychiatrist, was enjoying a weekend off playing beach volleyball with some friends. While flaunting his athletic prowess for a group of attractive beachgoers, he tried to block a spiked ball. Unfortunately, the spiker was also showing off, and the hurtling ball hyperextended Dr. Freiberg's left ring finger. Noticing no immediate deformity and that the motion of his proximal interphalangeal (PIP) joint was good (and not wanting to appear fainthearted in the eyes of his new fans), he decided to push through the pain. So following his teammates' advice, he took off his wedding band (for the swelling of course) and continued playing.

Now, 2 days later, he complains of a swollen, painful digit with limited motion and an unfortunate inability to get his wedding ring back in place. He denies having had similar problems in the past. His general health is excellent. Examination shows swelling of the digit centered at the PIP joint.

PRINCIPLE: Remove any constricting jewelry and clothing from injured limbs as soon as possible.

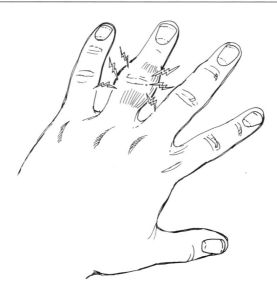

Swelling following a jamming injury of the proximal interphalangeal joint can persist for 6-12 months.

Active motion at the metacarpophalangeal and distal interphalangeal joints is normal. Active motion at the PIP joint is restricted, extension/flexion is 20/70, and passive excursion beyond the active range is too painful to test. The PIP joint collateral ligaments are stable to medial and lateral stresses. The fingertip demonstrates normal sensibility, color, and capillary filling. Findings from the remainder of the hand examination are normal.

Do you want to see an x-ray? Of course.

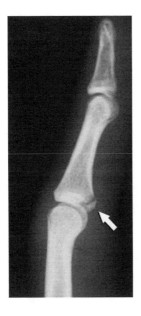

This x-ray, which reveals only a small chip fracture, poorly documents the extent of the injury to the proximal interphalangeal joint.

Do you want any other studies? What is your diagnosis? Would you tell Dr. Freiberg to give up volleyball? Knowing that immobilization risks joint stiffness and that motion risks delayed healing, what treatment do you recommend? Don't you dare proceed until you have answered these questions.

On the lateral x-ray did you note the small avulsion fracture at the base of the patient's middle phalanx? This bony fragment was pulled off during the sudden hyperextension of the digit. The thickened volar portion of the joint capsule, known as the palmar plate, attaches so securely to the bone there that an avulsion fracture, rather than a soft tissue disruption, often occurs.

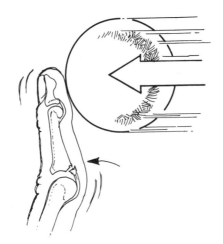

The stress of a forced hyperextension injury breaks the weakest link in the system, avulsing the palmar plate off its attachment to the middle phalanx.

With slightly more force, the volleyball might have dislocated the joint. The x-ray examination for this patient shows no evidence of dislocation or subluxation (partial dislocation).

Appropriate treatment is directed at avoiding the common complication from small-joint injuries. What do you believe that complication is: stiffness or instability? Think about it. Have you ever known anyone with a stiff finger? Probably. How about a chronically unstable finger joint, one that bends back too far or one that is wobbly from side to side? Doubtful. Stiffness is a far more common consequence of digital joint injury than instability, so we should direct our efforts at avoiding it.

PRINCIPLE: **See beyond the x-ray examination. Use your intuition to assess probable adjacent soft tissue injuries. Treat the patient, not the x-ray.**

Knowing that phalangeal fractures take 3 to 4 weeks to achieve clinical healing and longer to show healing on x-rays, you might be inclined to immobilize the injured joint for 3 to 6 weeks. But to do so would cause the patient to suffer the common consequence of such an injury—permanently restricted joint motion. Unseen on the x-ray is a substantial injury to the surrounding capsular and ligamentous supports. To immobilize these supple tissues for 3 to 6 weeks would allow random patterns of collagen deposition and cross-linking, which would decrease the ultimate functional strength of the healing tissues (collagen orients in line with applied stresses) and increase stiffness (collagen shortens as it matures).

Appropriate treatment is immobilization of the injured joint in a slightly flexed position for 7 to 10 days. This allows the acute inflammation and the associated pain to subside. After that, the joint still needs to be protected against further injury, but gentle motion will model the new collagen and preclude development of a severe joint contracture. To protect the injured tissues while allowing gentle motion, the ring and middle fingers are taped together. After 6 weeks the healing is sufficiently advanced to discontinue the buddy tape and resume full activity. Any residual contracture needs to be treated aggressively at this time with active and passive stretching exercises. These are best done while soaking the hand in warm water, which softens the tissues and reduces the pain. A mature PIP joint contracture cannot be corrected by even the most vigorous therapy and is unlikely to be completely corrected by surgical capsulotomy. Prevention trumps treatment.

Follow-up Note: Four months after injury, Dr. Freiberg has no aching or morning stiffness, but he is still unable to slide his wedding ring over the persistently thickened joint. He and his nervous wife seem relieved to learn that continued healing can be anticipated over an additional 4 to 6 months, and that the ring will eventually fit.

P R I N C I P L E :   Following an injury, surgical or otherwise, collagen remodeling and scar maturation are not complete for 2 years in soft tissues and longer in bone.

ADVANCED READING

Chinchalkar SJ, Gan BS. Management of proximal interphalangeal joint fractures and dislocations. J Hand Ther 16:117-128, 2003.

Glickel SZ, Barron OA, Eaton RG. Dislocations and ligament injuries in the digits. In Green DP, Hotchkiss RN, Pederson WC, eds. Green's Operative Hand Surgery, 4th ed. New York: Churchill Livingstone, 1999, pp 772-808.

Incavo SJ, Mogan JV, Hilfrank BC. Extension splinting of palmar plate avulsion injuries of the proximal interphalangeal joint. J Hand Surg Am 14:659-661, 1989.

Kuczynski K. The proximal interphalangeal joint. Anatomy and causes of stiffness in the fingers. J Bone Joint Surg Br 50:656-663, 1968.

Leibovic SJ, Bowers WH. Anatomy of the proximal interphalangeal joint. Hand Clin 10:169-178, 1994.

◆ *Can you fasten a button with your index PIP joint fixed in 90 degrees of flexion? Can you hold a tennis racket securely with your little finger PIP joint fixed in full extension? If you had to have a PIP joint fused, which position would be best?*

39

If the Shoe Hurts

Ronald K. Robinson ✦ *Scott A. Mitchell* ✦ *Roy A. Meals*

It was 5 AM. Even in his predawn stupor, he immediately recognized the squeaky voice of Scotland Yard's Sergeant Winer. "Sorry to wake you so early, Detective Holmes, but we've got another body."

"Same as the others?"

"Similar sir, very similar. In the shoe district again. Choked, on a wing-tip this time. Better bring a shoehorn . . . ha, ha, ha . . . shoehorn, get it? Ha, ha."

"Yes, Winer, very amusing. I'll be right there. Don't touch anything." As he groped to shut off his cell phone, he could still hear intermittent quakes of laughter from the somewhat imbalanced sergeant.

Dr. Watson was already at the scene when Detective Holmes arrived. Together they closely examined the black, size 12, wing-tipped shoe protruding from the mouth of its victim. Across the dusty warehouse floor, a large set of bizarre footprints led to a rear door, which was ajar. Instead of the crescentic shape of normal bare footprints, these were wide elongated blobs with toe impressions pointing slightly laterally. The same ones had been found at the sites of three other murders. "What do you make of all this, Holmes?" Watson asked, still kneeling on the floor.

"I think he probably stuck his foot in his mouth," squeaked Sergeant Winer. "Ha, ha, ha . . . foot? . . . the shoe? Get it? Ha, ha."

Sherlock rolled his eyes. "As usual, Sergeant Winer, very amusing." He pulled a magnifying lens from his coat pocket and examined the footprints more closely. "I once saw footprints like these, Watson, during my travels in Africa. They were those of a man with elephantiasis. I haven't got time to explain now, but I'll meet you Friday as usual."

As promised, Holmes visited his friend the following week. "As I started to explain before, Watson, I believe the culprit has elephantiasis, caused by a tiny parasite that blocks lymphatic drainage in the extremities. The feet, the legs, and sometimes the entire body can swell, sometimes to enormous proportions—although by the shape of the footprints, I would say our adversary is only mildly affected. The same worm also causes blindness, you know. My guess is that the chap has some sort of shoe fetish. It's interesting that all of the victims sold shoes, though only a coincidence, I suspect."

"Sounds pretty weak, I think," Watson responded, "What you're saying is that we should be searching for a blind pervert with elephant legs?"

"Stranger things have been known to happen," Sherlock snapped defensively.

"I think you're missing the boat here, sir." Even as the words left his lips, Watson regretted the comment.

"Watson, how dare you second-guess me! Surely you haven't forgotten how I embarrassed you recently in the case of Mrs. Houlihan's spinal stenosis. . . ."

Sherlock's impending lecture to Watson was put on hold by a telephone call from Sergeant Winer. "Holmes here. Another one. . . . Really? . . . No shoes this time? . . . Interesting. What exactly is different about the tracks? . . . Uh huh. . . . OK, we'll be right there. . . . Yes, Winer, I know. . . . Yes, that's very funny."

Sergeant Winer's cackling abruptly halted as Holmes snapped his phone closed. "What is it with the flatfoots in this city, Watson? They laugh at everything. It's really starting to annoy me. Let's go."

At the latest victim's apartment, the men found a somewhat familiar scene: no shoe this time, but a contorted body and bloody tracks. The left foot gave the customary elephant print, but the right side looked more like small intermittent patches of tire tread.

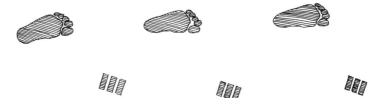

Prints noted at the scene of the most recent murder.

Holmes stooped to inspect the victim. "What's that in his mouth, Winer?"

"I don't know. Some sort of plastic scoop or something."

On close examination Dr. Watson recognized the object. "That's no scoop. It's an orthotic device normally placed in a person's shoe to alleviate pain from some sort of foot disorder. Is this man a shoe salesman like the rest?"

"From the business cards on his desk, it appears he's a podiatrist."

"Rest in peace," Watson mumbled to himself. "Any brilliant ideas, Holmes? Is it your pipe that's making you pensive?"

"Well, I'd like to alter my hypothesis a bit and suggest that our elephantiasis friend has a new peg leg but continues to kill people with items from their respective trades. For instance, perhaps the next victim will be an orthopedist slashed with his goniometer."

"Or maybe a detective bludgeoned with his magnifying lens," Watson replied sarcastically. "Listen, I have some ideas of my own. I'll call you if I come up with anything."

Two months passed without communication between the two old friends, until one day they both appeared at Scotland Yard almost simultaneously. Dr. Watson was leading a limping youth in handcuffs. Sherlock strutted over, shoving ahead of him a crooked old man with thick glasses and strangely enlarged extremities, evidence of his tropical disease. Dr. Watson took one look at Holmes's crippled captive and laughed. "You think your antique is the killer? He must be 85 years old."

"Yes, Watson, I have our culprit. You would do well to listen to me in the future. He's size 12, and, as you can see, he suffers from elephantiasis but with only mild derangement of his feet. The onset of his condition corresponds to the first murder just over a year ago. But here's the clincher: 50 years ago he was arrested for assaulting a butcher with a rancid Polish kielbasa, probably the start of his criminal tendencies."

"Holmes, let me ask the gentleman a couple of questions. Sir, when your disease began last year, what part of your body was primarily affected?"

"My arms, Dr. Watson."

"And at what point did your feet become involved?"

"Just a month ago, sir."

"He's lying, Watson. He's our killer!"

"That's ridiculous. Do you want to hear what I've discovered, Holmes, or would you prefer that we beat a confession from your helpless relic?"

"I think that I'd rather be beaten than suffer through your feeble logic."

"Well sir, admittedly it may be difficult for you, but see whether you can follow me. I must admit I owe you some credit. Until the fourth murder, I was as confused as you still are. It was only when you called Sergeant Winer a flatfoot that it dawned on me. The elephant tracks were those of someone with a pes planus deformity, which results from loss of a normal longitudinal arch of the foot.

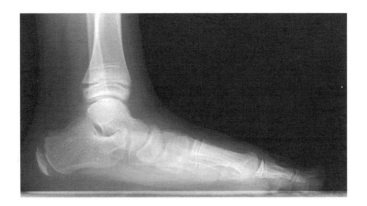

Lateral x-ray showing loss of longitudinal arch.

"Now a pes planus deformity causes more than just an isolated flat foot. Weakening and stretching of the stabilizers of the medial longitudinal arch allows several additional changes to take place that create the distinctive footprints we have been so mystified by. First, the entire foot moves into a position of eversion—in other words the heel shifts into valgus and the forefoot pronates. This causes the entire length of the foot to contact the ground with each stride, rather than just the heel, lateral border, and toes as occurs with a normal arch. Further, the resulting increased stresses on the midfoot from bearing weight in this everted position gradually stretches the talonavicular capsule and surrounding ligaments, causing an abduction deformity of the midfoot and the forefoot. This accounts for the laterally positioned toe prints our suspect left.

"Close inspection of the shoes that our culprit left behind revealed that each model offered progressively more arch support, consistent with . . ."

Holmes interrupted. "But flatfoot is very common, and in the vast majority of people it's asymptomatic. In many individuals the condition is so mild as to be considered a variant of normal. Don't we agree that the murderer's feet hurt?"

"I'm getting to that Holmes, just let me proceed. In the admittedly unusual event that flatfoot becomes symptomatic, the person suffers a diffuse, dull aching during prolonged weight bearing or increased activity. From the drastic actions of our culprit, I gathered that he was in pain and that increasingly rigid arch supports were not alleviating his symptoms. In a most violent and uncivilized manner, he vented his frustrations against the well-intended people who had sold him the shoes."

"So when he'd exhausted attempts to relieve the pain by shoes alone, he sought relief using orthotic shoe inserts?" Holmes grudgingly suggested.

"Precisely, and having failed an orthotic trial, his next step, so to speak, was a surgical solution. So I began questioning the local orthopedic surgeons. There are a number of different causes of flatfoot, many of which respond to surgery if conservative methods like arch supports and other orthotics fail."

P R I N C I P L E :   Before considering surgery for pain relief, alleviate all possible external causes.

"I thought all types of flatfoot were alike—and painless." Holmes conceded.

"Not so," Watson replied, gaining momentum. "Flatfoot is either flexible or rigid and either congenital or acquired. I'll start with the flexible type if you will kindly refrain from these incessant interruptions. *Congenital* flexible flatfoot is what you are thinking of, and it does account for the vast majority of flatfooted individuals. So our culprit would logically have fallen into this class, except that these people are most often asymptomatic. The rare person with a painful congenital flexible flatfoot can generally find relief with orthotic shoe inserts that help to distribute the body's weight along the entire foot. And because the assailant has recently resorted to surgery, his type of flatfoot is most likely of another variety."

"How can you be sure he has had surgery, Watson?"

"Elementary, my dear Holmes. The track at the most recent scene, made by what you called a peg leg, was actually made by the rubber heel of a walking cast. Now let me continue with my line of logic. The *acquired* type of flexible flatfoot is commonly caused by rupture of the posterior tibial tendon, which normally lends support to the foot's longitudinal arch. But this is more common in middle-aged women, unlikely assailants in the case at hand. Another cause of acquired flexible flatfoot is dysfunction of the subtalar joint as a result of a fracture such as a broken talus or calcaneus. Because the elephant tracks were initially bilateral, it is less likely that our suspect had either a ruptured tendon or a fracture. Generalized arthritis, polio, and other neuromuscular imbalances result in bilateral flexible pes planus, but because our quarry exhibited considerable strength, I excluded these causes."

Holmes fidgeted uncomfortably. Sergeant Winer stepped closer and began taking notes. Watson continued: "Now moving on to the rigid types of flatfoot, *congenital* rigid flatfoot is most often secondary to tarsal coalitions. Coalitions are abnormal fibrous, cartilaginous, or osseous bridges between tarsal bones, most often between the talus and calcaneus or the navicular and calcaneus. Such abnormal unions result from failure of synovial joint formation embryologically.

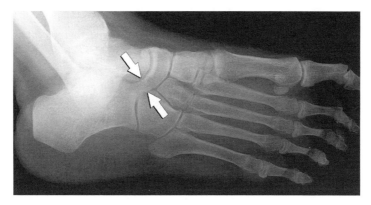

Calcaneonavicular coalition. Note the mature osseous bar connecting the anterior process of the calcaneus to the lateral aspect of the navicular *(arrows)*.

"It's important to realize that hindfoot motion—inversion and eversion of the heel—depends on synchronized movements of the subtalar, talonavicular, and calcaneocuboid joints moving in concert. The presence of a coalition across any one of these linked joints disrupts this coordination, severely restricting hindfoot motion. Most of these coalitions begin with a fibrous or cartilaginous bar between the affected bones that permits at least some degree of motion. In adolescence or early adulthood, however, these bars begin to ossify, further restricting hindfoot mobility and increasing the stresses on the unaffected joints within the subtalar complex. It is thought that both the ossifying coalition itself, as well as the increased stresses concentrated on adjacent joints, may result in significant pain. Because tarsal coalitions are often bilateral and painful, I felt confident that this was the killer's diagnosis. Such persons are less likely to be relieved by orthotics, and an attempt to surgically resect the bar of coalescing tissue is worthwhile. In a significant proportion of cases, however, degenerative changes will already have begun to appear in the adjacent joints by the time a coalition becomes symptomatic. In such situations, or following a failed bar excision, then a triple arthrodesis—fusion of the entire subtalar joint complex (talus, calcaneus, navicular, and cuboid)—must be performed."

Holmes withdrew his pocket watch, inspected it, tapped it, and held it to his ear rather conspicuously before replacing it in his vest pocket. Ignoring Holmes and now talking directly to Winer, the doctor added, "The last category, *acquired* rigid flatfoot, can be the result of a fracture, sprain, arthritis, tuberculosis—any process that scars and stiffens the joints of the midfoot and hindfoot. In fact, acquired flatfoot from most any cause may initially be flexible but becomes progressively rigid because of abnormal loading mechanics. Interestingly, this phenomenon is often not seen in the common congenital flexible flatfoot."

By this time Sherlock's annoyance erupted. "Watson, why don't you practice what you preach to your medical students and stick to the pertinent facts? Must you spew your entire knowledge of medicine?"

"Perhaps *you* could use a bit of education in practical medicine, Detective Elephant Man," Watson replied calmly, much to the delight of Sergeant Winer, who fought back a wave of laughter. "Let me finish. Obviously I couldn't check all young men with size 12 shoes for flatfoot."

"Even if you could, how would you differentiate a rigid from a flexible flatfoot?" Sherlock asked with slowly growing appreciation for his friend's crime-solving abilities.

"Rigid flatfoot is always flat, even when the feet are dangling from a table or when the patient stands on tiptoes. The most sensitive test is to check for motion at the subtalar joint by stabilizing the leg with one hand and trying sequentially to invert and evert the heel with the other hand. A rigid flatfoot will have little or no motion in this plane. Another easy way is simply to have patients stand up on their toes. In cases of flexible flatfoot, this maneuver will produce tension on the medial longitudinal ligament enough to reconstitute the arch, and the heel will shift from its everted position into varus. With rigid flatfoot, the heel remains immobile in its valgus position."

NOTE: *Having a patient with a flatfoot deformity attempt to rise onto his or her toes is also a common test for insufficiency of the posterior tibial tendon. Affected patients will not be able to initiate heel rise from the standing position.*

"So how did you apprehend this flatfooted suspect?"

"Well, for weeks I've been poring over operative records for tarsal bar excisions and triple arthrodeses, and looking through x-rays of tarsal coalitions. I actually found the scum, however, in the cast room."

"Well, Watson, I feel a bit foolish. I guess I should apologize for my behavior. You've handled this case masterfully. How exciting to examine a person and realize that he matches the killer's profile perfectly. Then to have him arrested without a doubt in your mind that he's the . . . "

Sergeant Winer exploded into laughter, and Sherlock noticed a reddening of Watson's complexion.

"Now what are you cackling about, Winer?"

"Well, you're right about having no doubt that he was the killer," Winer squeaked between hilarious gasps. "Dr. Watson never examined him though, never even laid a hand on him. The man had indeed undergone tarsal bar excision last month. By serendipity, Watson found him in the clinic's cast room trying to ram pieces of his postoperative cast down the cast tech's throat."

ADVANCED READING

Beals TC, Pomeroy GC, Manoli A. Posterior tendon insufficiency: Diagnosis and treatment. J Am Acad Orthop Surg 7:112-118, 1999.

Griffin P, Rand F. Static deformities. In Helal B, Wilson D, eds. The Foot. Edinburgh: Churchill Livingstone, 1988.

Huunnan W. Congenital foot and ankle deformities. In Coughlin MJ, Mann RA, eds. Surgery of the Foot and Ankle, 7th ed. St. Louis: Mosby, 1999.

Klaue K. Planovalgus and cavovarus deformity of the hind foot. A functional approach to management. J Bone Joint Surg Br 79:892-895, 1997.

Meehan RE, Brage M. Adult acquired flat foot deformity: Clinical and radiographic examination. Foot Ankle Clin 8:431-452, 2003.

Thometz J. Tarsal Coalition. Foot Ankle Clin 5:103-118, 2000.

Trnka HJ. Dysfunction of the tendon of tibialis posterior. J Bone Joint Surg Br 86:939-946, 2004.

Van Boerum DH, Sangeorzan BJ. Biomechanics and pathophysiology of flat foot. Foot Ankle Clin 8:419-430, 2003.

Vincent KA. Tarsal coalition and painful flatfoot. J Am Acad Orthop Surg 6:274-281, 1998.

◆ *What is happening when you crack your knuckles?*

40

The Weakened Pinky

A 27-year-old data analyst and unpublished poet struck her dominant right little finger against a cabinet door when reaching for her computer mouse. She notes pain, swelling, and an angular deformity. Her history and a review of her systems are entirely unremarkable.

Examination in the emergency room shows normal fingertip neurovascular status. The right little finger rests at a 40-degree abducted position. The base of the digit is swollen, tender, and ecchymotic. The joints allow active motion but are restricted because of pain. What does the x-ray show?

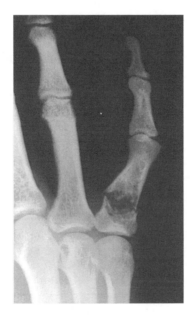

Proximal phalanx fracture resulting from minor trauma. Any concerns?

What is the diagnosis? When should the underlying problem be treated?

A minor blow to the hand has resulted in a fractured proximal phalanx. A fracture sustained from such a low-energy event suggests that the bone was abnormal before the injury. Scrutiny of the x-rays reveals that the fracture occurred through a lytic area in the proximal phalanx with a thinned cortical shell. The responsible tumor has been growing slowly, evidenced by the gradual distortion of the contour without violation of the cortex, and therefore it is likely to be benign. The bone has become sufficiently weakened that a minor injury has resulted in fracture, a scenario typical of enchondroma, the most common bony tumor in the hand.

PRINCIPLE: Malignant tumors have little respect for periosteum—or anything else for that matter.

These benign cartilaginous tumors occur most commonly in the metacarpals and phalanges of young adults. As a tumor grows it pushes against the bone, gradually expanding and thinning it. A patient may note a painless enlargement of the digit, but usually a pathologic fracture is the first problem experienced. The differential diagnosis also includes a giant cell tumor of bone, an aneurysmal bone cyst, and chondrosarcoma, all rarely occurring in the hand. Enchondromas are common in the hands and feet; solitary enchondromas are uncommon elsewhere.

Despite the patient's and the doctor's initial urge to deal with the tumor immediately, the preferred treatment is to reduce and splint the fracture when the x-ray examination shows signs characteristic of enchondroma. Several months later, when the bone is stabilized and soft tissue gliding is restored, the lesion can be curetted ("scraped out") and verified histologically. Then the cavity can be packed with cancellous bone graft. For a solitary enchondroma, this procedure should be curative. Rarely, a patient will have multiple enchondromas scattered throughout the long bones of the body, perhaps associated with hemangiomas. In these cases malignant degeneration of the bone tumors to chondrosarcoma is possible. Therefore anyone with an enchondroma should have both a bone scan to ensure that the tumor is solitary and a careful histologic review of any excised tissue to ensure the diagnosis.

PRINCIPLE: Time surgery to minimize adversity.

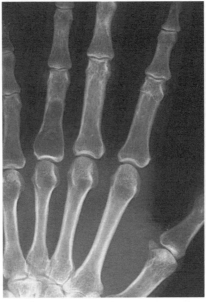 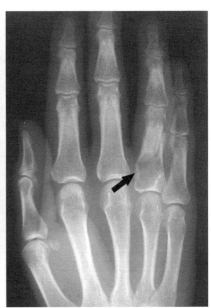

Examples of enchondromas. **A,** A thin cortical rim is preserved in this lesion. Faint intralesional calcification is also present. **B,** Pathologic fracture *(arrow)* through a similar lesion at the base of the ring finger proximal phalanx.

A　　　　　**B**

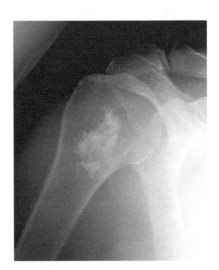

Enchondroma of the proximal humerus. The proximal humerus and distal femur are characteristic sites of long-bone involvement, although considerably less common than in the small bones of the hand. Note the stippled calcifications (also called "popcorn" calcifications) in this characteristic lesion.

Follow-up Note:　　The poet's fracture was splinted for 3 weeks, followed by 2 weeks of "buddy taping" the ring and small fingers. A technetium bone scan lit up over the pathologic fracture but was otherwise normal. Once full digital motion had been regained, the enchondroma was curetted and packed with allograft cancellous bone chips. The excised tissue was gritty, friable, and opalescent, and the diagnosis of enchondroma was confirmed histologically.

The patient, short of cash, offered to pay for my services by giving me poetry-writing lessons. Instead, I asked her to help me write the next chapter.

ADVANCED READING

Mirra JM. Intramedullary cartilage- and chondroid-producing tumors. In Mirra JM, ed. Bone Tumors: Clinical, Radiologic, and Pathologic Correlations. Philadelphia: Lea & Febiger, 1989.

O'Connor MI, Bancroft LW. Benign and malignant cartilage tumors of the hand. Hand Clin 20:317-323, 2004.

Weiner SD. Enchondroma and chondrosarcoma of bone: Clinical, radiologic, and histologic differentiation. Instr Course Lect 53:645-649, 2004.

41

Mary Had a Three-Year-Old

Mary had a three-year-old,
Her hair was blond as dough,
And everywhere that Mary went,
She took her child in tow.

Mother and her darling girl
Did errands one bright day.
Mary had her work to do.
The child knew only play.

At the crosswalk hand in hand,
Everything was fine.
Then the toddler spied a leaf
And stooped to call it "mine."

Car! A car, oh dear, oh dear,
But baby didn't know.
Mother wisely gave a yank
To keep the child in tow.

Tears and crying, wailing too,
The child in agony.
Arm held tight against her side
With palm faced toward her knee.

What have I done? the mother thought,
I saved her from the car,
But now I've broken my dear's arm.
Where is my lucky star?

"Dr. Eldridge, help this girl,
Before it gets too late.
Forearm's fixed in pronation,
It will not supinate."

The doctor listened carefully.
Nerves, vessels, she did check.
The x-rays showed no broken bones.
She stretched and rubbed her neck.

Elbow she did gently flex
With tyke propped on mom's lap.
And with a supinating turn,
She felt a gentle snap.

PRINCIPLE:
**When possible, examine and treat toddlers
from the security of a guardian's lap.**

The child looked up in startled fear,
Then stopped and thought again.
Checking then, she smiled and laughed
And kissed Doc on the chin.

She used both hands to wipe her tears.
"Let's go, I feel just fine.
Shopping waits us. I will help.
It's Doctor's time to dine."

"Nursemaid's elbow" doctor shrugged
(Although put off with rhyme).
"A sudden jerk on toddlers' arms.
This happens all the time.

"Tugging little arms through sleeves,
Or stifling tantrums' woes.
The elbow joint does then get stretched.
The weakest link first goes.

"From beneath its ligament,
The radial head slips out.
It's back in place, no splint required.
No reason more to pout.

"By the time the child turns five,
The ligament gets tough.
Carefully handle until then,
Pull gently, not too rough."

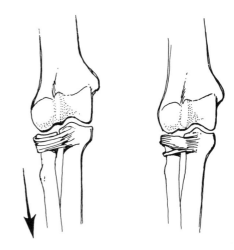

Longitudinal traction draws the radial head distally under a tear in the anular ligament. This causes a painful locking of the forearm in extension and pronation. Gentle, passive elbow flexion and forearm supination restore the normal ligament-bone relationship.

ADVANCED READING

Illingworth CM. Pulled elbow: A study of 100 patients. Br Med J 2:672-674, 1975.

Jerome J. The Poet's Handbook. Cincinnati: Writer's Digest Books, 1980.

Tachdjian MO. Pulled elbow (nursemaid's elbow, temper tantrum elbow). In Tachdjian MO. Pediatric Orthopedics, 2nd ed. Philadelphia: WB Saunders, 1990, pp 3148-3151.

◆ *What led to our specialty originally being spelled "orthopaedics"? No, the derivation does not come from "straight feet," it comes from straight _____, and the "ae" was thrown in to make that distinction.*

42

Johnny Mann

Johnny Mann is a 59-year-old painter and a former high school state champion weight lifter. I had treated him for a hand infection years ago and then lost track of him. He had been to see me five times over the past 2 years because of recurrent right shoulder pain. Initially it responded to nonsteroidal antiinflammatory drugs (NSAIDs) and then to one cortisone injection into the subacromial space—the space between the acromion and the humeral head. The pain has always been related to shoulder motion, primarily with overhead activities, and there has been no suggestion of referred pain from heart or gallbladder disease. About 6 months ago he had to stop taking the NSAIDs because of altered liver function tests. He reports that since then he has had trouble sleeping after a long day's work because of pain in his right shoulder. Last night, when lifting a 5-gallon bucket of paint into his pickup truck, Mr. Mann felt a "snap" and has subsequently been unable to raise his arm overhead.

PRINCIPLE: In the initial evaluation of shoulder pain, the patient's age is among the most important clues for diagnosis. With patients under 30, instability is the most common cause; for patients 30 to 50 years old, impingement syndrome is the most common cause; and with patients over 50, rotator cuff tears account for most complaints.

All patients on NSAIDs need to be warned about gastrointestinal bleeding and perforation. Other side effects include renal insufficiency, hypertension, and a risk of cardiovascular events. Those taking NSAIDs for more than a few months need to have hematopoietic, liver, and kidney functions evaluated periodically.

Inspection of the shoulders from the front, behind, and above showed bilateral symmetry with no evidence of muscle atrophy. Bony contours were bilaterally symmetric when palpated, and tenderness was restricted to the anterior border of the acromion. Both active abduction and flexion of the right shoulder were limited to 40 degrees, and although external rotation was full, the right shoulder was weak compared with the left shoulder. Mr. Mann kindly pointed out, however, that it was still much stronger than mine. A neurovascular examination of the hand revealed no abnormality. X-ray examination showed a slight narrowing of the space between the acromion and the humeral head, but no acute changes. After injecting 10 ml of 1% lidocaine into the subacromial area, I could move the shoulder through its full range of motion, but actively Mr. Mann could still abduct the limb to only 40 degrees. Despite the pain relief, external rotation of the shoulder was no stronger than before.

What do you think has been going on for 2 years? What happened last night? What should I do next?

Mr. Mann has sustained one of the most common tendon ruptures known. He demonstrates classic rotator cuff disease. The rotator cuff is the conjoined tendons of the **s**upraspinatus, **i**nfraspinatus, **t**eres minor, and **s**ubscapularis (SITS muscles), which envelop the joint capsule and assist in glenohumeral rotation.

✦ *The rotator cuff "sits" on the humeral head and inserts onto the greater and lesser tuberosities to abduct and rotate the humerus on the glenoid.*

Although the rotator cuff muscles are commonly associated with specific shoulder motions, perhaps their most important function is to provide dynamic stability to the glenohumeral joint by compressing the humeral head into the glenoid. Coordinated contraction of the cuff musculature holds the head securely in the relatively shallow glenoid cavity through the wide range of motion achieved at this joint.

The tendons of the supraspinatus and infraspinatus muscles pass beneath the narrow arch formed by the acromion, acromioclavicular joint, and coracoacromial ligament in route to their insertion onto the humeral head. And as Hamlet said, "There's the rub."

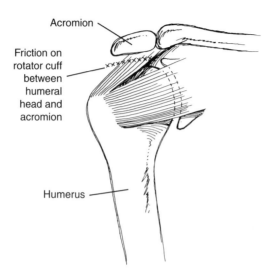

Acromion

Friction on
rotator cuff
between
humeral
head and
acromion

Humerus

Here's the rub.

With shoulder abduction, the subacromial space is narrowed further, compressing the cuff tendons against the undersurface of the acromion. Not only is this conjoined tendon gradually abraded by the undersurface of the acromial arch during repetitive activities, the tendon is also poorly vascularized in the region near its insertion. Thus whereas the initial manifestations of the impingement syndrome involve inflammation of the subacromial bursa, degenerative changes ultimately develop within the substance of the tendons, and these changes continue to progress with aging. Symptoms usually develop over years and are related to bouts of microtears, inflammation, and scarring. As with many forms of degenerative tendinitis, healing is insufficient because of the poor vascularity, particularly in the presence of continued insults from activity. The weakened tendon finally succumbs to a trivial force. Although active abduction and external rotation may be limited by pain from cuff tendinitis, instillation of a local anesthetic to block pain will typically restore strength and motion at least to some degree. The presence of a full-thickness tear, however, precludes active shoulder motion even with lidocaine.

PRINCIPLE: The commonly used yet nebulous term impingement syndrome refers to the mechanical irritation of the rotator cuff tendon beneath the anteroinferior portion of the acromion. It encompasses a spectrum of the degenerative process ranging from cuff tendinitis and subacromial bursitis to partial and complete thickness rotator cuff tears.

Although the diagnosis of rotator cuff degeneration is commonly made clinically, imaging studies are often helpful to localize the problem and differentiate tendinitis or bursitis from partial- and full-thickness tears. Plain x-rays are often useful for identifying the acromiohumeral distance (narrowed by large cuff tears) as well as inferior spurring of the acromioclavicular joint that may contribute to impingement. MRI is quite sensitive and specific in detecting the type and location of cuff abnormality. Ultrasound is an inexpensive and easily accessible technique that has also gained acceptance, though its accuracy is somewhat operator-dependent and may be less sensitive than MRI.

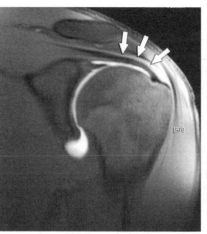 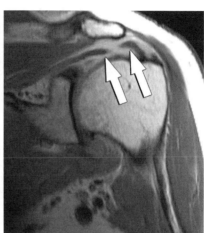

A, MRI arthrogram revealing an intact supraspinatus tendon *(arrows).* **B,** MRI revealing a large full-thickness tear of the supraspinatus *(white arrows).* Note the defect *(between arrows)* caused by retraction of the proximal musculo-tendinous unit.

A   **B**

Although rest and physical therapy will eventually relieve pain in most patients, operative intervention has gained acceptance in certain circumstances. Because nothing can be done to alter the tendon's vascularity or its natural tendency to degenerate, a well-timed subacromial decompression (thinning the undersurface of the acromion), often performed arthroscopically, may prevent further tendon abrasion and eventual rupture.

Operative repair of full-thickness rotator cuff tears has been shown to provide substantial relief from pain and improvement of motion to a lesser degree. Surgery can be performed openly or arthroscopically. Complete arthroscopic cuff repair is a technically demanding procedure—thus most surgeons combine the two approaches. The surgery and the subsequent rehabilitation must be carefully performed because sutures placed along the edges of the tear further strangulate the tissue that needs to heal. Passive exercises are prescribed to maintain joint motion and reduce scarring among normally gliding structures, but active abduction of the shoulder is avoided for 6 to 8 weeks after surgery to minimize risk of rerupture.

P R I N C I P L E :   Treating a tendon injury is only half completed in the operating room. The other half occurs with a carefully graded exercise program following surgery.

Follow-up Note: Mr. Mann's MRI revealed a full-thickness tear in the supraspinatus tendon. This was confirmed arthroscopically before a "mini-open" rotator cuff repair with an arthroscopic subacromial decompression. Because after surgery he had to alter his style for holding a roller brush while painting ceilings, similar impingement symptoms developed in the left shoulder. So far these have responded to a cortisone injection and several short courses of NSAIDs. He has also been encouraged to perform cuff strengthening exercises on both sides. It took some time to convince him that he didn't need to use the heavy weights he was used to—5 pounds is enough if done properly. He finally decided to give up weight lifting for good, and he gave his barbells to me. He said I needed them more than anybody he knew.

ADVANCED READING

Bigliani LU, Levine WN. Subacromial impingement syndrome. J Bone Joint Surg Am 79:1854-1868, 1997.

Herzog RJ. Magnetic resonance imaging of the shoulder. Instr Course Lect 47:3-20, 1998.

Mantone JK, Burkhead WZ Jr, Noonan J Jr. Nonoperative treatment of rotator cuff tears. Orthop Clin North Am 31:295-311, 2000.

McConville OR, Iannotti JP. Partial-thickness tears of the rotator cuff: Evaluation and management. J Am Acad Orthop Surg 7:32-43, 1999.

Yamaguchi K, Levine WN, Marra G, et al. Transitioning to arthroscopic rotator cuff repair: The pros and cons. Instr Course Lect 52:81-92, 2003.

◆ *Did you know that some people can voluntarily dislocate their shoulders?*

43

Iffy for Effie

"Hi, I'm Dr. Carlson. You must be Effie."

"Yes. I remember you from my surgery clerkship lectures last year. You really brought orthopedics to life for us."

"Thanks. So what happened to you?"

"Uh, it was really kind of stupid now that I think about it. I'd been on call and had finally gotten back home to my apartment. You know the feeling that all you want to do is crash onto the sofa and sleep? Anyway, I realized I'd forgotten my keys, so I had to pound on the window to wake up my roommate. Guess I was a bit overzealous, 'cause the glass broke, and, well, here I am."

"Well, let's have a look. How old are you, Effie?"

The transected median nerve *(black arrows)* lies superficially at the wrist. There is a tangential laceration in the palmaris longus tendon *(white arrow)*. All other structures were functioning during the preoperative examination and were found to be intact at surgery.

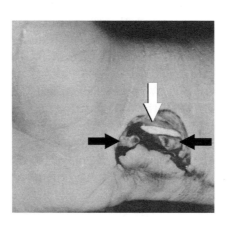

"Twenty-seven. Can you believe I wanted to go into Ob/Gyn? And now this happens to me!"

"How's your health in general?"

"Great—no meds, allergies, illnesses, or ops. Negative review of systems too. Healthy and just plain stupid."

"Come on, give yourself a break. Accidents happen. Do you feel me touching your fingers?"

"Yeah. The little one's fine. I can feel the middle and ring some, but the index and thumb are dead."

"I prefer the term 'numb.' But anyway, open and close your fist. I'm sure it hurts some, but see? All your flexor tendons are working. Now touch your thumb and little finger together. Let's compare it to the opposite side to look for any subtle differences. See? Normally when you oppose your thumb, the tip is well away from the palm, and the nail is parallel to the palm's surface. On the injured side here, the thenar muscles aren't working."

"So it looks like I bagged my median nerve, right? Are you going to explore the wound here in the emergency room to confirm it?"

PRINCIPLE: For soft tissue injuries, the distal physical examination should determine whether there is a need for operative intervention. Emergency room exploration of the wound for diagnosis risks further tissue damage and bacterial contamination.

"That's both unnecessary and meddlesome. The exam shows the nerve is at least partially cut, and that's all we need to know for surgical planning. How much do you remember about nerve healing?"

"Not enough, probably. Something about wallerian degeneration, right? The axon processes that are distal to the injury die and are engulfed by macrophages and residing Schwann cells. If the two ends are approximated, then new axons sprout across the laceration and grow distally into the residual connective tissue sheaths. If not, then a neuroma forms when the axonal sprouts don't find a distal target."

"That's pretty good. A nerve laceration is called neurotmesis— the nerve fibers and all their connective tissue supports are divided. By contrast, neurapraxia is where the nerve and sheath are anatomically intact but the nerve is nonfunctional from ischemia—such as when your foot goes to sleep. The intermediate degree of injury is axonotmesis—the sheath is still intact but the axons are disrupted, such as in long-standing, severe carpal tunnel syndrome."

PRINCIPLE: The ability of an injured nerve to regenerate depends highly on the continuity of the axons and their connective tissue sheath. Neurapraxia has the best prognosis because both the axons and the sheath remain in continuity. Axonotmesis has an intermediate prognosis because axons are disrupted, but the sheath remains intact. Neurotmesis carries the poorest prognosis for recovery (without surgical approximation) because all anatomic continuity is lost.

"So what does median nerve neurotmesis mean to a 27-year-old aspiring gynecologist? Don't nerve fibers regenerate about a millimeter a day?"

"Correct, and the completeness of regeneration is related to age. A 4-year-old with a carefully repaired sharp laceration at the wrist will have an essentially normal hand 2 years later. Anybody in middle age or beyond probably will recover protective sensation, enough to know when they're touching something hot or sharp but not enough for fine discriminations such as distinguishing denim from burlap."

"What about muscle function? Will I be able to oppose my thumb?"

"Probably. Again, kids do the best, elderly folks the worst. Even in the best of circumstances, only about 75% of motor function will be regained. Also, motor recovery is affected by the level of injury. Approximately 1% of the denervated motor endplates degenerate irreversibly each week. Because nerves regrow at a speed of 1 mm a day, it's a race to see whether enough intact motor endplates remain to be reinnervated when the axons finally arrive. For instance, if you had cut your nerve at the elbow, it would take a year for axons to regrow into the hand, and by then half the denervated thenar muscle fibers would have lost their hookups."

"That shouldn't be a problem with a laceration at the wrist, should it?"

"Fortunately no, because the thenar muscles are innervated only a couple of centimeters distal to the wrist."

"Good, but what can I expect over the next several months? I'm on radiology for the next 4 weeks, and then I'm supposed to have my resident interviews."

"Well, I recommend we get you to the OR this afternoon to fix the nerve. Then your wrist needs to be splinted in flexion for about 3 weeks to protect the repair site. So you'll be out of the splint in time for your interviews. In about 6 to 7 months, you'll start getting sense back in your fingertips. The timing should work out."

"That's good news. Another question: How do you get the nerve lined up so motor axons grow toward the muscles and sensory axons grow toward the skin?"

"That's a good question. Using an operating microscope, I align the nerve ends as carefully as possible. The fascicular pattern, the nerve's oval cross section, and any surface vessels help guide the alignment. People have tried various suture techniques, but the best seems to be a minimal number of coapting stitches placed circumferentially in the outermost epineurial covering. Further effort at fascicle-to-fascicle coaptation is technically possible but results in more scarring, which interferes with axon regrowth. In addition there are trophic and chemotactic factors for the sprouting neurons that we are just beginning to understand. These seem to direct motor and sensory axons to their appropriate targets. Now with that said, the process is far from perfect, and in fact some transposition of sensory and motor sprouts does inevitably occur. These are thought to form nonfunctional connections and may partially account for the incomplete recovery that we see even under ideal conditions."

"I remember reading about that. Really interesting."

"I'll go over to the OR and see when we can get started; then I'll stop back by, so think of some more questions. Remember not to eat or drink anything until we're done."

"OK. Thanks, Dr. Carlson. As much as I wish this hadn't happened, already I think I'm going to be a better doctor for it."

ADVANCED READING

Allan CH. Functional results of primary nerve repair. Hand Clin 16:67-72, 2000.

Dvali L, Mackinnon S. Nerve repair, grafting, and nerve transfers. Clin Plast Surg 30:203-221, 2003.

Lee SK, Wolfe SW. Peripheral nerve injury and repair. J Am Acad Orthop Surg 8:243-252, 2000.

Lundborg G. A 25-year perspective of peripheral nerve surgery: Evolving neuroscientific concepts and clinical significance. J Hand Surg Am 25: 391-414, 2000.

Steinberg DR, Koman LA. Factors affecting the results of peripheral nerve repair. In Gelberman RH, ed. Operative Nerve Repair and Reconstruction. Philadelphia: Lippincott, 1991.

44

To Bowl or Not to Bowl

Yong Sung ✦ *Roy A. Meals*

A 67-year-old Shakespearean actor of Welsh-Irish descent expresses distress over a progressive palmar thickening and associated "curling in" of his ring finger on his dominant left hand. The deformity does not interfere with his dramatic portrayals, and although he can no longer easily clap or wash his face without sticking his contracted finger in his eye, his main concern is lawn bowling. He cites Richard II: "What sport shall we devise here in this garden, to drive away the heavy thought of care? Madam, we'll play at bowls."

PRINCIPLE: Note handedness in patients with upper limb complaints; it may affect the treatment plan.

He has noticed the problem progressing gradually over several years, but now he cannot grasp and release the bowl properly to perform his cunningly contrived block shots. His club championship is therefore at risk. A similar fate befell his father and resulted in considerable loss of wager income and the family's eventual immigration to Boston. Your patient admits to "episodic alcoholic overindulgence" and denies epilepsy or any thickened areas on the shaft of his penis or on the soles of his feet. He wonders why you ask these delicate and seemingly unrelated questions.

Here are photographs of his hands. What is the diagnosis? What remedy can you offer?

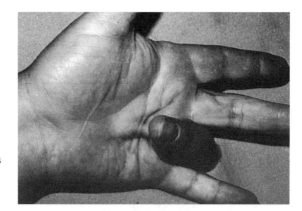

A dense subcutaneous cord markedly restricts extension of the metacarpophalangeal joints of the ring finger.

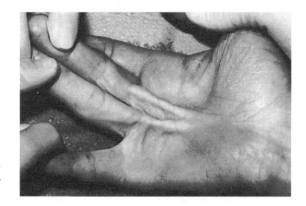

Palmar cords affecting both the ring and long finger metacarpophalangeal joint extensions.

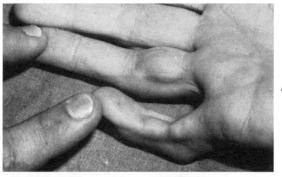

A

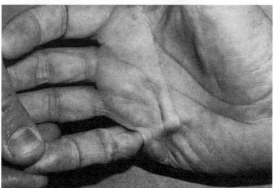

B

Dupuytren's fasciitis also commonly affects the small finger. As shown here, a cord extending into the digits restricts extension of the proximal interphalangeal joint **(A)**, and a palmar cord restricts extension of the metacarpophalangeal joint **(B).**

✦ ✦ ✦

In the palm and on the anterior surfaces of the digits, a layer of fascia stabilizes the skin so that gripping and pinching can occur without the skin and the grasped object sliding away. For reasons incompletely understood, this fascia sometimes becomes inflamed, then thickens and contracts, drawing the fingers into progressively more flexed positions. A powerful and arrogant Parisian surgeon named Dupuytren lectured about its treatment in the nineteenth century, and his name is still associated with it even though the condition and operative treatment had been described earlier.

Dupuytren's fasciitis is most often seen in individuals of northern European origin, especially those of Celtic ancestry. Penetrance is incomplete, however; so family members may or may not be affected. The predisposition may extend to other anatomic areas, accounting for occasional association with fibrous plaques in the shaft of the penis or a fascial thickening on the sole of the foot. The fact that men are affected far more commonly than women, coupled with the fact that alcoholic cirrhosis and chronic use of anticonvulsant medication are predisposing factors, suggests a hormonally affected enzyme abnormality. The fundamental abnormality seems to be a proliferation and overactivity of myofibroblasts, fibroblastlike mesenchymal cells that possess contractile elements and deposit an excessive collagen matrix in affected areas.

Nobody understands why the ring and little fingers are the most commonly involved digits or why the thickening can be quiescent for years and then can cause a symptomatic digital contracture in a matter of months. In the early phases of development the fasciitis presents as tender nodules in the palm. The tenderness gradually subsides as cords develop and then shorten. Because the fascia normally has cutaneous attachments, the digital contractures are associated with puckering and dimpling of the overlying skin. The patient may confuse the subcutaneously located cords with the more deeply located flexor tendons. The differentiation is easy, however, because the cords do not move with active finger motion.

During the nearly 2 centuries since Dupuytren first operated on these contractions, a myriad of other treatments have been tried, including cortisone and saline injections, percutaneous sectioning with needles or special blades, splinting, and electricity. Collagenase injections are under investigation and show some promise. Surgery, however, has proved the only effective treatment for Dupuytren's contracture, though even it has its shortcomings. The patient must understand the three major risks: (1) the surgical injury may itself generate scarring and joint stiffness, (2) the digital nerves are at risk for laceration because their course is frequently distorted by the contracted fascia, and (3) the disease may recur in the operated areas and even extend into a previously undisturbed portion of the hand. When told these realities, your patient cites Hamlet: "Diseases desperate grown by desperate appliance are relieved, or not at all."

Precisely. Because of the risks, surgery should be focused on the areas that are presently causing dysfunction and the areas that are known to respond poorly to late intervention. In other words, contractures of the metacarpophalangeal (MP) joints are best left untreated until functional limitations have developed. Otherwise the treatment may leave the patient with a worse hand than before. Simple transection of the palmar cord gives partial and temporary relief of the MP contracture. But more extensive fasciectomy, sometimes even with skin grafting, is required to fully relieve the condition at the MP joint. Proximal interphalangeal (PIP) joints contracted more than 50 degrees respond poorly to surgery; so in this case the best result comes from removing the fascia long before the joint becomes dysfunctional. For both MP and PIP joint corrections, patient compliance with a postoperative regimen of motion exercises and splinting over many weeks is paramount for an optimal outcome.

You explain the etiology, natural history, and surgical management of Dupuytren's contracture along with its risks, benefits, necessary aftercare, and anticipated outcome to your actor/bowler patient. He is in a quandary. To operate on both hands simultaneously would render him entirely helpless for self-care activities for weeks; therefore one side should be healed before treating the other. The patient is torn between having the contracted PIP joint on his right hand done first or having his currently dysfunctional left hand treated to hasten his triumphant return to the bowling green. With a flourish of his cape, he departs moaning, "'Whether 'tis nobler in the mind to suffer the slings and arrows of outrageous fortune, or to take arms against a sea of troubles,' . . . I'll call you on the morrow with my decision."

PRINCIPLE: Elective, bilateral, upper limb surgery should always be staged in adults. The same usually applies with lower limb surgery. For infants, who are totally dependent anyway, simultaneous bilateral corrections are desirable.

ADVANCED READING

Draviaraj KP, Chakrabarti I. Functional outcome after surgery for Dupuytren's contracture: A prospective study. J Hand Surg Am 29:804-808, 2004.

Dupuytren G. Permanent retraction of the fingers, produced by an affection of the palmar fascia. Lancet 2:222-225, 1834.

Godtfredsen NS, Lucht H, Prescott E, et al. A prospective study linked both alcohol and tobacco to Dupuytren's disease. J Clin Epidemiol 57:858-863, 2004.

Gudmundsson KG, Johsson T, Arngrimsson R. Guillaume Dupuytren and finger contractures. Lancet 362:165-168, 2003.

Qian A, Meals RA, Rajfer J, et al. Comparison of gene expression profiles between Peyronie's disease and Dupuytren's contracture. Urology 64:399-404, 2004.

Shakespeare W. Hamlet, King of Denmark.

◆ *What heritable disorder of connective tissue did Abraham Lincoln have?*

45

The Way It Really Happened

Nicholas E. Rose ✦ *Roy A. Meals*

Once upon a time, in a kingdom far, far away, there lived a beautiful young woman named Cinderella. From endless days and nights of housework, Cinderella's right foot had gradually become so painful that even standing and walking were extremely uncomfortable.

One day as she limped in from the mailbox she noted among the mail-order catalogues an invitation from the King addressed to all subjects of the realm. The King's son, Dr. Charming, had just finished his orthopedic surgery residency and was returning to the kingdom. The Prince was in need of two things: patients for his royal orthopedic practice and a wife. To help his son fulfill these dreams, the King announced a day of free orthopedic consultations at the palace clinic, followed that night by a formal ball during which his son would choose a wife from among the fairest maidens of the realm.

Cinderella's stepmother and stepsisters gathered up their multiple petty orthopedic complaints and rushed to the clinic, leaving Cinderella at home with an insurmountable list of chores. By afternoon Cinderella was limping badly, so her fairy godmother reluctantly finished the chores. Capitalizing on this rare occurrence, Cinderella threw rags over her head to disguise herself from her evil stepmother and sneaked into town.

Dr. Charming was struck by Cinderella's poise and gentle voice, though he was perplexed by her cloak of rags. He reviewed her chart, kissed her hand, and began, "My royal medical student assistant indicates that your past history, systems, and the rest of your physical examination are normal. How and when did the pain in your foot start, my dear?"

"I'm on my feet from dawn 'til midnight. The pain gets worse with each step as the day goes on, but I don't remember being struck there or stepping on anything sharp. I've been limping for at least a week."

"I noticed your antalgic gait as you came in. Show me where it hurts."

Cinderella pointed to her heel. Dr. Charming examined her leg and foot and compared them to her other leg and foot. She winced ever so slightly as his skilled hands deftly localized the point tenderness on the weight-bearing surface of her heel.

"The differential diagnosis of heel pain is extensive, but a thorough history and a careful examination looking for tender points helps narrow the possibilities. Tendinitis can occur medially, posteriorly, and laterally; bursitis can occur posteriorly; neuritis can occur medially; and fasciitis can occur inferiorly. And those are just the soft tissue considerations. Arthritis in the subtalar joint, a stress fracture, infection, and a tumor in the calcaneus itself also have to be considered, so I had the Grand Duke perform an x-ray examination."

"Here are my films, Your Highness."

So enchanted was Cinderella with Dr. Charming's intelligence and patience that she pleaded, "Do tell me more."

"Judging by the heavy calluses, you spend a lot of time on your bare feet. People who stand or walk a lot are predisposed to this type of inflammation, especially if they are obese and middle-aged or older." He peered momentarily into the tangle of rags and then continued: "See, your x-ray examination is fine except for this spur on the calcaneus. That's right where the plantar fascia attaches, and that's also where you're tender."

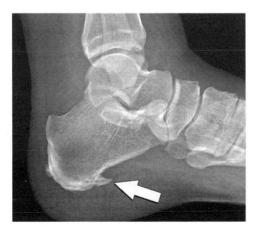

A large calcaneal spur may or may not be a source of heel pain.

"Oh my, is that spike causing my pain?"

"Calcaneal spurs are common and are frequently asymptomatic, but in view of your prolonged weight bearing and point tenderness, I think it's related."

"Is it curable, Dr. Charming? I'm afraid if I tried to rest it, I would be treated rather harshly by my stepsisters."

"You need to rest and ice the area as much as possible. Also, look at your shoes. They are too small, and small shoes can contribute to plantar fasciitis. You need to wear shoes with thicker, well-cushioned midsoles. Here, use these silicone heel cups and place them in your shoes. You'll also want to take nonsteroidal antiinflammatory medication with food or lots of water. You may have to continue the medication for several weeks before you notice some gradual relief from your pain."

"Is there anything else that would help?" asked Cinderella.

"I'd also like you to undertake a stretching and strengthening program and wear this night splint. The splint allows passive stretching of the calf and plantar fascia during sleep."

Cinderella, trying to think of excuses to return to the palace clinic, asked, "What if my heel still hurts after all that, Dr. Charming?"

"If your pain persists, we would proceed with a corticosteroid injection. Only about 5% of cases require surgery, which entails releasing part of the plantar fascia ligament. If you wish, I can explain more at the Royal Ball tonight." Cinderella smiled through her disguise of rags, thanked Dr. Charming, and limped out to the Royal Pharmacy.

That evening she was met by her fairy godmother who, with several waves of her magic wand, made Cinderella an exquisite gown and tiny glass shoes into which she inserted the orthotic heel pads. The shoes had heels high enough to shift her weight forward but not with such narrow toes as to predispose her to hallux valgus and bunion formation.

At the Royal Ball, Dr. Charming was enchanted with Cinderella's radiant loveliness, although she limped slightly. The two spent a magical evening together, and Dr. Charming was paged to the Royal Hospital only twice. Mistakenly thinking the prince was fascinated with Cinderella's limp rather than her beauty and charm, her stepsisters made quite a scene imitating various limps—Trendelenburg gait, stiff knee, short limb, and footdrop, to name a few—but they were unsuccessful in attracting his interest.

Cinderella's plantar fasciitis gradually subsided, and the rest of the story is pretty much as you remember it.

ADVANCED READING

Buchbinder R. Clinical practice. Plantar fasciitis. N Engl J Med 350:2159-2166, 2004.

Crawford F. Plantar heel pain and fasciitis. Clin Evid 10:1431-1443, 2003.

Schepsis AA, Leach RE, Gorzyca J. Plantar fasciitis: Etiology, treatment, surgical results, and review of the literature. Clin Orthop Relat Res 266:185-196, 1991.

Walt Disney's Cinderella. New York: Golden Books, 1986.

Young CC, Rutherford DS, Niedfeldt MW. Treatment of plantar fasciitis. Am Fam Physician 63:467-478, 2001.

46

Bozo Mania

Thomas L. Gautsch ✦ *Roy A. Meals*

"Nick, my man, you're not going to believe this. There are seven bozos from the Valley waiting to see you in the cast room, all with broken forearms."

"C'mon. Don't joke with me like that in the middle of the night. And you shouldn't talk about patients that way."

"I'm serious. Real bozos—noisy honkers, face paint, wild clothes, huge floppy shoes. They all fell off a unicycle. Come on, I'll introduce you. . . . Here he is, folks, the bone specialist I told you about."

"Hi, Doc. Are we glad to see you!"

"Wow, aren't you guys a ragged bunch? Who can tell me what happened?"

"Well, you see, we kinda fell down."

"What he really means is that he made us fall."

"Yeah! [honk-honk] And we hadn't even gotten to the hard part."

"And you call yourself a clown!"

"Ollie! Ulno! Skippy! Stop it! Doc, I'm Bobo the Clown, and this is my troop, 'Bobo's Buffoons.' Maybe you've heard of us. Mostly birthday parties, bar mitzvahs, weddings, and that sort of stuff. But we wanna get on *Letterman*, so we're working on a new stunt— all of us on a unicycle. My 10-year-old, little Bobo Junior here, was on my shoulders. I was on Gabby Galy's. . . ."

"Hi."

". . . he was on Merry Monty's. . . ."

"Hullo."

". . . who was on Smiley Skippy's. . . ."

"Yo."

". . . who was on Ollie's, who was on Unsteady Ulno here, who was on the unicycle."

"So what happened, Ulno?"

"Well, my foot sort of slipped off the pedal as we were coming 'round the barrel. We fell like a stack of donuts."

"Which way?"

"To the right. Did you see the x-ray film?"

"Not yet. Did anybody hurt their neck or back, bump their head, lose consciousness, or hurt anything other than their forearm? . . . No? OK then, I'll start from the top. Bobo Junior, you fell the farthest. Let's have a look. . . . Hmmm, your forearm definitely shouldn't be bent back like that. . . ."

"It doesn't hurt so much anymore. . . . DON'T MOVE IT!"

"OK. I'll be very gentle. Can you feel me touch your fingers here, and here, and here? Any numb areas? Can you wiggle all your fingers . . . and spread them out? Both pulses are good. No breaks in the skin . . . elbow's OK. . . . Judging by this sharp bend in the middle of your forearm, you've broken the shafts of both the radius and ulna. Kids heal so well though, that we'll almost certainly be able to treat your injury with a closed reduction and a cast from your armpit to your palm."

PRINCIPLE: To immobilize a fracture with casting, include in the cast the first joints both proximal and distal to the injury.

A, An acute forearm fracture of both bones in a child that is being appropriately treated with casting.
B, Appearance of the limb shortly after fracture healing. Anatomic realignment of the broken bones was not perfectly restored, and some limitation of forearm rotation is to be expected.
C, With normal bone growth over the next several years, the joints grow away from the fracture site and the bones remodel, thus restoring forearm rotation.

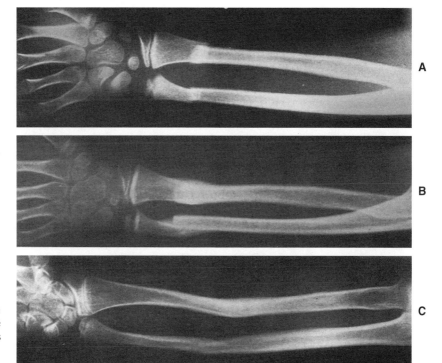

"After it heals, will the bone keep on growing normally? You can see I'm sorta short; I'd like to be as tall as my dad."

"Midshaft fractures are well away from the growth centers, so this shouldn't slow you down at all. Now Bobo Senior, let's see under your splint. . . . Well, look at that—like father, like son."

"I think Junior fell on my arm."

"That'd make sense, Bobo. I'm afraid you have a both-bones forearm fracture too. The good news is we can fix it, but it's going to require surgery."

A both-bones forearm fracture in an adult. Casting would allow healing, but the bony malalignment would preclude recovery of forearm rotation.

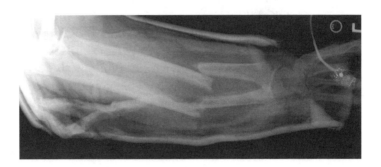

"S-s-surgery? Wait a minute! You said I had the same thing as the little guy. I want a cast too."

"Ah, that's the price of growing up. Your son has such a great capacity to remodel his bones as he continues to grow that almost all we have to do is get the fracture ends close together. His body will take care of the rest. With adults though, casting these fractures results in a very high percentage of bad results. Unless we keep the bones aligned almost perfectly while they heal, any deformity will be permanent. And that would prevent the radius from rotating around the ulna—pronation and supination, we say."

PRINCIPLE: Identical injuries in patients of different ages may require different treatments.

"So will I ever be able to juggle again?"

"You can see how important forearm rotation is. It's tough to do a lot of things without it—turn doorknobs, take change. During surgery I'll restore the precise alignment and hold the bones in place with plates and screws. Then you can get moving right away to prevent stiffness. Juggling will be great therapy."

"OK, I'll do whatever it takes. Monty, looks like you're next."

"Please be careful. And don't make me move my elbow. It really smarts."

"Your forearm looks funny too. It's curving backward—right here, not quite half way from your elbow to your wrist."

"Yeah, that's exactly where it hurts, there and all the way up to my elbow."

"Let me just carefully feel your shoulder and down to your elbow. OK, no pain along the humerus or at the epicondyles. Olecranon feels all right—not dislocated. Ah, but your radial head's sitting up here in your antecubital fossa."

"Is that bad, Doc? It's pretty sore there."

"Well, it can be, Monty. What I suspect is that a blow to the extensor surface of your forearm broke your ulna and pushed the radial head forward. Sometimes with the radial head dislocated, part or all of the radial nerve can get stretched, causing loss of finger and wrist extension. But your motor exam checks out."

NOTE: *Always be alert for concomitant injuries to the proximal and distal radioulnar joints with fractures of the radial or ulnar shafts.*

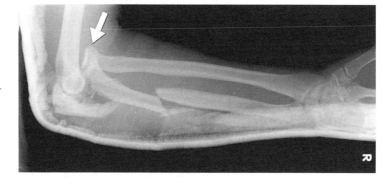

Monteggia fracture-dislocation. A blow to the forearm can fracture the proximal ulna and dislocate the radial head *(arrow)*.

PRINCIPLE: Subluxation or dislocation of the radial head can be subtle on x-rays, especially in children. Remember that the radial head should point directly to the capitellum on all views of the elbow.

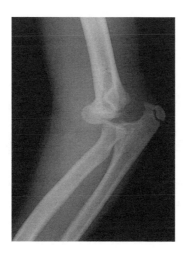

Which joint or joints are dislocated—radiocapitellar, ulnohumeral, or proximal radioulnar? Is there a fracture of the olecranon?

"Great! So how do we make the bones right?"

"What we need to do is straighten the ulna and hold it out to its full length. Usually this will reduce the radial head and keep it in place while the surrounding ligaments heal. Again, though, this means surgery to put a metal plate along the ulna. Even if we reduced the fracture and the dislocation perfectly and put on a cast, these deformities would tend to recur because of the strong pull of your forearm muscles. We need a plate and screws to counteract that tendency."

"After it heals, will I be able to play the calliope?"

"Ye . . . umm, wait, could you play it before?"

"Of course not."

"Funny guy!"

"Whadda yuh expect? I'm a clown." [honk-honk]

"Galy, you're next. What happened to you?"

"I fell with my arm stretched out and turned in. It hurts here just above my watch on the thumb side and just beyond my watch on the pinky finger side. And look at that huge lump on my wrist."

"Does it hurt your elbow when I move it or squeeze it?"

"No."

"Down here? Or here? Here?"

"You're getting closer. . . . Ouch! Right there, that's really tender."

"Hmmm. That's fairly far along your radius toward your wrist. Does this hurt here over the distal ulna?"

"Ouch! Yeah, it's real sore around that bump. Look how huge it is compared with my left side."

"Good comparison. That's the other end of your ulna dislocated off the radius. And here, above your watch, which I want you to take off, by the way, is a painful and swollen area where you've probably broken your radius. I can get it back in place just by manipulation, but you'll still need surgery."

Galeazzi's fracture-dislocation. The radius is fractured, and the distal ulna *(arrow)* is dislocated from its normal relationship with the radius and the carpus. With this injury, the radial fracture is typically more distal than shown here.

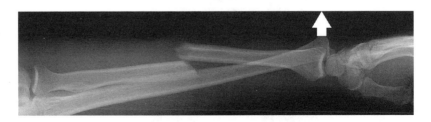

"Now wait a minute, Doc. Bobo Junior's bent forearm can be fixed with a cast; and I can understand surgery for his old man because the deformity is obvious and the fracture ends are probably overlapped. But you said you can line up my bones. Let's go with a cast."

"That's one banana peel that we don't want to slip on, so to speak. Galy, your injury consists of a radius fracture with a dislocation of the distal radioulnar joint—sort of the reverse of Monty's injury, which is an ulna fracture with dislocation of the proximal radioulnar joint. But it has the same problem. It really needs rigid internal fixation to counter the muscle forces. Without it, the healing radius gradually angulates, and the disrupted distal radioulnar joint persists. You'd lose a lot of pronation and supination and may have chronic pain in your wrist from an unstable distal ulna."

PRINCIPLE: The intricate mechanics of forearm rotation depend on motion proximally at the articulations between the radial head, capitellum, and ulna, and distally at the radioulnar joint. Disruption of any of these articulations or of the bony alignment between the radial and ulnar shafts can significantly limit pronation and supination of the forearm.

"OK, Doc. When you explain it like that, it makes sense. Go for it."

"Good. So, Skippy, you're next."

"Hey, Doctor Dude."

"Oh! Grow up in the Valley, did you Skip?"

"Yeah. Like, how'd ya know?"

"Uh, just a guess. You look like you managed to pull yourself through this pretty much unscathed."

"Yeah. And I didn't hardly get hurt neither. I felt it coming, just like getting caught inside by a big set. I didn't wanna get pitched by this big body wave, so I bailed. Way cool, huh?"

"Let me take a look at you anyway. Does anything hurt?"

"Nope. See? I can move everything. Well, I think I might have sprained my elbow. It hurts a little when I—whadda yuh call it—pronate. Opening that door killed me."

"Hmmm . . . no pain here at the wrist or along the forearm. It looks like you've got a bit of an effusion in your elbow though. When I hold my thumb over your radial head and rotate your forearm, does that hurt?"

"Whoa, yeah! Easy on the goods man! Is that like a pinched nerve or something?"

"No. But I want to see the x-ray because I think you may have a head fracture."

"No-o-o way! You guys are all the same. That other bogus doctor who brought you in here claimed I had a totally radical head fracture, but I didn't even hit my head."

"Did he see the results of your x-ray examination?"

"Yeah. That's when he said it."

"Ah, Skippy, I think what he meant was that you have a *radial* head fracture. The radial head is the end of this bone in your forearm. It adds to the stability of your elbow and lets you rotate your forearm. I bet you stopped your fall with your hand. That jammed the radius against the humerus with enough stress to break the radial head."

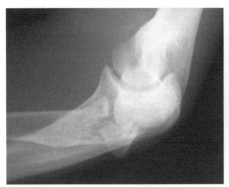 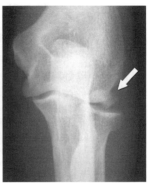

Displaced fracture of the radial head. This fracture is likely amenable to internal fixation. The associated capsular and ligamentous injuries are unseen but significant.

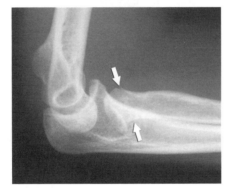

Angulated fracture through the radial neck. The articular surface of the radial head is well-preserved, although its alignment with the capitellum is significantly altered.

"Whoa, that's what I told 'em. I was like totally stressed, man. But hey, you're not gonna have to cut on me, are ya dude?"

"I don't think so, but I really have to see the x-ray results to tell with this one. If the shape of the head is reasonably preserved, you get a sling and early motion. If the head is displaced or shattered, then I'd recommend surgery to repair it if possible, or if it's too crunched, to replace it with a piece of metal. We used to simply remove the radial head when there were too many pieces to fix, but we have found that it plays an important role in load sharing as well as elbow and even forearm stability. A metal replacement can restore these functions and helps you get your full motion back."

"Whoa. Then I'd really be a metal-head. Gnarly."

"Totally. . . . So, Ollie, your elbow looks pretty darn swollen too."

"It hurts a fair amount, Doc. And it really feels weird when I straighten it out—like something's loose in there."

"Let me take a close look. Does your upper arm hurt when I squeeze it? How about over the epicondyles? Back here at the olecranon?"

"Ow! Ow! Right there, that's the spot."

"OK. I'm going to gently extend your elbow, now I'll flex it. Now forearm pronation. Supination. That all seems to work."

"It hurts a little."

"Now try extending your elbow as I try to flex it."

"I'm trying. Wow, that feels really strange . . . and hurts. But look, I can extend it some when you let go."

"Well, there's a good reason for that. You broke your ulna proximally, right where the triceps muscle attaches. So when your triceps contracts to extend your elbow against resistance, that fragment is pulled proximally, but the forearm doesn't move. That's what you're feeling."

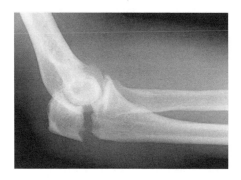

The pull of the triceps on the proximal fragment keeps an olecranon fracture distracted.

"Sounds really bad. You can fix it somehow, can't you?"

"You're actually pretty lucky. These can be a lot worse. If they break further into the joint, the elbow becomes unstable and can dislocate. The challenge here is to reconnect the olecranon to the shaft of the ulna, which we can do with a screw or with wires, and then we need to quickly get this elbow moving so it doesn't stiffen up."

"Have you ever done this before?"

"I've done it again and again. It's a more common injury than Bobo's, Monty's, or Galy's, but I haven't examined Ulno yet. So, Ulno, last but certainly not least, the clown who brought us all together."

"Very funny. You try riding a unicycle with six clowns piled on your shoulders. I could've managed it just fine if it wasn't for these silly shoes. But I think I came out OK, just some scrapes and bruises. I was the only one able to drive us here."

"Believe us, Doc, we wouldn't have ridden with him again if we could have helped it. Ha, ha, ha."

"You're a riot, Monty. Here, let me shake your hand. Ha, ha, ha. Seriously, Doc, I was falling right toward the tent pole, but I got my arm up in time to block it. I hit right on the middle of my forearm. See the big bruise?"

"Yes, definitely. Does it hurt to press on it, Ulno?"

"Of course. Bruises always hurt."

"How about if I squeeze your radius and ulna together down here away from the bruise?"

"Agh! That hurts too. Ow! It hurts when you rotate my forearm all the way into a palm-up position. Agh! And palm-down too."

"That tells me a great deal. I think there's a good chance that you have an isolated fracture of the ulna, Ulno."

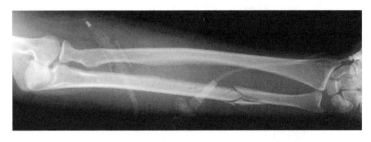

A direct blow to the subcutaneously located ulna can cause an isolated shaft fracture.

"It's sometimes called a nightstick fracture. If it's not displaced, all you'll need is a splint until the swelling goes down and then a cast. But if it's displaced, you'll need a plate like Bobo Senior, Galy, and Monty. Otherwise the bony malalignment and soft tissue scarring will preclude good forearm rotation."

"Sounds reasonable, Doc, but one question. I've got some friends who fell last winter, and they all got fractures around their wrists. Why all these different injuries when everybody just tried to stop their falls with their hands?"

"That's a good question. There certainly are quite a few injury patterns that can result from falls like yours. The nature of the injury depends on how hard you fall, the exact position of your trunk and limb, whether your hand slips along the ground, and things like that. And of course, it depends on your age and the relative strengths of the bones and supporting ligaments. As you've seen, slight variations in these factors can produce dramatically different injuries. Now, gentlemen, is that everything? To confirm my diagnoses, I'll go look at the x-rays. And of course I'll make sure that they include your wrists and elbows. Then we'll get this show on the road!"

"Ugh!" [honk-honk].

P R I N C I P L E :   To avoid overlooking an associated dislocation, fracture x-ray examinations must include the adjacent joints.

ADVANCED READING

Chambers HG. Fractures of the proximal radius and ulna. In Beaty JH, Kasser JR, eds. Fractures in Children, 5th ed. Philadelphia: Lippincott, 2001.

Hak DJ, Golladay GJ. Olecranon fractures: Treatment options. J Am Acad Orthop Surg 8:266-275, 2000.

Hotchkiss RN. Fractures of the radial head and related instability and contracture of the forearm. Instr Course Lect 47:173-177, 1998.

Morrey BF. Current concepts in the treatment of fractures of the radial head, the olecranon, and the coronoid. Instr Course Lect 44:175-185, 1995.

Noonan KJ, Price CT. Forearm and distal radius fractures in children. J Am Acad Orthop Surg 6:146-156, 1998.

O'Driscoll SW, Jupiter JB, Cohen MS, et al. Difficult elbow fractures: Pearls and pitfalls. Instr Course Lect 52:113-134, 2003.

Perron AD, Hersh RE, Brady WJ, et al. Orthopedic pitfalls in the ED: Galeazzi and Monteggia fracture-dislocation. Am J Emerg Med 19:225-228, 2001.

Price CT, Mencio GA. Injuries to the shafts of the radius and ulna. In Beaty JH, Kasser JR, eds. Fractures in Children, 5th ed. Philadelphia: Lippincott, 2001.

Richards RA. Fractures of the shafts of the radius and ulna. In Rockwood CA Jr, Bucholz RW, Heckman, JD, et al, eds. Fractures in Adults, vol 1, 5th ed. Philadelphia: Lippincott, 2001.

Ring D, Jupiter JB, Waters PM. Monteggia fractures in children and adults. J Am Acad Orthop Surg 6:215-224, 1998.

47

SER

Gary L. Zohman ✦ *Roy A. Meals*

Within 4 hours of finishing their surgery examination, Kevin, Nick, and Steve were wakeboarding. Unfortunately, by the following afternoon they were back in the emergency room. Steve had taken a dramatic, cartwheeling fall when jumping the wake in choppy water. His friends had to pull him into the boat and later had to support his weight on their shoulders as he limped into the hospital. Clearly there was something wrong with Steve's swollen and bruised ankle.

The emergency room physician, Samuel E. Rogers III, MD, satisfied himself that Steve had no head, neck, chest, or abdominal injuries. Then he turned his attention to the ankle. "Elevating his ankle was a good idea. Did you guys check the neurovascular status as well?"

"Uh, no, you see, we . . ." Nick stammered.

"Well, go ahead and tell me what you find. It's an extremely important part of evaluating ankle injuries. As you know, the primary neurovascular bundles to the foot pass directly anterior and directly medial to the ankle joint. If he has a fracture, a sharp bone fragment could easily damage these structures. Also, palpate the entire length of the fibula; I'll explain later."

Kevin and Nick carefully examined their friend, who was much more comfortable after Dr. Rogers gave him an injection for pain and placed his right lower extremity in a short posterior splint. "The splint will immobilize his ankle while we examine him and take him to x-ray," Dr. Rogers explained. "It's for protection as well as comfort. But we don't want him in a complete cast yet because there's bound to be more swelling, and an enclosed cast could cause not only terrible pain, but also potentially a compartment syndrome."

"The dorsalis pedis pulse is palpable," reported Nick. "But there's too much swelling over the medial malleolus for me to feel the posterior tibial pulse. He's got good capillary refill in his toes, and his leg compartments are soft and nontender. The foot's warm and pink."

Kevin added, "Sensation is intact for pinpricks in the distribution of the sural, saphenous, superficial peroneal, and deep peroneal nerves on the dorsum of the foot. It's also normal over the plantar aspect. His pain limits the motor exam, but he can wiggle all his toes. I deferred the ankle jerk," he continued, adeptly twirling the reflex hammer.

"He's exquisitely tender over both malleoli but nontender over the fibula more proximally. Why did you want me to palpate that far up, anyway?"

"To check for fractures, of course. I'll explain when we have more information. Meanwhile, tell me, Kevin, what is the sensory distribution of the deep peroneal nerve?"

"It innervates only a small patch of skin in the first web space. Its main function is nerve supply to the muscles of the anterior compartment."

"Precisely. The tibialis anterior, extensor hallucis longus, and extensor digitorum longus muscles, to be specific. And that's why diminished sensation in the first web space may be a clue of elevated anterior compartment pressures."

By this time the x-rays had come back, and Dr. Rogers stood before them stroking his chin. "Look fellows, Steve and I nearly have the same initials—I'm S.E.R. III, and he's Steven E. Randall IV. Very interesting—particularly in the face of the findings from his films.

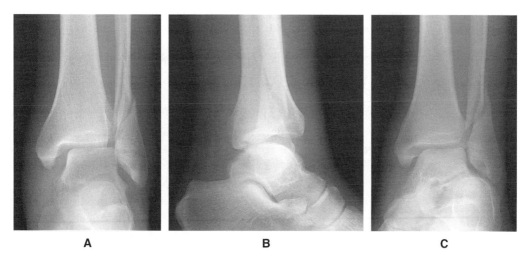

| A | B | C |

A, Anteroposterior, **B,** lateral, and **C,** mortise views demonstrating an oblique fibula fracture with a lateral shift of the talus, indicating deltoid ligament rupture. Although easily seen on this anteroposterior view because of the degree of displacement, medial widening can be subtle and may be apparent only on the mortise view.

"Nick, tell me why we have three views rather than just the anteroposterior and lateral."

"I believe the third film is a 'mortise' view."

"Right. The dome of the talus is snugly contained on three sides by the tibia and fibula, but the ankle mortise isn't aligned straight forward as you might think—it's actually a bit oblique. When Steve's leg is internally rotated about 15 degrees, the film shows us the joint space medially, superiorly, and laterally, usually without any bony overlap. So tell me what you see, Kevin."

"Looks like Steve broke his ankle. There's a spiral fracture of the distal fibula. The lateral malleolus is shifted several millimeters proximally and laterally."

"Anything else?"

"Well, the tibia looks fine. So does the talus."

"Nick?"

"Uh, I concur."

"Look at the widened space between the talus and the medial malleolus. Normally on the mortise view, the space on all three sides of the talus is equal, but here it is twice as wide medially as it is superiorly and laterally. Steve's talus has shifted laterally. Nick, do you know anything about the ankle ligaments?"

"Why, yes. Three principal groups of ligaments stabilize the ankle. The one from the medial malleolus to the tarsals is known as the deltoid ligament because of its shape. The lateral ligaments attach the fibula to the tarsal bones; they're relatively weak and commonly tear with an ankle sprain. Then there's the system of ligaments holding the tibia and fibula together; they keep the mortise narrow."

"Very impressive, Nick. Now tell me which ligament Steve tore."

"It must be the deltoid."

"That's right. Only a medial malleolus fracture or a deltoid ligament tear will allow the talus to shift laterally in the mortise. Think of the stable ankle joint as an intact ring consisting of the deltoid ligament, the medial malleolus, tibiofibular ligaments, the lateral malleolus, lateral ligaments, and the talus. Therefore, if the talus is shifted, the mortise ring must be disrupted in at least two places. The fibular disruption here is obvious, and we must infer the deltoid ligament tear from the position of the talus."

"That also explains the tenderness and swelling next to the medial malleolus," offered Kevin.

"OK, Kevin, since you're on a roll, why don't you tell me what position his ankle was in when he broke it."

"You're kidding, Dr. Rogers. He was moving pretty fast when he lost it. All I saw were a bunch of flying arms and legs."

"I'm sure. But by looking at the pattern of injury on the x-rays, we can deduce the direction of the forces. And that's important because when we go to reduce the fracture-dislocation, we want to apply forces exactly opposite to those that deformed the ankle. For instance, Steve's injury pattern implies that his supinated foot underwent an unpleasant external rotation. It's an extremely common mechanism and results in a spiral fracture of the fibula as the talus is twisted out of the mortise. Sometimes, though, the fibula fracture will be proximal and cannot be seen on ankle x-rays. That's why I had Nick palpate the entire fibula."

"Let's go tell Steve what we've learned."

"Okay, but just one more thing. The degree of injury from these **s**upination–**e**xternal-**r**otation (SER) injuries depends on the amount of force absorbed. The SER injury begins anteriorly and proceeds laterally around the ring. This makes sense when you imagine externally rotating your supinated foot. The first structure damaged is the anterior tibiofibular ligament, next the fibula, then the posterior tibiofibular ligaments, and finally the medial structures. Steve's deltoid ligament tore, but sometimes the medial malleolus is avulsed instead.

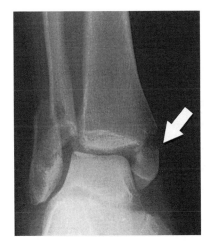

Example of a supination–external-rotation injury resulting in avulsion of the medial malleolus *(arrow)* rather than a deltoid ligament tear.

"Because the injury proceeded around the entire circumference of the ankle, it's called an SER IV. Most SER injuries don't get this far, but you said he was really blasting when he fell."

Dr. Rogers, Kevin, and Nick showed Steve the fractured fibula on the x-rays and explained about the torn ligaments. "Steve, you have an intraarticular fracture and an unstable ankle," Dr. Rogers said.

"So now what?"

"I'll try to reduce it by pronating and internally rotating your foot. If I can get everything perfectly repositioned, then cast treatment may work. But if there is any residual shift of the talus, even as little as 1 to 2 mm, then the contact stresses in the ankle joint are dramatically increased from the incongruity. Even if I get a perfect reduction today, as the swelling goes down things may still settle in a suboptimal position. Most orthopedists would agree that a bimalleolar fracture, especially one that is displaced like yours, would probably benefit from surgery. Yours is actually considered a bimalleolar equivalent because the deltoid ligament ruptured rather than the medial malleolus, but functionally they're similar. During surgery, the fibula is realigned and a plate is applied. This usually pushes the talus back into its anatomic position, and the deltoid ligament is allowed to heal on its own."

"Can't we just accept a general realignment like when I was 8 years old and broke both bones in my forearm? The doctor was right in predicting that those bones would remodel over time, although my mother practically went ballistic when she saw the x-rays with the fracture fragments incompletely aligned."

"No, for two reasons. Those were extraarticular fractures, and you were still growing then. The ankle bears more weight per surface area than any other joint in the body, and if perfect articular congruency is not restored, degenerative arthritis will ensue. Also, it's difficult to hold a spirally fractured fibula out to full length in a cast. That's important to prevent the talus from subluxating laterally during heel strike."

"What are the risks of casting versus open reduction and internal fixation?"

"Casting risks pressure sores, compartment syndrome, and ankle stiffness. Surgery, of course, risks infection and poor wound healing; but internal fixation allows earlier mobilization of the soft tissues, which helps prevent atrophy, edema, osteoporosis, and stiffness."

"So what are we waiting for?"

"Look Steve, you're no longer in the Big City. The orthopedic surgeon won't be here for an hour, and even if he decides to operate, he'll probably want to wait several days until some of the swelling subsides. Otherwise he might not be able to get the skin closed."

"Wait a minute," interrupted Kevin. "Aren't you an orthopedic surgeon?"

"No way. I'm the ER doc."

"Then how come you know so much about ankle injuries?"

"Because I just finished reading a book called *One Hundred Orthopedic Conditions Every Doctor Should Understand.*"

ADVANCED READING

Michelson JD. Ankle fractures resulting from rotational injuries. J Am Acad Orthop Surg 11:403-412, 2003.

Title CI, Katschis SD. Traumatic foot and ankle injuries in the athlete. Orthop Clin North Am 33:587-598, 2002.

Vander Griend R, Michelson JD, Bone LB. Fractures of the ankle and the distal part of the tibia. Instr Course Lect 46:311-321, 1997.

48

The New Tattoo

An 18-year-old man comes to your office for evaluation because he flunked his induction physical for the Marines. He was apparently told that he walked as though he had an "attitude," and was reprimanded for only being able to reach his kneecaps when told to bend forward and touch his toes. Once the drill sergeant caught wind of his unwillingness to stand at attention, he was promptly dismissed and told to get his back checked out. He insists it is OK. On further questioning, however, he does admit to a vague ache in his lower back extending to his buttocks and the posterior aspect of his thighs after working out at the gym, particularly after using the rowing machine. He adamantly denies any lower limb weakness, numbness, or bowel or bladder dysfunction. His history is unremarkable. He is adopted, so his family history is unknown.

You note as he walks down the hall that he has a stiff-legged gait with a short stride and that he rotates the pelvis forward with each step. During the examination you find a pronounced lumbar lordosis and tenderness when you palpate the low back.

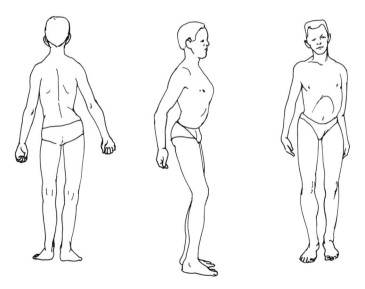

Lumbar hyperlordosis causes prominence of the lower abdomen.

When viewed from the front, the lower part of his abdomen is thrust forward—a posture not particularly appealing to boot camp drill instructors. You verify his gross inability to touch his toes when bending forward, and with him supine, you confirm hamstring muscle tightness by his inability to do a straight-leg raise more than 30 degrees. When tested individually, however, hip and knee motions are full.

What's wrong with this recruit? Is he fit for the Marines, or should his combat training be limited to computer games?

The lumbar hyperlordosis, local tenderness, and tight hamstrings all suggest a forward slippage of a lumbar vertebra. Collectively referred to as the *posterior elements* are the structures that form the neural arch and the contribution of each vertebra to the superior and inferior facet joints. Normally the overlapping orientation of the facet joints prevents the vertebral bodies from slipping anteriorly (anterolisthesis) or posteriorly (retrolisthesis). However, a stress fracture in the area between the superior and inferior articular processes unlinks the vertebral body from the stabilizing influence of these posterior elements. Failure in this region, known in Latin simply as the *pars interarticularis* (or just *pars* for short) allows the anterior structures to slide forward while the inferior facets maintain their normal anatomic relationship with the underlying vertebra.

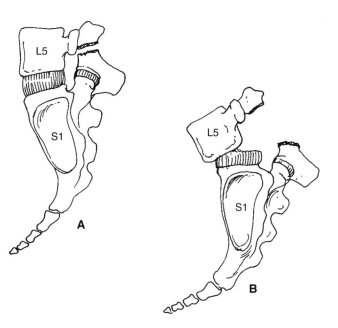

A, A pars interarticularis defect without slippage—spondylolysis. **B,** Spondylolisthesis with about 50% forward slippage of L5 on S1.

The L5 to S1 level is most commonly affected by this malady, and it seems to be a curse of upright posture, because it is unknown in quadrupeds. Although it is generally believed that a stress fracture is responsible, the condition has racial and gender variations as well as familial tendencies, suggesting an inherited predisposition. The defect in the pars interarticularis is known as *spondylolysis*—literally, "spine disintegration." Once the integrity of the posterior elements is disrupted, shear stresses are transferred from the facet joints to the intervertebral disc, and gradual slippage occurs. *Spondylolisthesis* means "slipped spine" and can begin at about age 8 in girls and age 12 in boys. Maximum slippage occurs during the adolescent growth spurt, and further movement after age 20 is rare.

Although the defect is present radiographically in 5% of people, and some slippage may occur in childhood, pain in children is uncommon, and pain in teenagers is usually not sufficiently bothersome for them to seek medical care. If pain does occur, it is usually related to activity. Strenuous, repetitive activities involving flexion and extension of the spine, such as gymnastics, diving, and rowing, are particularly irksome and possibly causative. The condition is also common in young football linemen, presumably because of increased loading of the spine in the hyperextended position. A youth may be brought to see a doctor because of abnormal posture and gait rather than complaints of pain. Such disturbances are related to the exaggerated lumbar lordosis and the tight hamstring muscles that frequently accompany a slip. The tight hamstrings prevent sufficient hip flexion for a normal stride and result in a stiff-legged, short-step gait with compensatory pelvic rotation—the so-called pelvic waddle. The hollow-back deformity and the associated prominence of the lower abdomen become more pronounced as the degree of slippage increases. Scoliosis, typically related to muscle spasm rather than structural changes, may also accompany spondylolisthesis. Nerve root compression is uncommon in children, so weakness and sensory or reflex changes are unusual.

Because more than 6% of white males have spondylolysis, the bony disruptions are only an incidental finding in some children and teenagers presenting with low back complaints. Therefore a pars defect with or without slippage should not be implicated as the cause of back pain or neurologic symptoms without a thorough search for other causes such as disc-space infection, bone or spinal cord tumor, or ruptured disc.

P R I N C I P L E :   Treat the patient, not the x-ray.

Because of the oblique orientation of the posterior vertebral elements, routine anteroposterior and lateral x-rays may not identify a pars defect before slippage has occurred. Thus spondylolysis must be carefully sought in young people with low back pain and tight hamstrings. Oblique x-rays, bone scans, and CT scans are all helpful.

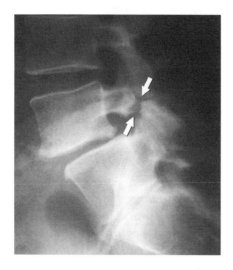

Spondylolysis defect in the pars interarticularis *(arrows)*. Also note the forward slip of L5 on S1. Compare the vertebral body alignment between L4 and L5 and between L5 and S1.

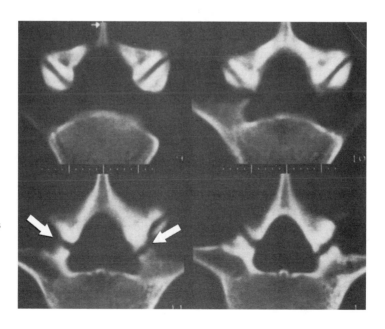

CT scan of the lumbar spine. The upper two images show the obliquely oriented facet joints and the vertebral body. The lower two images show bilateral pars interarticularis defects *(arrows)*.

The degree of slippage in spondylolisthesis is best determined from a standing lateral x-ray of the lumbosacral junction.

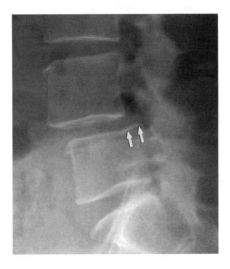

Low-grade spondylolisthesis of L4 on L5. As is commonly the case, the pars defect is difficult to see on this lateral projection. Oblique views, CT scans, and bone scans are often helpful.

If spondylolysis is identified shortly after an obvious injury, immobilization in a cast or brace can result in healing, particularly if the fracture is unilateral. For more common chronic bilateral defects, immobilization is unlikely to promote healing. Avoiding strenuous activities coupled with trunk-strengthening exercises can usually alleviate the mild backache and tight hamstrings. Any youth with spondylolysis should be followed to see whether slippage begins; but as long as pain is minimal and there is no more than a minor slip, no restriction of activities is required.

With moderate slips (>50%), participating in contact sports or other activities associated with a high risk of back injury should be very carefully considered. Additionally, the risk of low back pain in adult life is significantly greater in adolescents with symptomatic slips of a moderate or severe degree. Thus if conservative measures fail to relieve symptoms, or if there is evidence of slip progression or neurological deficit, fusion of the unstable vertebrae is appropriate. Even without reduction of the slippage, fusion is quite successful in relieving backache and hamstring tightness, although it does not correct the hyperlordosis. Methods of internal fixation have been developed that correct the slip and the postural deformity, but they carry an increased risk of nerve root damage during reduction. Use of such methods remains controversial.

Follow-up Note: With slippage of more than 50% noted on the office x-rays, your patient will likely need to avoid heavy lifting and contact activities. Therefore the Marines are out. He angrily asks you what he is to do about his new tattoo and then storms out of the office.

ADVANCED READING

Bono CM. Low-back pain in athletes. J Bone Joint Surg Am 86:382-396, 2004.

Debnath UK, Freeman BJ, Gregory P, et al. Clinical outcome and return to sport after the surgical treatment of spondylolysis in young athletes. J Bone Joint Surg Br 85:244-249, 2003.

Herman MJ, Pizzutillo PD, Cavalier R. Spondylolysis and spondylolisthesis in the child and adolescent athlete. Orthop Clin North Am 34:461-467, 2003.

49

The Obnoxious Sibling

"Hello, this is Dr. Rogers."

"Hi, Sam. This is Jim Honeychurch at the medical center. I thought I'd call and let you know how the man you sent down last week is doing—the one with the amputated left thumb and the nearly amputated right index finger."

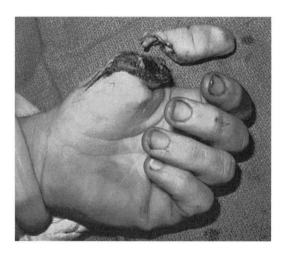

Typical electric handsaw "kickback" injury.

"Yeah. I'm glad to hear from you. That was one unfortunate power saw accident. I was in such a hurry compressing his wounds for hemostasis, getting his hands and the part x-rayed, and giving him his tetanus prophylaxis and antibiotics, that I almost forgot to cool the amputated part. Was it OK wrapped in gauze and in a plastic bag with the bag on ice?"

"That was perfect. Cooling slows the tissues' metabolic demands; it's especially important for more proximal amputations through the palm or forearm when muscle is included, because muscle tolerates ischemia so poorly. In those cases we've only got about 6 hours to get circulation reestablished, even when the part is cooled. We've usually got a bit longer with digital amputations, up to 12 hours if the part is properly cooled. However, you've also got to consider surgical time, especially with multiple digits, because it can take several hours to complete each replantation."

P R I N C I P L E :   Get amputated parts on ice as soon as possible.

"How did his thumb go? It was pretty chewed up. You told me once before that thumbs amputated through the interphalangeal joint or more distally have plenty of length to function well even without replantation. I also remember that very distal replantations are technically difficult because of the tiny blood vessels. But this guy's thumb was off through the base of the proximal phalanx."

"Well, you're right that more distal amputations of the thumb can often be treated with some type of soft tissue coverage, and replantation is typically avoided. However, you have to consider the unique function of the opposable thumb, which allows for gripping, pinching, and manipulation of objects against the remaining digits. So we are definitely more aggressive with thumb amputations, in general, than with other digits. In this patient's case, the tissue edges were sort of jagged, but by shortening the bone and fusing his metacarpophalangeal joint, we could trim off the frayed portions of his tendons, vessels, and nerves and make tidy repairs.

GUIDELINES FOR REPLANTATION:

Indications for Replantation

Thumb amputation

Individual digit distal to the insertion of the flexor digitorum superficialis (FDS) muscle (zone I amputation)

Metacarpal amputation

Multiple digits

Amputation at the wrist or distal forearm

Bilateral amputations

Almost any pediatric amputation

Relative Contraindications

Prolonged warm ischemia (>12 hours for a digit, >6 hours for wrist or proximal)

Crushing or avulsion injury (mangled extremity)

Diffuse arterial damage

Polytrauma

Amputations at multiple levels

Severe bony comminution and loss of joint integrity

"Unfortunately, 3 days later his thumb became engorged and blue, yet demonstrated very brisk capillary refill, which together are characteristic of outflow problems such as venous thrombosis. These findings are in contrast to the cold and white appearance of a digit with delayed capillary refill, which is typical of inflow problems such as arterial spasm or occlusion."

"Did you use the ugly suckers?"

"Their mothers don't think they're ugly, but yes, leeches can frequently save a failed venous repair. Once the leech feeds and falls off after about 30 minutes, its bite mark continues to ooze blood for at least 8 hours because of the anticoagulant agent it deposited. This decongests the capillary network and allows for perfusion."

"So his circulation is OK now that the granulation tissue has opened new channels? How's his sensation?"

"Not so fast. His circulation is probably OK, but even one cigarette could still spoil it. And patients with limb replantations complain of cold sensitivity for at least 2 years because of persistent relative ischemia. With nerves we can only sew the connective tissue coverings together. Then the sprouting axons advance about a millimeter a day. So it's going to be a couple of months before he gets any feeling back, and it will never fully return to normal."

"So do you wait until he has feeling in it before you let him start moving it?"

"The tendons would be impossibly scarred if we waited that long. We've already started him moving it a little, but replanted digits rarely recover full motion because of the inevitable scarring that surrounds both the flexor and extensor repairs. So our expectations have to be guarded."

"I don't get it. You say his replanted thumb is going to be short, numb, stiff, and cold intolerant. What's the point if it's not going to be perfect?"

"There's no way all those injured tissues are going to heal without some significant deficits. But the replanted thumb, even with these deficiencies, is better than an amputation. Just think about how difficult a simple task such as grasping and pinching would be without the presence of a thumb."

"I guess I see your point. So how about his incompletely amputated index finger on the right hand? That injury was transverse and sharp—right through his proximal phalanx. A tiny skin bridge was still intact. No crush or avulsion. It must have been a slam dunk to replant that one, especially compared with some of the mutilating injuries that I've heard about involving lawn mowers, snow blowers, and corn pickers."

P R I N C I P L E :   Replantation surgery is salvage surgery.

"Well, technically we could have saved the index finger, but experience has shown us that to do so in this case would be a disservice to the patient. So we completed the amputation and closed the stump."

"Whoa! Now I'm really confused."

"Well, think about it. If you had a normal thumb and three other normal digits, you'd have a pretty good working hand. But what if they had to work around another digit that was short, inflexible, numb, and always complaining about the cold?"

"Yeah, kind of reminds me of my younger brother growing up."

"With all types of replantation or limb salvage surgery, you have to consider the function that you are trying to restore. In the upper extremity, fine motor functions such as grasping and pinching are the primary considerations. These are quite difficult to provide using prosthetics because of their high dependence on sensation, so replantation surgery is often considered. However, aside from the importance of the thumb as I have mentioned, these functions can often be approximated with the loss of one or even two digits. Compare this with a lower extremity amputation, in which the primary functional consideration is stable weight bearing. Pain-free and efficient weight bearing can often be substituted nicely with a durable prosthetic device, because sensation and fine motor function are significantly less important there than in the upper extremity. So a lower limb prosthesis serves quite well, far better than a replanted leg that requires massive bone shortening to approximate the soft tissues."

PRINCIPLE: Let reason triumph over technique.

"So how about somebody who cuts off all five fingers?"

"That's obviously a devastating injury, and then even digits with major deficiencies are generally better than no digits at all. Also, in kids we can liberalize our indications for replantation because youngsters don't seem to get so stiff, and they recover nerve function better."

"Then what about hand transplantation? I heard recently about a few of those being performed."

"Well, I think it's fair to say that hand transplantation is still in the experimental stages. The first was performed in the late 1990s, and a small number continue to be done each year. Though I guess technically the surgery itself is quite similar to a replant near the wrist or distal forearm, there are a lot of other factors that need to be considered with a transplant. First and foremost is the need for immune suppression that must be continued indefinitely—certainly not without infectious and neoplastic risks. Then there's also the rejection process itself that can lead to stiffness, scarring, and even the need for amputation. Those issues aside, it appears that a transplanted hand can restore basic grasping functions and protective sensation. Again though, some degree of caution is necessary, because return of intrinsic musculature has not yet been demonstrated, and it is unlikely that fine two-point discrimination will be achieved."

"One last question. Do you know anybody who would want to buy a table saw? I think I'm going to defer my power woodworking until retirement. My hands are too important to my work."

"No. But I think that's a good idea—something fun to look forward to."

"Say, where can I read more about replantation surgery? We get the occasional patient in here with something crushed or cut off, and I have to advise them what the best treatment route is."

"I'll send you a couple of things, OK?"

"Great. Thanks for the call. Bye."

"Take care."

ADVANCED READING

Breidenbach WC III, Tobin GR II, Gorantla VS, et al. A position statement in support of hand transplantation. J Hand Surg Am 27:760-770, 2002.

Jones NF. Concerns about human hand transplantation in the 21st century. J Hand Surg Am 27:771-787, 2002.

Merle M, Dautel G. Advances in digital replantation. Clin Plast Surg 24:87-105, 1997.

Soucacos PN. Indications and selection for digital amputation and replantation. J Hand Surg Br 26:572-581, 2001.

Wilhelmi BJ, Lee WP, Pagensteert GI, et al. Replantation in the mutilated hand. Hand Clin 19:89-120, 2003.

◆ *To heighten your appreciation for your thumb, keep it taped to the side of your index metacarpal all afternoon.*

50

Sensible Shoes

August 9

Dear Mom and Dad,

Have I got some great news for you! Remember how I said I was going to get a part-time job this summer in addition to my cartilage research? There's this women's shoe store I like, and the owner asked me about working Saturdays. I get a discount on shoes, but that's not the best thing. I never knew so many things could go wrong with people's feet. It's incredibly fascinating. But don't worry, I'm not about to drop out of medical school yet—selling shoes will make it *more* interesting, not less.

Yesterday, for instance, this stylishly dressed lady and her teenage daughter came in, both wearing high heels with narrow, pointed toes—they said that's all they ever wear. When the mother took her shoes off I almost fell over. It was all I could do not to let out a gasp. Her big toes nearly crossed right under her second toes, and she had big red calluses where the shoes had been pushing on her skin. She was impossible to fit. She said that everything I showed her that was wide enough for comfort didn't fit her image. But all the trendy high heels made her feet hurt.

I kept thinking about those feet all night, so I went to the library today. That's why I didn't call. The mother's deformity is called hallux valgus—a lateral deviation of the big toe. Either as cause or effect, the first metatarsal also deviates medially, so, as we say in medical circles, she has metatarsus primus varus.

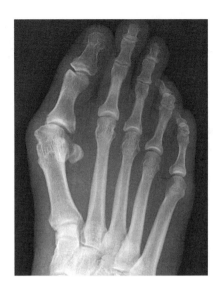

Varus deviation of
the first metatarsal
and valgus deformi-
ty of the hallux. Is
there evidence here
of hallux rigidus?

With the metatarsal going one way and the big toe going the other, the metatarsal head becomes prominent. When it pushes against a tight shoe, the bursa over the metatarsal head gets inflamed. That's what hurts. The inflamed bursa is called a bunion. Nobody is born with it. The deformity can be caused by ligamentous laxity from rheumatoid arthritis or by muscle imbalance from neuromuscular disorders, lumbar disc disease, spinal tumors, and so forth. But most of the time it's the shoes. Hallux valgus occurs nine times more frequently in women than men and often runs in families. There's a predisposition in people with flat feet and general ligamentous laxity. The deformity frequently begins in the preteen years and is greatly accelerated by chronic use of high heels, where the foot is forced into the wedge-shaped toe box. The second toe is pushed into a claw position (more about that later) and then fails to give lateral support to the big toe. Also, if the big toe is a little longer than normal, the shoe has a longer lever to push on.

What I found really interesting was that from both diagnostic and treatment points of view, hallux valgus and other toe deformities must be approached from a regional perspective. Malalignment or stiffness at the knee or ankle, hindfoot abnormalities, and a variety of tendon imbalances, for instance, may be causative. These conditions have to be addressed for adequate treatment. Conservative treatment includes improved shoe selection, splints, and pressure-relieving pads. But once the deformity progresses far enough, the altered pull of the affected tendons accelerates the collapse.

Surgery is directed at restoring alignment of the first ray and reducing pain. Although a successful correction improves the appearance, disfigurement alone should not be used as an indication for surgery. I found more than 100 operations described on the internet to correct hallux valgus. All of them have failure rates of at least 10%, partly related to choosing the wrong operation for the specific problem. The operations usually involve some combination of soft-tissue realignment and a corrective metatarsal osteotomy. But sometimes osteotomy of the distal phalanx or fusion of the medial cuneiform–first metatarsal joint is needed as well. Unfortunately, none of these surgeries are without complications. Recurrence of the deformity is probably the most common complication, especially when performed on adolescent patients. Overcorrection or undercorrection can also occur if the wrong type of surgery is selected. Persistent pain, most often caused by the presence of unrecognized hallux rigidus—degenerative arthritis of the first metatarsophalangeal (MTP) joint—is another common cause of failure. This degeneration is likely underestimated by most x-rays, so it's important to inspect the joint carefully at the time of surgery. A fusion across the joint should be performed if the hallux rigidus is severe enough.

PRINCIPLE: When multiple operations are available for a given condition, chances are good that none of them are totally effective.

August 16

I didn't have time to finish my last e-mail because I was waiting for Trevor to come over, but he didn't show up—again. What's up with guys and these disappearing acts? I'll tell you who did show up, though. That woman and her daughter came back to the store yesterday. As I suspected from my reading, the daughter already has a mild hallux valgus deformity; and fortunately the mother doesn't have hallux rigidus. Her first MTP joint shows a full range of motion, and her foot doesn't hurt when walking barefoot or rising up on her toes. I finally told them I was a medical student because they've become a bit wary of my apparent foot fetish. Kind of funny, but I assured them that my interest was purely professional. I've got to stop now; I'm going to go by Trevor's place.

August 23

The summer has really gone quickly. Yesterday was my last day at the shoe store, which is good because I probably would have been fired—I can't stop asking people about their crooked toes. Today I saw two more people with bunions. One of them was getting a stodgy pair of oxfords with low heels and a wide toe box. She said they made her feet feel great. I also spotted some more claw toes, a hammer toe, and a mallet toe.

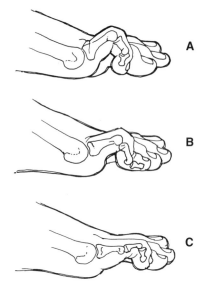

A, Claw toe.
B, Hammer toe.
C, Mallet toe.

Modified from Alexander IJ. The Foot: Examination and Diagnosis. New York: Churchill Livingstone, 1990, pp 68, 70-71.

Claw toes can result from an imbalance of the intrinsic muscles, just like claw fingers, but claw toes are more commonly related to tight shoes. There is hyperextension at the metatarsophalangeal joint and flexion through the interphalangeal (IP) joints—making the toe look kind of like a claw. A hammer toe is like a boutonniere deformity in a finger: excessive flexion at the proximal interphalangeal (PIP) joint and hyperextension at the distal interphalangeal (DIP) joint. Its usual cause in a foot is, surprise, a tight shoe. A mallet toe is like a mallet finger: the DIP joint droops from an extensor tendon disruption. I can spot them now from clear across the store.

I start my surgery clerkship tomorrow. Medical school should get more interesting now. I hope so. I'm tired of sitting in classes all day. Because I'm going to be on my feet a lot more now, and because I didn't make much money this summer, can you send me a little for some better shoes? If I'm busy next Sunday I'll try to call you at the shop during the week.

Love,
Sheri

P.S. Trevor is history.

ADVANCED READING

Coughlin MJ. Hallux Valgus. Instr Course Lect 46:357-391, 1997.

Coughlin MJ. Lesser toe abnormalities. Instr Course Lect 52:421-444, 2003.

Nyska M. Principles of first metatarsal osteotomies. Foot Ankle Clin 6:399-408, 2001.

Vanore JV, Christensen JC, Kravitz SR, et al. Diagnosis and treatment of first metatarsophalangeal disorders. Section I: Hallux valgus. J Foot Ankle Surg 42:112-123, 2003.

✦ *Could you stand on your toes with your first metatarsophalangeal joint fixed in 10 degrees of flexion? Could you comfortably wear shoes if your first MTP joint was fixed in 30 degrees of extension? If you had to have your first MTP joint fused, what position would be best?*

51

A Day in Court

J. Scott Smith ✦ *Roy A. Meals*

"Your Honor, I now call my client, Milo Oldenbuchs, to the stand.

"Dr. Oldenbuchs, please inform the court of the circumstances under which you and the plaintiff's son first met."

"Andrew first came to my office 3 years ago. He had just turned 18 and was headed for college. His right knee had been hurting for a couple of weeks, and although Andrew was extremely active in sports, he was certain that he had not injured it. A few days before he came in, the lad noticed swelling at the site of the soreness, and that initiated the visit."

"So where did things go from there?"

"His history was unremarkable except for what I have just related. Examination showed a tender, fixed mass just distal to his knee joint. The overlying skin was hot. I took an x-ray of his knee."

"Dr. Oldenbuchs, is this the x-ray you are referring to?"

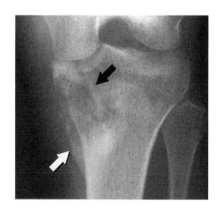

When present simultaneously, irregular bone erosion *(black arrow)*, periosteal reaction *(white arrow)*, and intralesional new bone formation are ominous signs.

"I believe so. You can see the mixed osteolytic and osteoblastic lesion in the proximal tibia. There is cortical destruction with new bone formation in both the medullary cavity and the soft tissues. Distally there is a triangle of new bone, which is caused by the tumor rapidly lifting the periosteum away from the cortex."

"What were your thoughts at this point?"

"The findings on the x-ray examination, coupled with the history and the physical, made me certain that this was an osteosarcoma. That's the most common malignancy in this age group, and the metaphyses of rapidly growing long bones are the most common sites. I guess a subacute osteomyelitis, syphilis, or another tumor might rarely have a similar presentation. We immediately scheduled Andrew for a technetium bone scan and a chest x-ray examination to determine whether the tumor had spread. The chest x-ray was clear, and the bone scan was negative for metastases. His serum alkaline phosphatase level was sky high though."

"How did Andrew react to all this?"

"He and his parents were obviously frightened and extremely discouraged when I explained to them the nature of the disease and the prognosis. They worked through the characteristic phases of denial, anger, bargaining, and so forth. I convinced them that immediate radical surgery would offer Andrew the best chance for survival. After an incisional biopsy confirmed the diagnosis, I performed an above-knee amputation without difficulty."

"How did things go after the surgery?"

"Andrew did extremely well. His wounds healed rapidly, and he adjusted as well as could be expected. He managed OK on crutches, but he was looking forward to wearing a prosthesis. Follow-up consisted of monthly examinations, chest x-ray examinations, and testing for alkaline phosphatase levels. Unfortunately 9 months postoperatively, his chest x-ray showed multiple metastases through both lung fields. There was nothing we could do for him. If the metastases had been unilateral, perhaps we could have attempted a pneumonectomy, but in this situation there was just nothing left for us to do. He survived only another 6 months. We were all extremely saddened by his death."

"Looking back, Doctor, is there anything you would do differently given the same situation?"

"No. We arrived at the diagnosis quickly and proceeded with surgery. Unfortunately this tumor is a bad actor. He received the standard textbook treatment."

"Nothing further, Your Honor."

"Would the prosecution care to cross-examine the defendant?"

"Yes, Your Honor. Dr. Oldenbuchs, when was the last time you cared for a patient with a bone tumor?"

"Well, Rose Rose passed on about 2 years ago, I guess. She had multiple myeloma. I practice in a fairly small town—mostly trauma, you know, and an occasional artificial joint. Primary bone tumors are just not that common. The only other osteosarcoma I've seen was during my residency almost 30 years ago. Metastases to bone are far more common than primary bone malignancies."

"Thank you, Doctor. That will be all. You may step down. The prosecution now calls Dr. Nosistuf to the stand.

"Dr. Nosistuf, you are a specialist in musculoskeletal tumors at University Medical Center, are you not?"

"That's right."

"And how long have you been caring for patients with orthopedic tumors?"

"Well, I guess it's been about 20 years by now."

"After hearing the defendant's testimony, how would you describe the medical treatment rendered to Andrew?"

"Dr. Oldenbuchs seemed to do the best he could, but a lot has happened with the treatment of malignant bone tumors since he moved here."

"Could you explain your answer, Doctor?"

"Of course. Optimal management of osteosarcoma requires both surgical control of the primary tumor and chemotherapeutic control of any metastases. Unfortunately, it is estimated that as many as 80% of patients who present with localized osteosarcoma, even without clinically detectable metastases, will have micrometastatic disease, usually involving the lungs. Tumor resection fails to address this systemic disease, thus accounting for the survival rates of only 20% with surgery alone. However, as we have also discovered, osteosarcoma is a malignancy that is often quite sensitive to chemotherapy. The addition of a combination chemotherapy regimen to a complete surgical resection boosts survival rates to as high as 75%. So although above-knee amputation may have been an appropriate part of therapy for the young man, amputation alone certainly limited Andrew's chances for survival."

"In your opinion, Doctor, did Andrew receive the current national standard of care for osteosarcoma?"

"I'm afraid not, ma'am."

"Given the same situation, how would you have proceeded?"

"Well, the history, physical exam, and x-ray exam all pointed toward a diagnosis of osteosarcoma as Dr. Oldenbuchs appropriately surmised. Although somewhat rare, osteosarcoma affects mostly adolescents and young adults. Patients typically present with pain, a mass, or a painful mass, as in Andrew's case. X-ray examinations reveal an aggressive mixed lytic and blastic lesion in the metaphysis of a long bone. The distal femur, proximal tibia, and proximal humerus account for two thirds of all locations. Andrew's x-rays show a predominately lytic variant, but I've also brought along some examples of primarily blastic osteosarcoma for comparison.

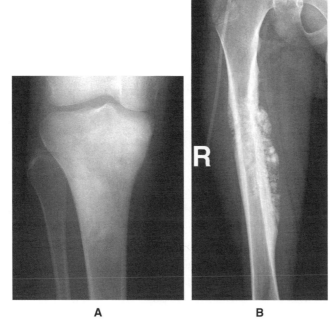

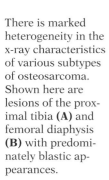

There is marked heterogeneity in the x-ray characteristics of various subtypes of osteosarcoma. Shown here are lesions of the proximal tibia **(A)** and femoral diaphysis **(B)** with predominately blastic appearances.

A   **B**

"Besides the studies Dr. Oldenbuchs obtained, I would have sent the patient for a CT scan of the thorax. CT scans are vastly superior to x-rays for defining pulmonary metastases and evaluating the response to chemotherapy. In addition, an assessment of the primary tumor site using either CT or MRI delineates the extent of the tumor far more accurately than conventional x-rays. Among the most important information regarding a patient's prognosis is the stage of the tumor. The tumor stage primarily relates to two factors: the grade of the tumor cells themselves and the extent of the disease, which is to say whether it is intracompartmental (confined to the bone) or extracompartmental (spread into soft tissues). The information provided by these scans, combined with the histologic grade of the tumor determined by biopsy, can provide a reasonable estimate of the patient's chances for survival and help guide treatment options.

"Dr. Oldenbuchs appropriately obtained a biopsy to confirm the diagnosis before proceeding with amputation. I should point out that a biopsy is not the benign procedure that many practitioners believe it to be. It needs to be well planned and meticulously performed, preferably by the tumor surgeon himself. The biopsy tract will be automatically seeded with malignant cells and will need to be excised en block with the tumor at the time of resection. Also, because sarcomas like to spread through the bloodstream, meticulous hemostasis is required during biopsy to prevent hematoma formation and consequent spread of the tumor into adjacent soft tissues. Because limb salvage is often undertaken, the biopsy site and approach need to be carefully chosen to not interfere with definitive resection.

P R I N C I P L E : Tumor biopsy is best left to the surgeon who will plan the definitive procedure.

"Before definitive surgery, systemic chemotherapy is used in an attempt to eliminate both macro- and microscopic metastatic disease that we now know are exceedingly common with osteosarcomas. Admittedly, chemotherapy has some major side effects, but the benefits justify the risks. In addition, chemo often shrinks the primary tumor, and that increases the feasibility of limb salvage. And in selected cases a thoracic surgeon can remove persistent or subsequent pulmonary metastases."

"What do you mean by limb salvage?"

"It's when we attempt to preserve a useful limb while removing the cancer. In the old days, pretty much the only operations performed by tumor surgeons were amputations. Now, however, limb salvage has become an attractive option for many patients. If the tumor can be removed with clear margins of normal tissue, either an allograft bone replacement or endoprosthesis can replace the resected bone. We attempt limb salvage when it appears that this will leave the patient with a functional and cosmetic result superior to amputation and prosthetic fitting."

"Are all of these patients candidates for limb salvage?"

"Unfortunately, no. If the tumor has invaded the major neurovascular structures or if adequate surgical margins cannot otherwise be achieved, limb salvage is not an option. Functional and cosmetic considerations are always secondary to tumor removal and survival. Limb salvage presents the additional problem of lower limb-length discrepancy for growing children, although extendable endoprostheses and limb-lengthening procedures are being tried. In very young children amputation may be the best and only course."

"Don't limb-sparing procedures jeopardize the patient's chance for a cure?"

"Local recurrences may be slightly more common in salvage procedures, but they can be treated and are not as ominous as the appearance of metastatic disease. Overall, there seems to be no major difference in long-term survival compared to amputations."

"In your book, Dr. Nosistuf, you stress the importance of sending the resected tumor specimen to pathology. The original biopsy reveals the diagnosis. What's the big deal with microscopic evaluation of the whole thing?"

"Prognosis. The degree of chemotherapy-induced necrosis predicts survival better than patient age, gender, tumor size, location, and histology combined. Confluent fields of viable tumor cells seen under high-power magnification indicate an incomplete response, and further chemotherapy should be administered with different agents. Only scattered foci of viable tumor or total necrosis constitute a near complete response."

"If proper chemotherapy had been included in Andrew's treatment, do you believe that he would be alive today?"

"That's impossible to say. Despite our best efforts we still lose too many patients. However, patients with newly diagnosed osteosarcoma without documented metastatic disease can expect cure rates of up to 75% after chemotherapy and surgery."

"What are you trying to say, Doctor?"

"Hmmm. With the treatment I have outlined, I guess the odds would have been in Andrew's favor rather than against him."

"Does the defense wish to cross-examine Dr. Nosistuf?"

"Uh, no, Your Honor. I do, however, request a recess until tomorrow morning in order to confer further with my client."

ADVANCED READING

Arndt CA, Crist WM. Common musculoskeletal tumors of childhood and adolescence. N Engl J Med 341:342-352, 1999.

Dicaprio MR, Friedlaender GE. Malignant bone tumors: Limb sparing versus amputation. J Am Acad Orthop Surg 11:25-37, 2003.

Eckardt JE. Newest knowledge of osteogenic sarcoma. Clin Orthop Relat Res 270:272-277, 1991.

Gibbs CP Jr, Weber K, Scarborough MT. Malignant bone tumors. J Bone Joint Surg Am 83:1728-1745, 2001.

Marina N, Gebhardt M, Teot L, et al. Biology and therapeutic advances for pediatric osteosarcoma. Oncologist 9:422-441, 2004.

Peabody TD, Gibbs CP, Simon MA. Current concepts review: Evaluation and staging of musculoskeletal neoplasms. J Bone Joint Surg Am 80:1204-1218, 1998.

Wittig JC, Bickels J, Priebat D, et al. Osteosarcoma: A multidisciplinary approach to diagnosis and treatment. Am Fam Physician 65:1123-1132, 2002.

52

Kevin

October 1

Dear Mom and Dad,

You're probably wondering what's happened to me. I've gotten all your text messages, but I've just been so busy. My surgery clerkship is going well, except the hours are incredibly long. It's hard finding time to spend with Kevin. Wait. I guess I haven't told you about him. Kevin Bone is an orthopedic surgery resident and a really fantastic guy. He came up to me in the cafeteria last week and out of the blue asked what was wrong with my right ankle.

Remember when I sprained my ankle last spring? It finally quit hurting, but I've been on my feet so much since beginning my clerkship that it's started to ache some. Kevin said he noticed me limping and followed me down the hall to figure out why. He described my gait as antalgic—that means pain relieving. He's so funny. He imitated my limp right there in the cafeteria. Kevin explained that to keep painful weight bearing to a minimum anyone will instinctively take quick, soft steps to shorten the stance phase of the gait on the affected side. If the pain is really bad they'll also kind of flap their arms like wings to further unweight the painful limb. I remember doing that right after I sprained my ankle when I tried to move around the apartment without my crutches. Kevin says he can even identify an antalgic gait just by listening to its rhythm: light-**heavy,** light-**heavy,** light-**heavy.**

When Kevin found out I didn't know anything about gait, he offered to meet me for lunch to explain it. Now I know that each step is divided into two phases: stance and swing.

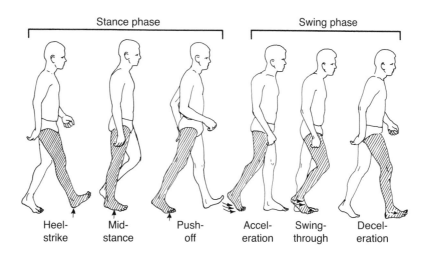

Stance phase | Swing phase

Heel-strike | Mid-stance | Push-off | Accel-eration | Swing-through | Decel-eration

Phases of gait.

During stance phase the foot is in contact with the ground and is bearing part or all of the body's weight. Stance is divided into heel-strike, midstance, and push-off. The swing phase begins when the toes leave the ground after push-off and ends when the forward swing of the limb stops at heel-strike. Swing is therefore divided into acceleration, swing-through, and deceleration. So, for instance, with every step my right foot goes like this: speed up, swing-through, slow down, heel-strike, full weight, push-off, speed up, swing-through, and so on. Kevin can say all that while walking at normal speed. He's phenomenal.

P R I N C I P L E :   To understand any complex motion, break it down to its component parts.

October 4

I was on call last night and got to hold retractors on a long case. Couldn't see much, though. It gave me time to think about what Kevin told me over dinner. Simple walking—we never give it a thought, but it's a beautiful concert of muscles and joints as far away as the shoulders. They all work together to propel us forward efficiently. Kevin explained that when we walk smoothly, we raise and lower our center of gravity very little and waste very little effort in side-to-side motions. Muscles, weak or tight, and joints, stiff or painful, can be compensated for, to an extent, by other regional joints and muscles. But when a gait abnormality occurs, the cause is usually discernible to a trained eye.

P R I N C I P L E : Take time to marvel at the normal functioning of the human body.

Analysis of pathologic changes begins with an understanding of normal structure and function.

When we were in the cafeteria the other day an elderly man shuffled in. Without staring Kevin pointed out his widely spaced feet, forward-leaning and rigid posture, very short stride length, and upper limb tremor. He even drew a sketch, which I've enclosed to let you see some of his talent.

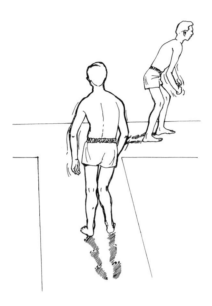

He won't tell me the diagnosis until after a movie on Saturday.

October 9

This has been even better than working in the shoe store last summer. I finally feel like I know what I want to do. It really makes studying a lot easier because I'm not just memorizing facts and wondering whether they're useful. Kevin is literally a walking encyclopedia. While waiting in line for the movie, a man limped by. Kevin said "stiff knee" before I hardly even had time to look. Then he explained: During swing-through the knee normally flexes so the foot doesn't drag on the ground. When the knee is stiff, one of three compensations is necessary.

(1) The person can tilt the pelvis up on the stiff side to lift the limb and prevent stumbling, but this makes the trunk list to the opposite side. (2) The person can rise on his toes on the good side to allow clearance of the stiff limb, but this means lifting the body's center of gravity a couple of inches with every step. (3) The person can swing the stiff leg out and around, but this also obviously requires spending more energy than usual. Kevin's sketches are enclosed.

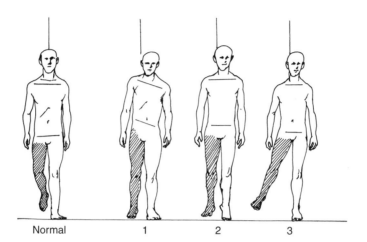

Gait alterations to compensate for a stiff right knee.

Normal   1   2   3

Then as we were walking out of the movie we saw a woman lurching from side to side. I thought she might be drunk, but we followed her at a discreet distance for over a block. Kevin called it a Trendelenburg gait related to weak gluteus medius muscles. Normally when we stand on one leg, the gluteus medius muscle on that side rotates the pelvis up to shift the weight of the trunk over the supporting limb. That's how we balance on one foot. If this important hip abductor is weak, then the weight of the trunk actually causes the pelvis to tilt downward in the opposite direction during a single-leg stance. The only way to keep from falling over is to throw the hip out to the side and shift the upper body over the weighted limb to bring the body's center of gravity back over the foot. The same thing happens when a person with dysfunctional hip abductors walks—lurching first to one side to keep from falling, then lurching back to the other. It's been called a waddling gait when both hips are affected. More sketches. Can you believe how talented Kevin is?

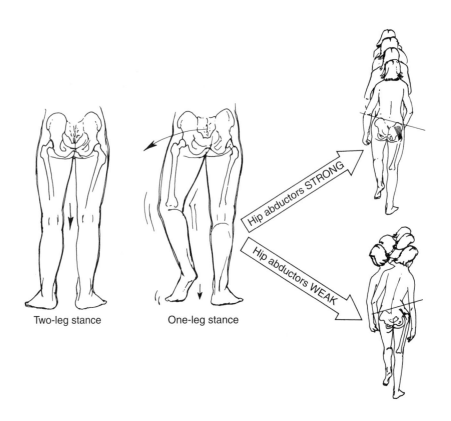

Two-leg stance   One-leg stance

Hip abductors STRONG

Hip abductors WEAK

Effect of gluteus
medius function
on gait.

Later he showed me a book with the x-rays of a person who had congenitally dislocated hips that were never treated. Because the femoral heads had ridden proximally, the hip abductors were shortened and couldn't function effectively. That may have been what was wrong with the woman at the movie. Kevin is amazing. He said he could. . . .

October 20
You see how busy I am. I can't seem to finish an e-mail. It's going to get worse now that my surgery exams are coming up. But before I go study, I want to tell you what I just discovered about Kevin. He was walking barefoot around my apartment kind of funny last night, and at first I thought he was imitating another limp. I'm pretty good at analyzing gait now, so I secretly watched him. Normally during swing-through we dorsiflex our ankle to keep our toes from dragging on the ground. Well, he wasn't dorsiflexing his ankle, so his foot dropped down with every step. He didn't drag it,

however, because he compensated by lifting it higher off the ground with more hip and knee flexion. Then the whole foot would sort of slap down at heel-strike. I'm not such a good artist, but I've sketched it for you.

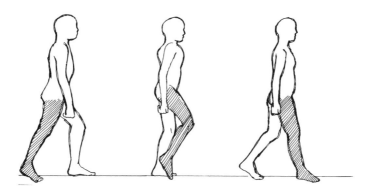

Drop-foot gait of peroneal nerve palsy.

After he left I read about it. It's called a drop-foot gait, and it's related to weakness of the ankle dorsiflexor muscles, all innervated by the peroneal nerve. Polio used to be a major cause, but peroneal nerve injury is far more common now. Poor Kevin. I'd never noticed it before because people with a peroneal nerve palsy usually wear a molded polyethylene shell (called an ankle-foot orthosis—AFO for short) inside the sock. This prevents the foot from dropping during swing-through.

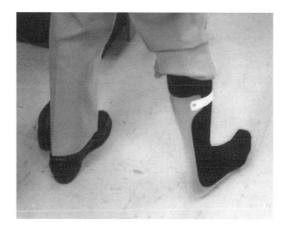

Polyethylene ankle-foot orthosis used to compensate for weak ankle dorsiflexors during swing-through.

I'm going to ask him about it tomorrow because I don't want this interfering with our relationship. Then when I bring him home with me at Thanksgiving he won't be embarrassed about it and can show all his limps to you. Do you think the neighbors would be interested? I'll give you a call after exams.

Love,
Sheri

P.S. Remember how upset I used to be about my intoeing? (Dr. Eldridge called it femoral anteversion.) Well, it must have gotten better because Kevin hasn't said anything about it, and he certainly notices such things.

FEATURES OF COMMON GAIT ABNORMALITIES:

Gait Abnormality	Characteristic Features	Causes
Antalgic gait	Stance phase shortened	Pain with weight bearing located anywhere from toes to pelvis
Trendelenburg gait (waddling gait if bilateral)	Pelvic tilt, trunk shift	Gluteus medius weakness, developmental dislocation of the hip, coxa vara, short femoral neck
Short leg limp	Head bobs up and down through gait cycle	Congenital limb length discrepancy, premature femoral/tibial physeal closure, bone loss from fracture
Stiff knee gait	Decreased knee flexion during swing phase	Intraarticular knee pathology that is painful with flexion, knee fusion, knee brace
Quadriceps avoidance gait	Knee locked in hyperextension during stance phase, difficulty with stairs	Quadriceps weakness, often seen with knee abnormality
Ataxic gait (propulsive gait)	Widely spaced feet, stooped posture, neck flexed to look at ground	Proprioceptive or neurologic disorders
Steppage gait (drop-foot gait)	Increased hip and knee flexion through swing phase to compensate for foot drop (toes pointing down)	Weakness of anterior compartment muscles of leg (TA, EDC, EHL)

EDC = Extensor digitorum communis; EHL = extensor hallucis longus; TA = tibialis anterior.

ADVANCED READING

Chambers HG, Sutherland DH. A practical guide to gait analysis. J Am Acad Orthop Surg 10:222-231, 2002.

Ducroquet R, Ducroquet J, Ducroquet P. Walking and Limping: A Study of Normal and Pathological Walking. Philadelphia: JB Lippincott, 1968.

Ounpuu S. The biomechanics of walking and running. Clin Sports Med 13:843-863, 1994.

Simon S. Gait and neuromuscular disorders. In Poss R, ed. Orthopaedic Knowledge Update III. Park Ridge, Ill: American Academy of Orthopaedic Surgeons, 1990.

Trendelenburg F. Uber den Gang bei angeborener Hilftgelenksluxation. Dtsch Med Wochenschr 21:21-24, 1895.

53

The Grinch Who Steals Cartilage

Roy A. Meals ✦ *Scott A. Mitchell*

ANCHOR: Coming to you live, **ORTHO** News brings you our exclusive, behind-the-scenes investigation that has uncovered a plot that may imperil your very own child. This scheme threatens to deprive our children of their precious articular cartilage, forcing them down a spiraling path to pain, dysfunction, deformity, and ultimately degenerative arthritis. We have now for the first time discovered the identity of the mastermind behind these devastating afflictions. He now joins us for an exclusive first-look interview.

REPORTER: I introduce to you today, reporting from a confidential, undisclosed location, a human menace well known for his past exploits, but only now revealing himself as the architect of this vast conspiracy. Tell me Grinch, you've already been forced to make restitution for your infamous holiday stealing, but now we understand that you have developed an even more diabolic and nefarious plot to thwart human happiness.

GRINCH: Yes, and you left out "insidious," too. Looking back, holiday theft was for amateurs. I was just a rookie then. Too blatant, too predictable, and yeah, I guess I got busted. But I'm wiser now—my schemes are more deceptive and better disguised. They'll never be able to pin this one on me—heh heh heh. Hip disease—it's brilliant. I do my work in childhood, but the complete crippling doesn't show up until years, maybe decades later. By then I'm long gone. Just a myth. And they hate me forever. Hip pain, limping, canes, crutches, surgery, revisions, suffering—oh the suffering! And not just for a measly holiday or two but for every day of their lives. Every time they try to get out of a chair, climb stairs, or take a step, they think of little ol' me and how I got the best of 'em. Terrible I am.

REPORTER: Can you give us your modus operandi?

GRINCH: Well, I don't like to divulge too many of my trade secrets, but just this time I think I'll boast a bit. I like to start early, so I get the hips dislocated at birth, or even before—especially with girls. I like to get the first-born too, because the family's so unsuspecting then. Capsular laxity is the key—from either genetic or hormonal influences. Also, the acetabulum may be genetically defective. Sometimes it's mechanical factors—abnormal uterine positioning or just insufficient space can do it. Oh so many places to strike—hee hee. Then when the hips are extended—especially if they're held in extension—whoopee! The femoral head slips right out of the socket. That's why breech deliveries are great. The doctor grabs those little feet and pulls—does the job for me. Now in some cultures babies are carried with their hips abducted; then my best work is stymied because that position tends to reduce the dislocation and let the capsule tighten. But in other societies the babies are wrapped and carried with their hips extended and adducted, which of course is great for me—it perpetuates the problem. All I have to do is sit back and watch.

Developmental dislocation of the hip, called DDH for short, can be diagnosed by a careful physical examination—not so easily done on those little tykes when they get crabby. And because the femoral head is not radiopaque for many months (and maybe not even for a year if it's dislocated—hee hee), the dislocation is not easily diagnosed using x-rays, and by then it may be too late. One of my favorite things is fooling high-tech doctors who do a sloppy physical and rely on x-ray studies.

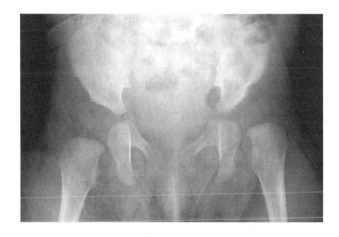

Which hip is dislocated? Because the femoral heads are not ossified at this age, radiographic diagnosis of developmental dislocation of the hip is difficult.

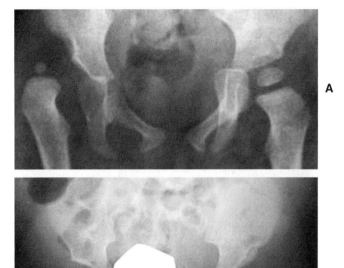

A, Developmental dislocation of the right hip. **B,** A more subtle radiographic presentation of DDH. Note the delayed ossification of the left femoral epiphysis, the lateral and superior displacement of the proximal femur, and the shallow acetabulum.

REPORTER: So what happens if you get away with it?

GRINCH: The muscles crossing the hip joint pull the femoral head upward and backward so it rests against the iliac wing. Eventually a false acetabulum develops there from the pressure of the femoral head against the pelvis. Without the growth stimulation normally provided by the femoral head, the true acetabulum remains small and flat. And the longer the head is out, the harder it is to get it back in. The muscles and soft tissues around the hip become increasingly contracted and the acetabulum gets more dysplastic.

REPORTER: Then what?

GRINCH: When the child begins to walk, her hip abductors are weak because of the shortened distance from origin to insertion. She can't stand or walk on that leg without her pelvis tilting down.

REPORTER: We call that Trendelenburg's sign.

GRINCH: Right. If one side is affected, she limps. If both sides are dislocated, she walks like a drunken duck—lurching from side to side to keep her trunk balanced over her weak hips. I think I've heard you guys call it a waddling gait.

REPORTER: What else?

GRINCH: The longer the hip stays dislocated, the less likely it will ever be normal. If neglected into adulthood, the cartilage finally erodes away and the pain gets worse.

And even if the docs do get the hip back in place, the acetabulum might not develop normally, leaving a large portion of the femoral head uncovered. This accelerates wear on the areas remaining in contact and can still cause painful arthritis down the road. See, here's a good example. Oh, what's in store for this one.

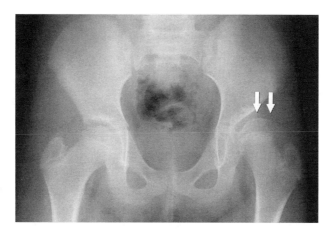

Acetabular dysplasia. Note the incomplete coverage of the femoral head on the *left*, indicated by the region between the *two arrows*.

REPORTER: So what's your biggest concern about DDH?

GRINCH: That it's diagnosed and treated early. If DDH is picked up in infancy and treated properly, the hip can develop entirely normally, no surgery required. But if care is delayed just 18 months, even prolonged traction and abduction splinting may not achieve a closed reduction and may even cause avascular necrosis of the femoral head due to the excessive pressure. Then the real fun starts with palliative treatment: open reductions, corrective osteotomies of the pelvis or femur, total joint replacements—all possibly complicated by avascular necrosis, redislocation, fracture, and nerve paralysis. Agonizing for the patient and frustrating for the doctor, especially if he or she's the one who missed the diagnosis early on.

REPORTER: Well, how can we diagnose it early?

GRINCH: I'd rather not go into that.

REPORTER: Uh . . . uh . . . OK.

GRINCH: Instead, let me tell you how I get young boys. My ancestors have known about this disease for centuries, but because three humans, Legg, Calvé, and Perthes, independently described it in 1910, their names are attached. You also call it coxa plana—in other words, flat hip. Nobody has to be a rocket scientist to see that a flat femoral head won't work in a round socket—ha ha. Boys, 4 to 10, are my favorite. Once again a nice, slow, insidious onset. A little pain, increasing with activity, decreasing with rest, maybe a history of trauma, but humans that age are always getting bumped. The neat thing is that the pain is usually felt at the knee, and unsuspecting clinicians can go down in flames focusing their attention there. There's just nothing like that feeling of bamboozling all those overeducated doctors.

PRINCIPLE: Hip disease may be the source of symptoms for patients, especially children, complaining of knee pain.

REPORTER: What might a perceptive doctor find?

GRINCH: An antalgic gait pattern and limited hip motion, especially in abduction and internal rotation.

REPORTER: So what happens to flatten the femoral head?

GRINCH: Avascular necrosis. Even I'm not sure of the exact mechanism. It's possible that a synovitis increases intraarticular pressure, or maybe there's an initial venous obstruction, either of which can create a tamponade off the vessels supplying the femoral head. Then part or all of the femoral head dies. Over a matter of months, the necrotic bone softens as revascularization occurs, but the overlying cartilage keeps the femoral head round.

REPORTER: I thought you said "flat hip."

GRINCH: I'm getting to that. Capillaries and osteoblasts gradually creep in from the margins to revitalize the femoral head, and the dead bone is slowly resorbed. These cellular changes lead to a temporary weakening of the subchondral bone and a fragmented appearance of the femoral head on x-rays.

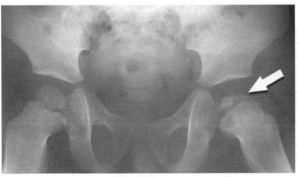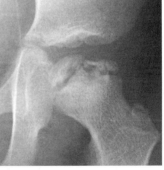

A   B

Legg-Calvé-Perthes disease. **A,** Disruption of the blood supply to the immature femoral head leads to sclerosis and fragmentation. **B,** Flattening and distortion of both the femoral head and the acetabulum can follow.

If the head is not completely protected within the acetabulum during this time, a pathologic fracture through the weakened bone allows a gradual distortion of its spherical shape. Eventually the femoral head flattens out. Then, even though normal bone trabeculae eventually reform and circulation redevelops, the damage is done. The misshapen head alters the development of the acetabulum secondarily, and degenerative arthritis is inevitable. Which reminds me, I've got work to do.

REPORTER: Wait, Grinch. You said you had three ways to cripple hips.

GRINCH: Oh yes, I nearly forgot: Slipped capital femoral epiphysis. Here again, I prefer boys, but this time I strike a bit later, ages 10 to 14; many are obese, and some may have subtle endocrine changes as causative factors, but others may have normal builds. The physeal junction between the femoral head and neck weakens; and as a result of weight-bearing forces and muscle pull the femoral head slips down and back—sort of like a scoop of ice cream sliding off the cone. Nice and quiet; you know?

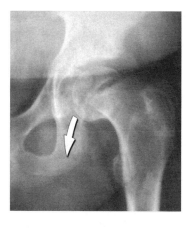

Slipped capital femoral epiphysis of the left hip. The femoral head slips inferiorly *(arrow)*.

Left undisturbed, the femoral head heals to the neck in this abnormal position, and joint incongruity leads to eventual osteoarthritis.

REPORTER: What will the patient and the doctor notice when the slip first occurs?

GRINCH: Limping. And knee pain—hee hee—sometimes for many months. Because the femoral head is slipping down and behind its normal location, hip adduction and external rotation movements are accentuated because those motions bring the femoral head into its normal relationship with the acetabulum. Flexion, abduction, and internal rotation are restricted for the same reason. A lateral x-ray will show even a subtle slip, but if the doctor doesn't know that, I win.

REPORTER: It must be like a fracture. Can't it just be put back in place?

GRINCH: That's the beauty of it—I win again. Misdirected efforts at reduction by forceful manipulation or surgery spoil the blood supply to the femoral head, making a bad situation impossible—avascular necrosis and collapse, you know. Sometimes a relatively recent slip can be partially corrected by skeletal traction with an internally rotating force, followed perhaps by gentle manipulation. But whether or not any reduction can be achieved, the epiphysis has to be secured on the femoral neck to prevent further displacement. This usually involves placing one or more steel pins up the neck of the femur and into the head. And if the pins are placed incorrectly they can damage the joint cartilage or disrupt the head's blood supply, and I guess you know what those injuries mean.

REPORTER: I'm afraid I do. What other diabolic features are present?

GRINCH: Hmm, I like the way you think. First, while everybody's attention is focused on one hip, the femoral head on the other side might just slip right off too. And second, some impatient surgeons have tried an immediate osteotomy of the femoral neck to correct the head-neck relationship, but that too may cause avascular necrosis. So any severe slip should be pinned in situ, with a corrective osteotomy planned later when the head is securely healed to the neck. Of course, the osteotomy is a complex, three-dimensional reconstruction and full of pitfalls. But I've raised your anxiety levels enough for 1 day, and I must be getting back to work. Lots of nice healthy cartilage out there just waiting for me. Tallyho.

REPORTER: I think that just about says it all. Back to you, Jane.

ANCHOR: Wow, you sure *are* a mean one, Mr. Grinch. We have just witnessed an incredible interview with one of the world's all-time scumbags. Here with me now in the studio are three experts on pediatric hip conditions to comment on the Grinch's conniving. Dr. Eldridge, as a noted pediatrician and self-appointed chief Grinch buster, what advice can you give to our audience regarding developmental dislocation of the hip?

DR. ELDRIDGE: Unfortunately, Jane, everything the Grinch said is true. Hip dislocation is one of the most common developmental deformities. Six girls are affected for every boy. One third of the cases are bilateral. Unless dislocation of the hip is specifically sought in infancy, the condition may not be recognized until the child walks. Walking may be delayed, and then it may be too late for the development of a normal hip even with prompt and thorough treatment. So early diagnosis is critical.

ANCHOR: Dr. Barlow, some years ago you described a maneuver to identify dislocation or subluxation of a hip in infancy. Can you demonstrate it on this doll?

DR. BARLOW: Sure. The examiner supports and steadies the pelvis with one hand—thumb in front, fingers in back. With the infant's hip flexed 90 degrees, the examiner's other hand alternately pushes the proximal femur posteriorly and pulls it anteriorly.

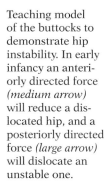

Teaching model of the buttocks to demonstrate hip instability. In early infancy an anteriorly directed force *(medium arrow)* will reduce a dislocated hip, and a posteriorly directed force *(large arrow)* will dislocate an unstable one.

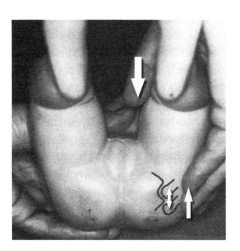

When applying anterior pressure with the fingers, the dislocated femoral head may be felt and even heard to clunk back into the acetabulum; with posteriorly directed pressure from the thumb an unstable joint will dislocate. This can be misleading in older infants, however—a point that I think even the Grinch forgot to make. As the muscles and capsular structures contract, the hip may simply be out and stay out. This absence of instability can deceive even me sometimes. If this is the case and it is unilateral, shortening of the limb may be noted when the hips are flexed and the knees are brought together. But even if it's bilateral, each affected hip will have a limited range of abduction in flexion.

ANCHOR: Dr. Eldridge, that all sounds good, but somewhat subjective. Can't you just perform an x-ray examination?

DR. ELDRIDGE: The bones around the newborn's hip are insufficiently calcified to show up on x-rays. At about a year of age or so, the femoral heads should be sufficiently ossified to cast an x-ray shadow, but even then the images can be difficult to interpret. And let's not forget that it's getting pretty late in the game by 1 year of age. The earlier appropriate treatment is begun, the better. Ultrasound and magnetic resonance imaging, on the other hand, do not rely on the ossification of these structures and show promise for improved imaging in equivocal cases.

ANCHOR: Tell us, Dr. Stanford, what treatment do you recommend?

DR. STANFORD: Well you can see that many hips thought to be unstable in the newborn nursery will tighten up on their own in a couple of weeks using gentle positioning in flexion and abduction. The easiest way to do that in these little tykes is to keep them in double diapers. But this should only be used as a temporary measure until they can be examined in the office within a couple of weeks. For hips that remain unstable, protection in moderate abduction for 3 months is recommended. This is best achieved using the so-called Pavlik harness, which keeps the hips in a position of moderate flexion and abduction while not completely immobilizing them as a spica cast would. It also allows mom and dad to change the little one's diapers without too much difficulty, and it can even be removed briefly for bathing once a day. Now these little ones need to be followed for up to a year of age or more to make sure that the femoral head remains properly located and that the acetabulum is developing appropriately.

ANCHOR: As Grinch alluded, late diagnosis and treatment are fraught with difficulties. I'm sure there's much more the three of you could say about developmental dislocation of the hip, but before we take a station break, I want to ask Dr. Stanford how he treats Perthes' disease in his own orthopedic practice.

DR. STANFORD: I'm sure the subtleties are well beyond the grasp of the typical layperson, but I'll do my best to simplify things for you. There's really no universally satisfactory treatment method, and I tell all of my patients and families that this will never be a truly normal hip, even in the best of circumstances. Now back in my day we used to place these boys on bed rest for as long as 2 years to reduce deforming forces on the softened femoral head, but trying to keep a 7-year-old boy in bed is like trying to keep a cobra in a paper bag. Not only that, but the forces on the hip joint from the muscles themselves, regardless of weight bearing, are sufficient to deform the softened head. The buzz words for current therapy are motion and containment. The acetabulum serves as a mold to hold the femoral head's spherical shape. Therefore if only a portion of the head is affected and the entire head is contained within the acetabulum, a few weeks of rest will usually allow the inflammation to subside enough to recover full range of motion. For more extensive involvement without complete containment, abduction splinting has given way to corrective osteotomy of either the pelvis or femur to bring the involved regions of the femoral head under the protective roof of the acetabulum.

ANCHOR: Dr. Barlow, in the 30 seconds we have left can you summarize what we've heard?

DR. BARLOW: Sure. Three conditions, occurring at different times in childhood and at slightly different locations, can all result in significant and permanent disability.

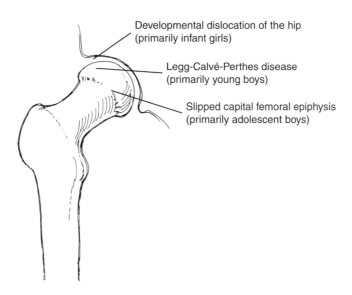

Pediatric hip conditions.

Their presentations may be subtle, but if identified and treated early; the damage can be minimized. We'll get you yet, Grinch.

ANCHOR: Thank you, Doctors, for being with us today. We'll be right back after these words from our sponsors.

ADVANCED READING

Dobbs MB, Weinstein SL. Natural history and long-term outcomes of slipped capital femoral epiphysis. Instr Course Lect 50:571-575, 2001.

Dr. Seuss. How the Grinch Stole Christmas. New York: Random House, 1957.

Harcke T, Kumar SJ. Current concepts review. The role of ultrasound in the diagnosis and management of congenital dislocation and dysplasia of the hip. J Bone Joint Surg Am 73:622-628, 1991.

Herring JA, Kim HT, Browne R. Legg-Calvé-Perthes disease. Part II: Prospective multicenter study on the effect of treatment on outcome. J Bone Joint Surg Am 86:2121-2134, 2004.

Hoppenfeld S. Physical Examination of the Spine and Extremities. New York: Appleton-Century-Crofts, 1976.

Legg AT. An obscure affection of the hip joint. Boston Med Surg J 162:202, 1910.

Loder RT, Aronsson DD, Dobbs MB, et al. Slipped capital femoral epiphysis. Instr Course Lect 50:555-570, 2001.

Thompson GH, Price CT, Roy D, et al. Legg-Calvé-Perthes disease: Current concepts. Instr Course Lect 51:367-384, 2002.

Weinstein SL, Mubarak SJ, Wenger DR. Developmental hip dysplasia and dislocation: Parts I and II. Instr Course Lect 53:523-542, 2004.

Uglow MG, Clarke NM. The management of slipped capital femoral epiphysis. J Bone Joint Surg Br 86:631-635, 2004.

◆ *What two tissues in the body have no blood supply and survive by diffusion of nutrients from adjacent fluid-filled cavities?*

54

A Leg to Stand On

Robert Eric Carlson ✦ *Scott A. Mitchell* ✦ *Roy A. Meals*

"Welcome to the oral portion of your surgery finals, Ms. Hyzer—Sheri, is it? I'm Dr. Jeffrey. Have you had an oral examination before?"

"Not in medical school."

"Very well. What orthopedic conditions did you encounter on your rotation?"

"Oh, various things. Carpal tunnel syndrome, rotator cuff tears, hip fractures, bunions, osteoarthritis, and a few other things that seem to have escaped me at the moment. Gait analysis fascinates me."

"Huh, how appropriate. Look at this x-ray and tell me what you think is going on. It's a 60-year-old man with knee pain who can't walk more than two blocks."

"Before I assess the x-ray, I'd like to get some history and do an examination. I mean, has he had any injuries? How long has he had this pain? What kind of pain does he have, and when does he have it—there might not be anything wrong with his knee at all. It could be neurogenic or vascular claudication, you know. Are any other joints involved? And what's his knee motion like? Is there any tenderness, effusion, malalignment, or instability?"

PRINCIPLE: Interpret radiographic data only in the context of a patient's history and physical examination.

"Humpf. No acute injury. He's worked all his life as a letter carrier. Good general health. Findings from back, hip, and neurovascular exams are normal. Knee motion is full, no effusion."

"Then judging from the x-ray, he's probably tender along the lateral and possibly the medial joint lines, and it looks like he has a valgus deformity—knock-kneed, you know. Based on what little information I have, I think he's got primary osteoarthritis."

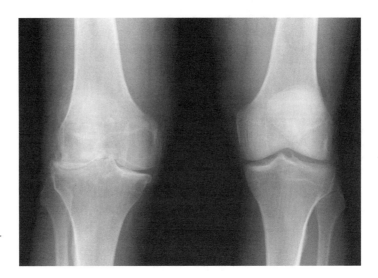

Pronounced joint space narrowing in the lateral compartment of the right knee.

"Osteoarthritis. Tell me about that."

"Well, as common as the disorder is, and as extensively as it's been studied, the etiology of osteoarthritis, or OA, remains unclear. It's a form of noninflammatory arthritis, as opposed to, say, rheumatoid arthritis, which is a characteristic inflammatory arthritis. OA has traditionally been thought of as simply a wear-and-tear phenomenon in which cartilage is gradually worn away. However, it now seems that the degeneration stems from a combination of both mechanical and biochemical processes. The degeneration begins primarily within the articular cartilage itself, though it is still debatable whether the cause is excessive stress on normal tissue or an inadequate chondrocyte response to normal forces. Either way, it appears that there is a net imbalance between the synthesis and breakdown of the cartilage matrix—in effect it's a failed attempt of chondrocytes to repair and maintain their biochemical environment. The combination of enzymatic matrix destruction and decreased proteoglycan and collagen synthesis renders the cartilage less resistant to external forces, which in turn further disrupts the cartilage matrix and accelerates the catabolic process. This ultimately leads to the softening, fibrillation, and erosion of the articular cartilage as the disease progresses.

"Osteoarthritis has been categorized as either primary or secondary, though there do not seem to be clear differences in the degenerative processes between these types. It's primary when there's no discernible cause. Obviously, if the mechanics of the joint have been altered by trauma, loose bodies, ligamentous instability, congenital malformation, or systemic disease, then the arthritis is considered secondary."

"What kind of systemic diseases?"

"Things like hemophilia, growth hormone disorders, or metabolic disorders that alter the health of the cartilage."

"What findings would you expect in this man when conducting a more-detailed history and physical?"

"Several points. Primary osteoarthritis is typically not seen before late middle age; age alone is not causative, but it may reduce the tissues' capacity for repair. Pain that worsens with activity progresses insidiously over many months or years. Unlike the inflammatory types of arthritis, the osteoarthritic joint is usually neither warm nor swollen, although it can at times develop quite an effusion during flare-ups, and morning stiffness is less prominent. When the cartilage erosion is severe enough, a grinding referred to as crepitus may be felt and even heard during joint motion."

"How would you describe his x-ray?"

"Classic for OA: Joint space narrowing, subchondral bone sclerosis, and marginal osteophyte formation. The osteophytes are a little hard to see in this film, but your Heberden's nodes are fine examples."

"Let's stay focused on knees. What treatment would you offer this postman . . . er, uh, letter carrier?"

"Thank you. Well, as with most orthopedic conditions, I'd take it in steps. First, advice and assurance. Many patients seek medical help not because they're particularly disabled, but they're concerned about having some horrible disease or that ignoring their early symptoms will lead to disaster. In these cases education alone often suffices. If he's obese, maybe get him to lose some weight."

"He's already skinny. What now?"

"Then I'd try conservative measures such as physical therapy. I'd also suggest using a cane and taking nonsteroidal antiinflammatory medication. If possible, I would see whether he could change to a more sedentary job. If ligament instability is contributory, I'd get him a brace. At some point I'd begin to consider an injection, either a corticosteroid or one of the hyaluronic acid derivatives. Though evidence is lacking that either of these truly alters disease progression, they can make some patients more comfortable for 6 months or even a year."

"He's tried all that. Now what?"

"Surgery. Osteotomy, arthroplasty, or arthrodesis. A realignment osteotomy corrects a varus or valgus deformity of the knee, unloading the degenerating compartment and transferring weight-bearing forces to the unaffected side of the joint. For him a closing wedge osteotomy of the distal femur would improve the valgus alignment, though it looks like he's already got some degenerative changes on the medial side as well. So, for that reason, it's probably a bit too late for either an osteotomy or a unicompartmental arthroplasty. As far as his alternatives go . . . wait, how tall is this fellow?"

"Why do you ask?"

"A tall person with a knee fusion has difficulty sitting in airplane and theater seats. A total joint arthroplasty is more functional but may require revision sooner or later because of implant loosening, infection, or persistent pain. An arthrodesis, on the other hand, is very durable. However, an arthrodesis might not be indicated if he's got disease elsewhere, particularly the ipsilateral hip or ankle. After a fusion, forces would be redistributed to the joints above and below, and in that case may hasten their deterioration. All things considered, total knee arthroplasty has a remarkably high success rate, even at 10 to 15 years of follow-up, and would be my recommendation for this patient."

P R I N C I P L E :   Don't fuse joints in patients with polyarticular disease.

"Fine. We must be moving along. Here's another patient, about the same age, in the ER having just been struck by a car while crossing the street. For the sake of time, his only injury is at his knee. What are your concerns?"

"Possible fracture, ligamentous injury, neurovascular damage. This scenario of car versus pedestrian is classic for producing tibial plateau fractures—bumper fractures."

"What's its mechanism of injury?"

"Either from a motor vehicle accident or a fall, the knee is forced into valgus angulation. In younger people the ligaments tear. In older people the lateral plateau of the tibia collapses. It depends on the relative strengths of the tissues, and these strengths are age related. First, I'd check his feet for sensation, motor control, and circulation. I'd also feel his calf for tightness suggestive of compartment syndrome. Then I'd look for ecchymosis, swelling, and tenderness around his knee. I'd get an x-ray before I tested his knee motion and ligament stability."

"So here it is. What do you see?"

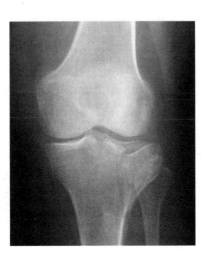

Depression fracture of the lateral portion of the tibial plateau.

"He has a depressed, lateral tibial plateau fracture. Though it's fairly obvious in this case, sometimes it's tough to estimate the degree of joint surface incongruity caused by these fractures, so a CT scan with specially reconstructed images can be helpful. But even with advanced imaging techniques, unseen ligamentous injury may also be present, so I'd want to check his joint stability—under anesthesia, of course. Both of these factors—the degree of articular step-off and any evidence of instability—along with the patient's age and physical demands, would help determine the best treatment strategy."

Coronal **(A)** and sagittal **(B)** CT reconstructed views showing the degree of articular step-off.

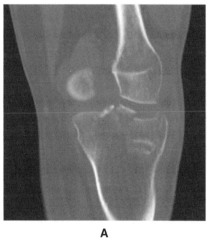
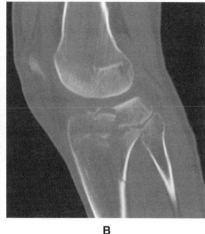

A   **B**

"What's the goal of treatment?"

"A well-aligned, stable, movable, pain-free joint."

"How do you achieve that?"

"The trick is to obtain and maintain a congruous joint surface without prolonged immobilization. Early motion is critical to cartilage nourishment and to prevent debilitating posttraumatic knee stiffness. Unfortunately, early motion also risks fracture displacement."

"What are your treatment alternatives?"

"First, I'd have to consider the patient's age, general health, and activity level, plus the fracture pattern, any associated injuries, and the surgeon's skill. For older patients who don't make great demands on their knees, some joint surface depression can be accepted providing the collateral ligaments are stable. For these patients early motion and protected weight bearing in a hinged-knee brace usually suffice. For younger, more active individuals, particularly those with major ligamentous instability, open reduction and internal fixation of the fracture and ligament repair are best."

"How important is anatomic alignment of the joint surface?"

"Fracture malalignment creates an incongruent joint surface, resulting in unequal distribution of weight-bearing forces across the joint. In effect there is decreased surface area available to transfer forces, leading to a concentration of stress across the regions that remain in contact. This ultimately leads to accelerated degenerative changes—secondary osteoarthritis, you know."

PRINCIPLE: Intraarticular fractures in weight-bearing joints should be reduced anatomically.

"Even the best surgeon can't always get things back together perfectly. Are these people doomed to eventual osteoarthritis?"

"Well, in the long term, probably, but not necessarily right away. Even though cartilage has a very limited healing capacity, the body does manage to fill in any gaps or depressions with fibrocartilage. As its name implies, this tissue has some of the elastic and shock-absorbing properties of cartilage, though it's certainly not as durable. A patient can have excellent functional results even with less than optimal x-ray findings.

"Uh, Dr. Jeffrey, there's another student at the door. I think our time is up."

"So it is, Ms. Hyzer. Your knowledge and poise are commendable. Quite impressive for your first oral examination."

"This is my first one in medical school. I had to defend my thesis in graduate school, of course."

"Oh. What was your subject?"

"Cartilage mechanics."

ADVANCED READING

Carter DR, Beaupre GS, Wong M, et al. The mechanobiology of articular cartilage development and degeneration. Clin Orthop Relat Res 427:67-77, 2004.

Cole BJ, Harner CD. Degenerative arthritis of the knee in active patients: Evaluation and management. J Am Acad Orthop Surg 7:389-402, 1999.

Coventry MB. Current concepts review. Upper tibial osteotomy for osteoarthritis. J Bone Joint Surg Am 67:1136-1140, 1985.

Delamarter R, Hohl M. The cast brace and tibial plateau fractures. Clin Orthop Relat Res 242:26-31, 1989.

Guyton JL. Arthroplasty of the ankle and knee. In Canale ST, ed. Campbell's Operative Orthopaedics, 9th ed. St Louis: Mosby, 1998, pp 232-295.

Hutchinson CR, Cho B, Wong N, et al. Proximal valgus tibial osteotomy for osteoarthritis of the knee. Instr Course Lect 48:131-134, 1999.

Meek RM, Masri BA, Duncan CP. Minimally invasive unicompartmental knee replacement: Rationale and correct indications. Orthop Clin North Am 35:191-200, 2004.

Mills WJ, Nork SE. Open reduction and internal fixation of high-energy tibial plateau fractures. Orthop Clin North Am 33:177-198, 2002.

Stevens DG, Beharry R, McKee MD, et al. The long-term functional outcome of operatively treated tibial plateau fractures. J Orthop Trauma 15:312-320, 2001.

◆ *In what century were plaster-impregnated cotton bandages first used for fracture immobilization?*

55

Mortality and Immortality

The disease is one of the most interesting and at the same time most sad of all those with which we have to deal: interesting on account of its peculiar features and mysterious nature; sad on account of our powerlessness to influence its course. . . . It is a disease of early life and of early growth. Manifesting itself commonly at the transition from infancy to childhood, it develops with the child's development, grows with his growth—so that every increase in stature means an increase in weakness, and each year takes him a step further on the road to a helpless infirmity, and in most cases to an early and inevitable death.

Thus began William Gowers' 1879 monograph. Then 34 years old, he had lived in London his entire life and had excelled at medical school. He would eventually become professor of medicine at University College. Gowers introduced into medical parlance terms such as "knee jerk" and "fibrositis," and outside the field of medicine he was a noted artist and an authority on mosses. His 1879 monograph detailed the clinical features of a recently delineated disease and gained him medical immortality through his description of the maneuver illustrated on the next page. Individuals with weak hip and knee extensors use it when rising from recumbency, and it is now widely known as Gowers' sign. When getting up, these persons perform the following movements:

. . . first [they] put the hands on the ground (1), then stretch out the legs behind them far apart, the chief weight of the trunk resting on the hands. By keeping the toes on the ground and pushing the body backwards, they manage to get the knees extended so that the trunk is supported by the hands and feet, all placed as widely apart as possible (2). Next the hands are moved alternately along the ground backwards so as to bring a larger portion of the weight of the trunk over the legs. Then one hand is placed upon the knee (3), and a push with this and with the other hand on the ground is sufficient to enable the extensors of the hip to bring the trunk into the upright posture.

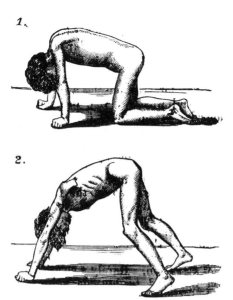

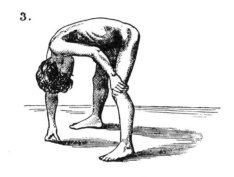

From Gowers WR. Clinical lectures on pseudohypertrophic muscular paralysis. Lancet 2:74, 1879.

Gowers emphasized that this was a disease of muscle rather than nerve. He also observed that a woman could have affected sons by different fathers, but that there were no instances in which the disease affected members of the fathers' families. He concluded that the mode of inheritance was the same as with hemophilia, though it would be another quarter century before the genetic mechanisms behind X-linked recessive disorders were well understood.

Although the unusual method of standing carries Gowers' eponym, the disease in its most common form carries the eponym of a Frenchman whose writings preceded those of Gowers by several years. Guillaume Duchenne spent his professional career in Paris making significant contributions to the understanding of neuromuscular diseases, although he did not have an official hospital or academic appointment. His obituary, published in *Lancet* in 1875, included the following observations:

His features were familiar to all who visited habitually the wards of the Paris hospitals. Every morning Duchenne was to be seen in one or other of the hospitals, studying cases, examining specimens, drawing his photographs of microscopic appearances, in which he was extraordinarily skillful. For a long time Duchenne's invariable presence in the wards, his incessant moving about, his ardent interrogation of patients, caused him to be looked upon with a somewhat suspicious and anxious eye by many hospital physicians. But his consummate experience of disease, his wonderful keenness and ability in making out a diagnosis in cases of paralysis, the sincerity and earnestness of his manner, the honesty of his proceedings, the authority which he gained by the publication of his original researches, the services which he rendered daily in the wards of the hospitals, brought him the esteem and appreciation of all, and made him a welcome guest everywhere.

Through the observations of Duchenne, Gowers, Erb, and others, we have a clear picture of the disease's clinical course. Although it is one of the most serious and common genetic disorders, the onset is insidious. Early symptoms may be recognized only in retrospect: developing head control, sitting unsupported, crawling, and walking are all delayed. Abnormal locomotion—toe walking or a wide-based waddling gait—may finally bring the boy to medical attention. The child stands with shoulders back, abdomen protruding, and marked lumbar lordosis. Frequent falls without noticeable tripping or stumbling are also common. The child then begins to have difficulty getting up and begins to manifest the Gowers' sign when rising. The calves and other muscle groups are paradoxically enlarged, but this is pseudohypertrophy caused by an accumulation of fat in the deteriorating muscles.

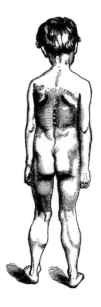

From Gowers WR. Clinical lectures on pseudohypertrophic muscular paralysis. Lancet 2:2, 1879.

Serum creatine phosphokinase levels may reach 50 to 100 times normal and then gradually decline as muscle mass diminishes. Electromyography shows a myopathic pattern, and muscle biopsy shows fiber size variation, degenerative and regenerative fibers, and fibrous tissue deposition.

The proximal muscles are the most severely weakened. Ineffective hip abduction (gluteus medius) accounts for the waddling Trendelenburg gait. Weakened hip extension (gluteus maximus) and knee extension (quadriceps) account for difficulties in stair climbing and rising from recumbency. The intercostal and cardiac muscles eventually become weak, which, combined with the scoliosis that often progresses rapidly after patients become wheelchair-bound, classically predispose the affected person to cardiorespiratory complications and death before age 20. With assisted mechanical ventilation, patients can now live much longer despite profound, diffuse muscle wasting.

Although little yet can prevent the progressive weakness, several things can be done orthopedically to keep these patients functioning as long as possible. Joint contractures develop when one muscle group is weaker than its antagonists. By this mechanism the ankle is susceptible to plantar flexion deformity, which accounts for toe walking that may be observed early on. Passive stretching exercises and corrective orthoses prolong the duration of the child's ability to walk and stand. This is important because once he is restricted to a wheelchair, scoliosis progresses rapidly along with hip and knee flexion contractures. The flexion contractures limit whatever limb movements remain and make dressing difficult. The thoracic deformities compound respiratory problems brought on by weak intercostal muscles.

P R I N C I P L E :   Orthopedics generally deals with quality of life issues rather than life-threatening issues.

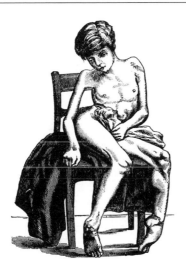

From Gowers WR. Clinical lectures on pseudo-hypertrophic muscular paralysis. Lancet 2:37, 1879.

Lightweight, long-leg splints facilitate standing when antigravity muscles at the knees are weak. Addition of a pelvic band and hip hinges to the orthoses compensates for weak hip extensors. Heel cord tenotomy may be required to maintain the foot in a plantigrade position. Unlike patients with typical adolescent idiopathic scoliosis, spinal fusion is advocated for patients with muscular dystrophies at the first signs of curve progression to maintain the skeletal structure required for pulmonary function. The considerable risks of surgery, however, must be weighed carefully against the anticipated benefits.

If you have read this far, you deserve to have your suspicion confirmed. This is muscular dystrophy in its common form. Numerous other forms have been recognized, varying by their pattern and severity of muscle involvement, age of onset, and mode of inheritance. Both Duchenne and Becker types of muscular dystrophy share a common mutant gene located on the X chromosome that codes for the protein dystrophin. The dystrophin gene product is a large cytoskeletal protein widely distributed throughout skeletal muscle as well as cardiac and smooth muscle. Duchenne type muscular dystrophy is caused by a variety of mutations that inactivate or produce nonfunctional forms of the dystrophin protein, whereas the less-severe Becker type results from mutations that produce less-active but still functional forms. Eponymic immortality awaits other industrious investigators as the search for a cure for these molecular defects continues.

ADVANCED READING

Biggar WD, Klamut HJ, Demacio PC, et al. Duchenne muscular dystrophy: Current knowledge, treatment, and future prospects. Clin Orthop Relat Res 401:88-106, 2002.

Bogdanovich S, Perkins KJ, Krag TO, et al. Therapeutics for Duchenne muscular dystrophy: Current approaches and future direction. J Mol Med 82: 102-115, 2004.

Dressna J. Neuromuscular disorders. In Lovell and Winter's Pediatric Orthopaedics, 5th ed. Philadelphia: Lippincott, 2000.

Gowers WR. Clinical lectures on pseudo-hypertrophic muscular paralysis. Lancet 2:1-2, 37-39, 73-75, 113-116, 1879.

Sussman M. Duchenne muscular dystrophy. J Am Acad Orthop Surg 10:138-151, 2002.

◆ *With what orthopedic disease, against which we are now immunized, was Franklin D. Roosevelt afflicted?*

56

Nursery School

"Dr. Bone, there's a baby in the newborn nursery they've asked you to see. Something's wrong with his hands. I've already talked to his parents."

"Webs, extras, or something really rare?"

"Webb? No, the family's name is Green—not that rare."

"Black or white?"

"No, Green. Baby Boy Green."

"You're not getting my drift. I was just trying to guess what young Green has before we see him. Let's go. Have you talked to his mother?"

"Yes. She's 28, so's the father. Both totally healthy and no family history of congenital anomalies. This is her first pregnancy. No problems really, a little first-trimester nausea, but she didn't take anything for it. No tobacco, alcohol, or other drugs. They actually live about a block from me. City water supply; no toxic dumps nearby. The boy's full term; labor and delivery uneventful, Apgar score of 9 at 1 minute. They're waiting to see us so they can go home."

"That's a good history. As you may know, some anomalies like cleft hand and Apert's syndrome are inherited, and others result from some insult during development, although we rarely can identify the exact cause."

"Thanks. Here he is."

"OK, you examine him and tell me what you find."

"Dr. Bone, you were right. Webs between his middle and ring fingers. What do you call this?"

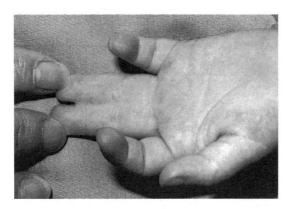

Syndactyly most commonly affects the cleft between the middle and ring fingers.

"I call it webbed digits, but doctors often resort to Greek to sound highfalutin. *Syn-* means 'together,' like synchronize, syncopate, syndrome, synthesis, s . . ."

"I remember. Syndactyly—together digits. How unusual!"

"Not in ducks. And it's actually the most common congenital anomaly seen by hand surgeons. Roughly one person in 2000 is affected. How do you suppose it happens?"

"Well, I'm amazed that anyone turns out right considering we start from one microscopic cell. But from what I remember, limb formation occurs between about the fourth and eighth weeks of gestation. It all starts as a swelling—the apical ectodermal ridge—that stimulates the longitudinal growth of the primitive limb. Initially, the hand itself looks like a little paddle."

"That's right. In the seventh week of development the webs between the five digital rays in the paddle normally recede, and presto, digits. Nobody knows why the web recession occasionally doesn't occur, but syndactyly is most common between the middle and ring fingers. What else do you find with this boy?"

"He looks fine to me. Just the syndactyly."

"Shame on you. We're supposed to be musculoskeletal system experts. You haven't even taken off his shirt and diaper. Think about all the amazing differentiation that is occurring during that 7th week when some minor insult keeps the webs from receding. It's embarrassing to have the pediatrician or the mother tell me about absent forearm rotation, an absent pectoral muscle, or extra toes. I will, however, leave internal possibilities such as cardiac septal defects to the pediatrician's expertise. Radial clubhand, for instance, has quite a list of organ anomalies that can accompany it. See, look at his toes. Simple, incomplete syndactyly between the second and third digits. This is so common, though, it's hardly an anomaly."

PRINCIPLE: When a child has one congenital anomaly, there's a high likelihood that others are present.

"I see why you call it incomplete because the web doesn't extend out to the tips like in the fingers, but why do you call it simple?"

"Good question. *Simple* means that it's only the soft tissues—skin and maybe nerves and arteries—that are shared. Complex means the phalanges are also joined, making for a much more difficult reconstruction."

"So when do you separate these? I can see that technically it would be quite difficult in a newborn. And of course there would be considerable anesthetic risk by operating before the pediatrician could be certain that the kidneys and other internal organs were OK. But wouldn't leaving them untreated affect the development of the digits as well as the child's manual dexterity?"

"You make good points. That's why we normally wait until the child is about 2 years old. Then it's technically easier to sew in the requisite skin grafts and safer for both the child and for his digital nerves, which also may have to be separated. The only reason to start earlier is when a shorter digit such as the thumb is tethering the adjacent one and forcing it to grow crooked. Both sides can be done on the same day. You probably have some more questions, but young Green is crying so loud I can hardly think. See if you can get his diaper on. I'll go explain all this to his mom, and I'll meet you in my office later to show you photographs of some other types of syndactyly."

PRINCIPLE: Elective bilateral upper limb surgery is appropriate for totally dependent individuals; otherwise the procedures should be staged so that one hand will be free to perform self-care activities.

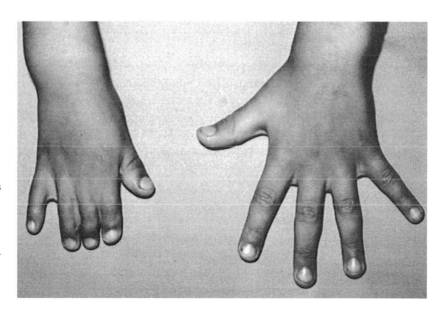

Simple, incomplete syndactyly affecting all four digital clefts along with hypoplasia of the hand. This form of syndactyly is usually associated with partial absence of the pectoralis major muscle.

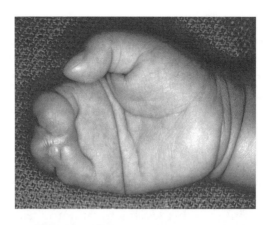

In this type of syndactyly the digits and clefts form normally, but then an amniotic band causes an injury that heals with distal webbing.

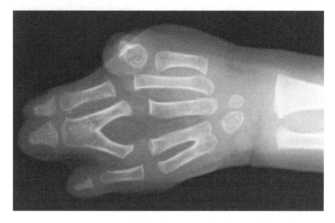

Complex syndactyly between the phalanges of the middle and ring fingers and between the metacarpals of the small and ring fingers.

One Week Later

"Hi, Dr. Bone. Welcome back from your trip. Do you have time to see another patient in the newborn nursery? This one has 11 fingers."

"Sure, but let me finish my coffee. How about it—black or white?"

"No thanks, I don't drink coffee."

"I mean the kid. Black? White?"

"No, Brown, Kelvin Brown."

"You don't get my drift. I'm trying to find out what this extra digit means to young Brown's general health even before we see him. Let's go. Nice to see you in a clean lab coat this morning. Maybe people can't judge a book by looking at the cover, but first impressions are important, especially when you're trying to establish rapport and credibility. Do you have a history on the boy?"

"The parents are both black. The father is 28; the mother is 26. This is their third child. Normal full-term pregnancy, no illnesses, medications, or use of tobacco. The mother drank a glass of wine three to four nights a week but quit when she knew she was pregnant. Kelvin's brother and sister are normal, but the mother and the maternal grandfather both had extra little fingers. The mother's were apparently tiny and were removed when she was an infant. Her father's were about half the size of his little finger, were never removed, and made wearing work gloves a little difficult."

"Nice history. Do you think the alcohol ingestion is relevant here?"

"I know about fetal alcohol syndrome, but usually the mother's alcohol intake is much heavier. The recognized orthopedic manifestations of fetal alcohol syndrome include absent forearm rotation, intercarpal fusions, and short or crooked fingers, but I don't remember extra digits being associated. Kelvin's problem sounds more hereditary to me."

"I agree. Check Kelvin out and tell me what you find."

"I already have. He's a normal-appearing infant. Neck motion's full. Shoulder girdles are normal in appearance and normal to palpation, no asymmetry of muscles or bones. Upper limbs are of equal length. Shoulder, elbow, and wrist motions are full passively, and he seems to move all the joints actively. He has this tiny extra digit just barely attached next to the metacarpophalangeal joint of the little finger. It doesn't move, and it's so tiny I can't say whether it contains any bone. The other digits are well-formed and show both active flexion and extension. He clasps his thumbs with his other digits, and my roommate said this is normal for newborns. Kelvin's spine is straight. The pelvis and thighs are symmetric, hip abduction is full bilaterally, and I can't sublux them. The knees and ankles show normal motion and stability. Heel cords aren't tight, and feet aren't adducted. Toes look fine, five per side. No lumps, abnormal skin creases, or discolorations anywhere on his trunk or limbs. He looks fine except for the extra digit. What do you call it?"

"I call it a damn good evaluation except you didn't check for forearm rotation. Sometimes kids can have a bone bridge between their radius and ulna with loss of forearm rotation that may not be picked up for years."

"I meant, what do you call the extra digit? It must have a fancy name."

"Extra digit is concise and precise, but you know doctors—why use two syllables when five will do? *Poly* means 'many,' like polygon, polyester, polygamy, polychrome, poly . . ."

"I get it, I get it. This must be polydactyly!"

"Right. And because the ulnar border of the limb is the postaxial portion of the limb bud, and because the extra digit is quite hypoplastic, I hereby dub it postaxial vestigial polydactyly. It's quite common in blacks, occurring perhaps once in every 300 children. Usually it's vestigial like this and can be easily tied off in the newborn nursery by the obstetrician or pediatrician. You were also right about its inheritance: autosomal dominant."

"So why did you keep asking me 'black or white'?"

"Well, in African-Americans it usually occurs as an isolated anomaly. It isn't a tenth so common in Caucasians, but when it does occur it's associated with a wide range of internal organ anomalies."

"If this is postaxial polydactyly, what's preaxial polydactyly?"

"That refers to thumb duplication. It's not nearly so common as postaxial. It doesn't seem to have any racial variation, nor is it particularly associated with any internal organ derangements. However, it can be rather dysfunctional, depending on the degree of duplication. In mild cases the thumbnail is merely widened. In extreme cases the entire phalangeal skeleton and all the soft tissues are duplicated. These require some careful surgical planning to improve the function and appearance of the thumb. I'll show you some pictures of these when we get back to the office. Thanks for bringing me by."

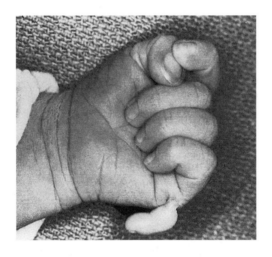

Vestigial postaxial polydactyly.

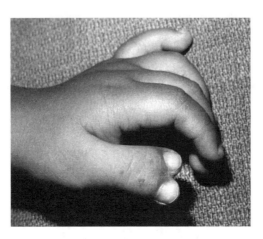

Partial duplication of the thumb.

ADVANCED READING

Daluiski A, Yi SE, Lyons KM. The molecular control of upper extremity development: Implications for congenital hand anomalies. J Hand Surg Am 26:8-22, 2001.

Dao KD, Shin AY, Billings A, et al. Surgical treatment of congenital syndactyly of the hand. J Am Acad Orthop Surg 12:39-48, 2004.

Flatt AE. The Care of Congenital Hand Anomalies. St. Louis: Mosby, 1977.

Kozin SH. Upper-extremity congenital anomalies. J Bone Joint Surg Am 85:1564-1576, 2003.

Ruby L, Goldberg M. Syndactyly and polydactyly. Orthop Clin North Am 7:361-374, 1976.

57

Sic Transit Gloria Mundi

Our U.S. senator, Marcus Thompson Jr., is a 40-year-old former Rhodes scholar in mythology who recently resumed playing tennis after a 15-year hiatus. While rushing the net this morning in a doubles match with the governor and his wife, he felt an excruciatingly sharp pain in the back of his right calf. He thought somebody had kicked him, but his wife was innocently standing at the baseline. The senator could not finish playing, and his partners brought him to your office. His past medical history is entirely unremarkable.

The back of his right leg is tender and ecchymotic. When sitting on your examining table with his feet hanging he is able to plantar flex his ankle, but he is in too much pain to try to rise on his right toes from a standing position. When he is prone you notice that the bulge of the right calf muscles is more proximally located than on the left. When palpating you can feel a defect in his right Achilles tendon approximately 4 cm above its insertion on the calcaneus. This is distinctly different from the uniform thickness of the left heel cord. When you compress the calf muscles between your thumb and fingers on the left, the ankle plantar flexes. When done on the right, the ankle does not move.

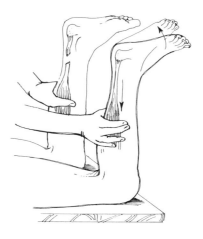

Compressing the calf causes ankle plantar flexion unless the heel cord is ruptured.

What's wrong with Senator Thompson? Are there any tests you need to order? What are the treatment options, and which do you recommend?

The paradox here is that something appears to be wrong with his Achilles tendon, yet he can still plantar flex his ankle. This persistence of active ankle flexion often misleads clinicians and delays the diagnosis of Achilles tendon rupture. The senator presents classic findings for this injury. It most often occurs in middle-aged individuals who indulge in an unaccustomed and strenuous athletic activity. The rupture occurs when excessive tensile force is applied to the tendon; it is accompanied by sudden, sharp, and severe pain and even at times by an audible snap. After several days the pain abates, and the patient can often plantar flex the ankle against minimal resistance by using other muscles—the tibialis posterior, flexor hallucis longus, and flexor digitorum. These secondary ankle flexors, however, are too weak to let him stand on tiptoes.

The diagnosis can be confirmed immediately by squeezing the gastrocsoleus muscle bellies. This shortens the motor unit and pulls the ankle into plantar flexion when the heel cord is intact. This is a passive contraction, and it eliminates any influence that the secondary ankle flexors have during the patient's effort to move the joint actively.

PRINCIPLE: When testing the integrity of muscle tendon units, consider which other muscles might be performing the same function.

✧ *What is the tendon that travels alongside the gastrocsoleus musculotendinous unit that may remain intact following an Achilles rupture?*

Over the years the pendulum has swung several times with respect to the enthusiasm for operative versus nonoperative treatment of heel cord rupture. The tendon ends are often frayed and avascular, and surgical exposure with suture placement further robs the tendon of its blood supply. Wound infections and skin sloughs are also well-known complications of operative treatment. If an infection is severe enough to require operative debridement (often including portions of the Achilles tendon itself) such complications can be disastrous. These considerations would naturally lead one to contemplate nonoperative treatment. In the senator's case, the ankle is cast in plantar flexion for roughly 2 months, and after that the patient is instructed to wear shoes with raised heels for another month. This method allows healing but is associated with a rerupture rate of about 10%, nearly twice that of operative treatment. Also, because the tendon will heal with the gastroc-soleus muscle in a shortened position, some residual weakness is common (remember the force versus length curve for muscle). In keeping with the trend toward minimally invasive surgery, recent "mini-open" techniques have been developed to minimize surgical trauma to adjacent soft tissues, and suture systems have been designed to provide strength while minimally damaging the blood supply. As such, operative treatment is now often favored, particularly for active patients.

Using terminology any layperson could understand, you give the senator your usual thorough explanation of the pathophysiology, diagnosis, and treatment of his condition. Both he and his wife ask only the most common questions regarding operative planning and subsequent rehabilitation. You conceal your disappointment that someone in his position is not interested in the nuances of fibroplasia.

PRINCIPLE: A patient's intelligence and social status bear no relationship to his or her understanding of medical problems.

Follow-up Note: During his convalescence, which proceeds smoothly, the senator stumps you on the mortality rate of heel cord injuries. He reminds you that Achilles' mother held him by his heel and dipped him in the River Styx to render him invulnerable. Achilles was subsequently raised by a centaur who fed him bear bone marrow and lion innards. Because of, or in spite of, this diet, he became the bravest, handsomest, and swiftest soldier in Agamemnon's army. A poison-tipped arrow hitting his unprotected heel, however, eventually undid him. (Arrow injuries to the heel cord are quite unusual these days, and therefore they are not covered in this book.)

ADVANCED READING

Arctinus of Miletus. Aethiopis.

Barnes MJ, Hardy AE. Delayed reconstruction of the calcaneal tendon. J Bone Joint Surg Br 68:121-124, 1986.

Homer. The Iliad. Fagels R, trans. New York: Penguin Group, 1991.

Khan, RJ, Fick D, Brammar TJ, et al. Interventions for treating acute Achilles tendon ruptures. Cochrane Database Syst Rev 3:CD003674, 2004.

Lawrence SJ, Grau GF. Management of acute Achilles tendon ruptures. Orthopedics 27:579-581, 2004.

Rippstein PF, Jung M, Assal M. Surgical repair of acute Achilles tendon rupture using a "mini-open" technique. Foot Ankle Clin 7:611-619, 2002.

58

The Surgical Letter
ON OPERATIONS AND THERAPEUTICS

Published by The Surgical Letter, Inc. • 1001 Main Street, New Rochelle, NY 80108 • A Nonexistent Publication

Vol. 47 (Issue 1199)
January 25

Orthopedic Management of Achondroplasia

Since the last *Surgical Letter* review of achondroplasia, the clown BoBo Jr. has won the hearts of people worldwide and brought new attention to this most common bone dysplasia. Many features of achondroplasia are now better understood, and several new surgical considerations are noteworthy.

PATHOLOGY — Achondroplasia is an autosomal dominant condition, but most cases are results of new mutations. It is the most common type of dwarfism and occurs in approximately 1 of 10,000 births. The disease is characterized by a defect in endochondral bone formation resulting in short stature with disproportionately short limbs. On epiphyseal growth plate biopsy, the normally active zone of cartilage proliferation shows a relative lack of cartilage production. Intramembranous bone formation, however, is unaffected. The condition existed as long ago as ancient Egypt and is not singular to humans. Dachshunds have an equivalent bone dysplasia.

The underlying cause of achondroplasia has been attributed to mutations in the fibroblast growth factor receptor (FGFR-III) gene locus. The mechanism by which mutations in the FGF receptor ultimately cause achondroplasia remains speculative, though this gene locus has been associated with several different clinical forms of dwarfism. Though somewhat counterintuitive, mutations in the FGFR-III gene product causing achondroplasia are gain-of-function mutations, producing unusually active forms of the receptor. Presumably, fibroblast growth factor normally plays a role in inhibiting cartilage proliferation and endochondral ossification, and this role is exaggerated by these activating receptor mutations.

CLINICAL FEATURES — The characteristic features of achondroplasia are present at birth: normal truncal height with disproportionately short limbs, a bulging forehead, and a depressed nasal bridge. Hypotonicity is evident for the first several years, and walking may be delayed. Intelligence is normal. Standing height at skeletal maturity is 75 to 120 cm (2.5 to 4 ft), and the fingertips reach no further than the hips. Even within the short limbs, the proximal segments (humerus and femur) are shorter than their distal counterparts. Hands are short and broad with splayed digits. Shortening of the middle finger in combination with an inability to juxtapose the long and ring fingers gives the appendage its so-called trident hand appearance.

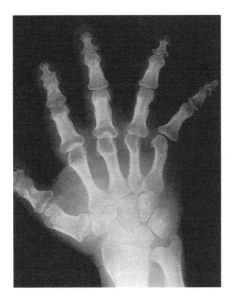

Increased lordosis of the lumbar spine gives prominence to the abdomen and buttocks and greatly reduces the anteroposterior dimension of the pelvic inlet.

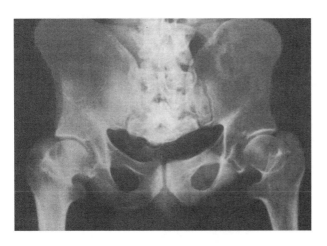

Characteristic "champagne-glass" appearance of the pelvic inlet in anteroposterior projections.

Lumbar lordosis and the bowed legs yield a waddling gait. The chest is also flattened from front to back because of short ribs.

DIFFERENTIAL DIAGNOSIS — The physical and radiographic findings are typically pathognomonic, but infants with cretinism, rickets, mucopolysaccharidoses, and other skeletal dysplasias may have a superficial resemblance.

RADIOGRAPHIC FEATURES — The calvaria of the skull is large, but the base is small. The lumbar vertebrae have short pedicles in a lateral view, which on an antero-posterior film are spaced progressively closer from L1 to L5. This narrowing of the interpedicular distances in the lumbar spine is considered pathognomonic for achondroplasia. The pelvis is typically broad and short, with radiographs showing widely flared, square iliac wings and small sciatic notches, giving rise to a characteristic "champagne-glass" appearance. Short femoral necks are also typical. In the lower extremity, there is metaphyseal flaring of the long bones with an inverted-V–shaped distal femoral physis. Bowing of the tibia and femur typically produce a genu varum deformity.

ADVERSE EFFECTS — Besides the obvious risks of psychological maladjustment, the bony abnormalities create multiple mechanical problems. The flattened chest predisposes these individuals to respiratory distress. The distorted pelvic inlet virtually precludes vaginal delivery. The diminished size of the spinal canal and intervertebral foramen, however, is the most common cause of serious problems. Spinal stenosis, with symptoms of neural claudication, impotence, and progressive neurologic deficit, may begin in early adult life.

P R I N C I P L E :   Bone growth anomalies have ramifications far beyond the musculoskeletal system.

SURGICAL CONSIDERATIONS — Symptoms of spinal stenosis need to be addressed promptly by evaluating the lumbar spinal canal with magnetic resonance imaging or computed tomography. *Surgical Letter* consultants universally advise extensive decompressive laminotomy to provide adequate space for the spinal cord and cauda equina.

Far more controversial is the consideration of lengthening the femurs and tibias for increased stature. Bone lengthening for correction of limb-length discrepancies has been available for some time and has been previously reviewed (Vol. 34, p. 432). With the advent of rigid yet expandable external fixation systems that use fine wires to minimize soft tissue damage, distraction-lengthening of the femurs and the tibias by 7.5 cm each (3 inches) in achondroplastic individuals is possible in about 10 months. By first letting a fracture callus form at the osteotomy site before beginning gradual lengthening, new bone forms in the gap, eliminating the need for subsequent bone grafting. Complications are frequent and include infection, joint stiffness, dislocation, and neurovascular compromise. To bring the upper limbs into proportion with the trunk and lengthened lower limbs, some *Surgical Letter* consultants advocate humeral lengthening as well. The psychological stress accompanying such a complicated, prolonged treatment is great, particularly when it does not address the commonly occurring and devastating pulmonary and neurologic complications of the condition.

CONCLUSION — The basic bone growth defect underlying achondroplasia is a genetic mutation that impairs the process of endochondral ossification. Advanced imaging techniques allow for more accurate diagnosis and provide the basis for more timely spinal decompression. Current bone-lengthening techniques allow for some increase in stature, but further experience will be required to determine whether this time-consuming, complicated procedure is more than a triumph of technique over reason.

ADVANCED READING —

Baitner AC, Maurer SG, Gruen MB, et al. The genetic basis of the osteochondrodysplasia. J Pediatr Orthop 20:594-605, 2000.

Birch JG, Samchukov ML. Use of the Ilizarov method to correct lower limb deformities in children and adolescents. J Am Acad Orthop Surg 12:144-154, 2004.

Herring JA, Tachdjian MO, eds. Tachdjian's Pediatric Orthopaedics, 3rd ed. Philadelphia: Saunders, 2001.

Tolo VT. Spinal deformity in short-stature syndromes. Instr Course Lect 39:399-405, 1990.

◆ *Did Tom Thumb have achondroplasia?*

59

Uncertainty

Kevin G. Shea ✦ *Roy A. Meals*

"Dr. Andre, I'm Jill Hill, third-year medical student. Do I have a great case to present! I'd like to help put the cast on a 19-month-old boy with osteogenesis imperfecta. He rolled off his parent's bed this evening and has a tibia fracture."

"Sounds interesting, Jill. Have you ever seen a patient with osteogenesis imperfecta before? How common is 'brittle bone disease'?"

"No, he's the first. I gather it's rare, but the mother has a tattered letter from their pediatrician in Europe confirming the diagnosis. The father's been here 6 months as an executive trainee."

"What else did you find out in the history?"

"After the boy had several fractures with minimal trauma, the condition was diagnosed almost a year ago. Mom says his growth and development have otherwise been normal. His past history is otherwise unremarkable, and his immunizations are up to date."

"How about his examination? Does he have blue sclerae? How do his teeth look?"

"No, his sclerae are white, but his conjunctivae are inflamed—from crying, I guess. I didn't think to look at his teeth though. As you'd expect, he won't move his left leg. The knee's tender. Sensibility and circulation to his foot are good. He has a couple of bruises on both shins. He keeps stumbling over toys in their small rental apartment. Accident prone, mom says."

"Any lab data? How about a urinalysis?"

"I didn't think of that, but the urine's normal in osteogenesis imperfecta, isn't it? I can't wait to tell my brother I've seen a case of OI; he probably doesn't even know what it is."

"Not so fast there. You're telling me a child with multiple bruises and a long-bone fracture sustained from a trivial injury has osteogenesis imperfecta. You said his sclerae are normal. When you hear hoofbeats, think horses, Jill, not zebras."

"But I did a PubMed search and everything—I even printed up some review articles. It says right here, 'osteogenesis imperfecta can present in many different ways, with some children having multiple intrauterine fractures and poor survival. Others have minimal physical findings except for an increased incidence of fractures.' And he's had a workup in Europe. His mother has the letter."

"If it weren't for the letter, would osteogenesis imperfecta be your working diagnosis?"

"I guess not. It should be in the differential, but child abuse probably comes to mind first."

"Precisely. Solid figures are hard to come by, but more than 1 million cases of child abuse are substantiated annually. In fact, it is estimated that as many as 10% or more of pediatric fractures are the result of some type of abuse. So for any child presenting with an injury, you must include abuse in the differential. On the other hand, osteogenesis imperfecta is so rare that even most orthopedists never see a case. So let's think about this case a bit differently. What features of this boy's presentation suggest a diagnosis of child abuse?"

"Well, a fracture from a seemingly trivial injury—either that or a history that is inconsistent with the type and severity of injury. Multiple bruises. I'm not sure about the inflamed conjunctivae. I know retinal and conjunctival hemorrhages occur in children who are shaken forcefully, but these are usually seen in young infants. Social isolation and family stress can contribute. The mother is not at all happy about living here."

"OK. What features are working against a diagnosis of battered child syndrome?"

"The mother brought the child in right away. Her story is consistent during repeated questioning. She and the boy seem to comfort each other, and her level of concern seems appropriate—neither detached nor overprotective. Both of them are dressed well. His immunizations are up to date. He's in the sixtieth to seventieth percentiles for height, weight, and head circumference. Except for the bruises on his shins, his skin's normal."

"Good. All useful points. Abused children may not be brought for treatment right away. The history may vary, contain discrepancies, and not fit the physical findings. The child also may show signs of neglect such as failure to thrive, abnormal behavior, or poor hygiene. Burns are very common, either from hot liquids or hot objects that leave a 'brand.' All kids get scraped and bruised but usually not on the buttocks, abdomen, or other soft areas. You implied that their socioeconomic status was pretty high. Be careful there. Family violence can certainly transcend economic status. What do you know about fractures associated with child abuse?"

"I know that spiral fractures of long bones and epiphyseal-metaphyseal "corner" fractures in infants are virtually pathognomonic of abuse. It's difficult to generate the pulling-twisting forces required to produce these injuries by accidental means, especially before the child starts walking. A femur fracture in an infant under 1 year of age is a classic example of a child abuse fracture. Multiple, unexplained fractures at various stages of healing without underlying systemic disease are also indicative, but we can't be sure about that in this boy. Rib and skull fractures can be suggestive too."

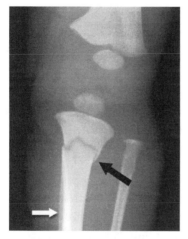

Recent metaphyseal fracture in the proximal tibia *(black arrow)* in a 6-week-old infant. The subperiosteal new bone along the medial border of the tibia *(white arrow)* suggests previous injury as well.

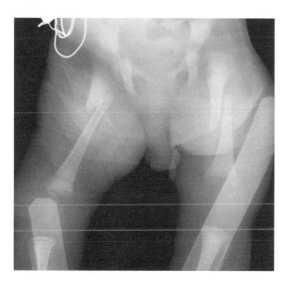

Bilateral femur fractures in a 2-month-old infant.

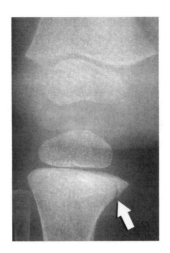

Metaphyseal corner fracture of the proximal tibia in an 11-month-old child. Avulsion injuries such as this require great force.

"All good points. What do you want to do now?"

"I guess we should get a radiographic skeletal survey. Of course if he does indeed have osteogenesis imperfecta, this could also show multiple fractures at various stages of healing. Though there is quite a bit of variability, x-rays of children with osteogenesis imperfecta tend to reveal thin bones with thin cortices. Deformities of long bones from multiple fractures (as well as the poorly understood, exaggerated bone turnover often seen in this disorder) may also be apparent. A bone scan will help identify nondisplaced fractures and subperiosteal hematomas, but it's not much good around the epiphyses because those areas usually show increased activity related to normal growth. Even with a thorough workup, however, it can sometimes be a difficult distinction between osteogenesis imperfecta and abuse. This is compounded by the fact that the definitive diagnosis of osteogenesis imperfecta requires a skin biopsy that may take as long as 6 months to yield a conclusive result."

"Excellent. Jill, what do you know about the legal aspects of reporting child abuse?"

"I know there's a state law mandating a report, and there are also laws that protect reporting physicians against liability."

"In fact, Jill, all 50 states have such laws. Many states also have significant sanctions against physicians who do not report suspected child abuse. It's very difficult to know what to do in cases in which child abuse is in the differential. But in questionable circumstances, the child abuse investigation team should be given the responsibility to distinguish between abuse and accidental trauma. Although an investigation is always traumatic for the family, we have to protect the child. Failure to do so has severe implications for these children. Otherwise 40% to 50% will suffer repeated abuse, and many of these will be left with permanent injuries. Ten percent die. Also, children who are abused tend to become abusers as adults."

"Dr. Andre, we've got to hurry. Shouldn't we contact the child abuse investigation team right away?"

"Let's first talk to the mother again and also see whether she has a local pediatrician we can talk to. Then we'll call the doctor who wrote the letter. It's almost 9 AM in Europe now. Jill, have you considered that the boy might have osteogenesis imperfecta and *also* be abused?"

ADVANCED READING

Carty, HM. Fractures caused by child abuse. J Bone Joint Surg Br 76:849-857, 1993.

Chapman S, Hall CM. Non-accidental injury or brittle bones. Pediatr Radiol 27:106-110, 1997.

Dent JA, Paterson CR. Fractures in early childhood: Osteogenesis imperfecta or child abuse? J Pediatr Orthop 11:184-186, 1991.

Kocher MS, Kasser JR. Orthopaedic aspects of child abuse. J Am Acad Orthop Surg 8:10-20, 2000.

Kocher MS, Shapiro F. Osteogenesis imperfecta. J Am Acad Orthop Surg 6:225-236, 1998.

60

For Some Strange Reason

Robert Gutierrez ✦ *Scott A. Mitchell* ✦ *Roy A. Meals*

"... in the physician or surgeon no quality takes rank with imperturbability ... coolness and presence of mind under all circumstances, calmness amid storm, clearness of judgment in moments of grave peril. ..."

Dr. William Osler's address to graduating
University of Pennsylvania medical students, 1889

It's Friday, well past midnight in the emergency room on the last night of your orthopedic trauma rotation. Weary from a long day's work, your body drained and scrubs splattered with plaster, you finally head off to the call room in hopes of catching a few moments rest. But wait! The paramedics are calling in from County Line Road at Grover Bypass. That's midway between the region's trauma center, where you are, and a community hospital with a sleepy emergency department. There are at least seven injured persons, including a toddler and her great-grandmother, a motorcyclist with an apparently isolated open tibia fracture, his girlfriend complaining of abdominal pain, a van driver with chest wall contusions complaining of hip pain, and his passenger who is conscious but has a large bump on her forehead. You look around. For some strange reason you are alone. The paramedics are desperate for guidance to triage these patients. Which ones should you accept?

a. The child, the great-grandmother, and the girlfriend
b. The van driver and his passenger
c. The patients with open wounds
d. The patients with head, chest, or abdominal injuries

PRINCIPLE: Patients who require immediate, multidisciplinary care are those who have sustained high-energy injuries; those who were previously fragile; and those with closed head or chest injury, penetrating injury to any body cavity, shock, or a dysvascular limb.

Even two of these patients arriving simultaneously at an emergency room can tax its resources, so the patients with the most life-threatening conditions must be brought to the trauma center, and the others can be managed in the community hospital. One half of civilian trauma deaths occur within the first hour from either central nervous system injury or exsanguination, and an additional 30% occur within the next several hours from internal bleeding. Therefore patients with any of the following dire indicators need a trauma center: automobile-induced abdominal trauma in a motorcyclist or pedestrian, penetrating injuries to a body cavity, blunt chest injury with low blood pressure or flail chest, and anyone who has fallen more than 15 feet or demonstrates no spontaneous eye opening. Additionally, young children less than 5 years old and elderly patients more than 65 years old require specialized treatment in a trauma center.

The motorcycle passenger arrives at the trauma center complaining of lower abdominal pain. The paramedics indicate that she was unconscious when they arrived at the accident scene. Following initial evaluation and stabilization, x-rays are obtained. Which screening films do you order?

a. Lumbar spine series, anteroposterior (AP) pelvis, and femoral arteriogram
b. Lateral cervical spine, supine AP chest, and AP pelvis
c. Lateral cervical spine, upright AP chest, AP pelvis, and skull series if history of loss of consciousness
d. Lateral cervical spine flexion-extension views, skull series, and AP pelvis

Although a meticulous physical examination takes precedence over routine x-ray studies, any multitraumatized patient needs to have the screening films listed in answer *b*. X-rays should be reviewed before repositioning the patient for detailed physical examination or special studies. For example, precautions for cervical spine injury must be maintained until the stability of the neck is confirmed radiographically.

Shown on the following page is the patient's pelvic x-ray.

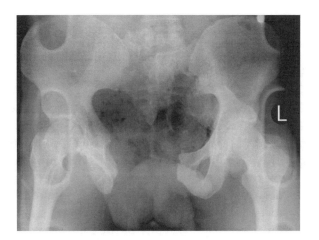

What should be done to control shock associated with this injury?

Her other x-rays reveal normal findings. Despite absence of external bleeding, she remains hypotensive. Peritoneal lavage is negative. You look around. For some strange reason everyone has disappeared from the trauma bay and you are alone. Which treatment do you choose?

  a. Additional fluid replacement
  b. Application of a pneumatic antishock garment
  c. Reduction and percutaneous fracture stabilization
  d. Under angiographic control, embolization of any bleeding vessels

Life-threatening loss of blood into the retroperitoneal space commonly follows major pelvic fractures. The bleeding is internal and unseen, so the development of shock can be insidious. Though blood loss from pelvic fractures may be severe, in most cases it is caused by venous bleeding from the fractured bony surfaces rather than arterial hemorrhage. By reducing the volume of the pelvis in this "open-book" type of fracture, the low-pressure bleeding will tamponade. The best treatment is a rapid application of external skeletal fixation for fracture reduction and stabilization.

NOTE: *An easily performed temporizing maneuver to reduce an unstable open-book injury such as the one shown here is to wrap a folded sheet around the patient's pelvis and apply traction while an assistant pulls in the opposite direction from the other side of the stretcher.*

As you are preparing the patient for the operating room, the nurse asks whether the minimally displaced pubic ramus fracture accounts for this patient's bleeding. You politely tell her that:

  a. The fractured ramus of the ischium accounts for the shock.
  b. Another site is present but unseen on this film.

c. Yes, the pubic ramus fracture requires immediate reduction.

d. The disrupted pubic symphysis is also bleeding.

The pelvis is a rigid bony ring. A disruption at one site must be accompanied by another break in the ring, even if unseen, to allow for the displacement. Anterior lesions involve either disruption of the symphysis pubis or fracture of the rami of the pubis and ischium. Associated posterior lesions involve fracture of the ilium or sacrum and/or dislocation of the sacroiliac joint. In addition to bleeding complications caused by displaced pelvic ring injuries, gastrointestinal, gynecologic, urologic, and neurologic injuries are often present.

Following application of the pelvic fixator, your patient's hypotension begins to resolve with fluid resuscitation. Had she not stabilized hemodynamically within an hour, you were prepared to apply selective embolization of the ruptured vessels under angiographic control. But before leaving the operating room, you find a small laceration next to the patient's right patella. Using a sterile technique, you inject a solution containing methylene blue into the knee joint from a location remote from the laceration. As you are injecting the knee, you see a trail of blue liquid begin to drip from the laceration, indicating communication with the knee joint. You look around, but for some strange reason the entire OR has been vacated. You decide to:

a. Extend the wound and irrigate the joint.

b. Put a stitch in the skin for loose closure.

c. Put a suction drain in the joint.

d. Apply a protective dressing and irrigate the joint later when she is more stable.

Open joint injuries, like open fractures, are prone to infection because bone has a relatively sparse blood supply and cartilage has none. Bacteria introduced into an open joint can thrive in the nutrient-rich synovial fluid. The cartilage is thereby deprived of its normal source of nourishment and is exposed to the degradative enzymes produced by the proliferating and dying bacteria as well as the body's inflammatory response. A 2-day course of intravenous antistaphylococcal antibiotics reduces the risk of infection following open bone and joint injuries, but thorough irrigation and debridement remain the mainstay of treatment. Additionally, the presence of shock in a trauma victim results in a suppression of the immune system, increasing the likelihood of infectious complications. This makes early irrigation and debridement all the more imperative.

Before leaving the operating room, the anesthesiologist informs you that the patient's vital signs are stabilizing but that she remains hypovolemic. What should you give her?

a. Typed whole blood
b. Lactated Ringer's solution
c. 5% human serum albumin solution
d. A vasoconstrictive drug

Probably because lactated Ringer's solution contains less chloride than a normal saline solution, it's seen by most surgeons as the most physiologic crystalloid solution. In practice, however, the two are often used interchangeably. Every hypotensive trauma patient should receive a 2 L bolus of one of these crystalloid solutions in the trauma bay. This temporarily increases intravascular volume, though it does not restore oxygen-carrying capacity provided by red cells. In a trauma patient who remains hypotensive despite initial crystalloid boluses, particularly in cases of ongoing hemorrhage, typed blood products are required.

PRINCIPLE: What is the best measure of a patient's response to fluid resuscitation? Remember the Foley catheter that you placed in the trauma bay?

You now refocus your attention on the emergency room. After a thorough evaluation, the great-grandmother's injuries seem limited to a chest wall contusion with two cracked ribs, a closed femoral shaft fracture on the left, and a proximal tibia fracture on the right. Pedal pulses are absent on the right, so you have wisely requested an arteriogram.

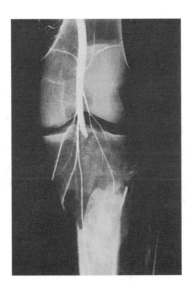

What are the sequence and timing for repairing these injuries?

You look around, and for some strange reason you are alone; what should you do next?
a. Wait until the cracked ribs heal before operating.
b. Fix the vessel and both fractures now.
c. Fix the vessel and tibia now and the femur next week.
d. Fix the vessel now and the fractures next week.

The physiologic status of a polytrauma patient rapidly deteriorates from the moment of injury. Hypoxia, poor cardiac perfusion, anemia, malnutrition, renal failure, immune system alterations, and skin breakdown are common components of multi-system failure, which can continue for many weeks. So even though these patients are not good candidates for emergency surgery, they are almost always better candidates shortly after injury than they will be for a long time. The revascularization of this patient's foot requires immediate surgery. Although the fractures could appropriately be fixed anytime in the first 24 to 48 hours after injury, they can be done efficiently during the same anesthetic period as the revascularization, and stabilizing the tibia will help protect the arterial anastomosis from further injury. Prompt, rigid fracture fixation allows early patient mobilization. This greatly enhances pulmonary toilet and intestinal motility, prevents bedsores, and generally aids the patient in reestablishing homeostasis.

P R I N C I P L E :   In multiple-trauma cases treat the patient's injuries without waiting for the body's response to the injuries.

As you finally reach the call room at 5 AM, you flop down by the radio. Ah, it's Charlie Parker's alto sax playing "A Night in Tunisia" by Dizzy Gillespie. Your mind's racing is gradually lulled. A half hour of cherished sleep intervenes before morning rounds.

Awakened with a start by your pager, you rally for your morning rotation in the intensive care unit, where, as luck would have it, you already know several patients. The great-grandmother seems to be doing pretty well and is extubated after the rounds. Her feet are warm and pink. You go back to talk to her later that afternoon, but now she seems disoriented and restless, and she doesn't recognize you. Her respirations are rapid and shallow. You look around, and wouldn't you know it, for some strange reason you are alone again. You decide first to:
a. Increase the flow of her nasal oxygen.
b. Order a pulmonary arteriogram.
c. Draw an arterial blood gas.
d. Repeat her ECG.

On a hunch you choose to do a blood gas while you are waiting for her ECG. Her P_{CO_2} is low normal, but the P_{O_2} comes back at 55 mm Hg even though the F_{iO_2} is 50%. You set about to look for petechiae on her conjunctiva, chest, and anterior axillary folds. This and an examination of a spun urine sample are aimed at diagnosing:

a. Pulmonary embolus
b. Malignant hyperthermia
c. Expanding subdural hematoma
d. Acute myocardial infarction
e. Fat embolus

Although any of these conditions could occur in this setting, the presence of petechiae and fat in the urine would indicate fat embolism as a cause of her respiratory distress. Fat embolisms usually occur 1 to 3 days after injury and may be fatal in 10% to 15% of cases. It is frequently associated with multiple long-bone fractures, although it can occur with massive trauma in the absence of fracture. It may also follow total joint replacement. The exact cause of fat embolism remains unclear. The two competing theories are (1) direct inoculation of marrow fat into the bloodstream following bone damage and (2) stress-induced metabolic alterations in the stability of circulating fatty acid complexes. Regardless of the mechanism, the results are fever, tachycardia, acute respiratory distress with tachypnea, low P_{CO_2}, and arterial hypoxemia. These changes lead to restlessness, confusion, and incoherency. The microemboli also manifest themselves as petechiae during physical examination and as diffuse, bilateral parenchymal infiltrates on chest x-rays. Which of the following is the most dangerous consequence of fat embolism?

a. Hypocapnia
b. Hypoxia
c. Hyponatremia
d. Hypokalemia

You look around. You are still alone, so you:

a. Increase IV fluids
b. Turn up the nasal oxygen and add nasal carbon dioxide
c. Intubate the patient
d. Give a diuretic to increase urinary output

The most dangerous consequence of fat embolism is hypoxia. Because it is urgent to correct this deficit, intubation and mechanical ventilation are required, keeping the Po_2 more than 60 mm Hg with the lowest possible Fio_2. Application of positive end-expiratory pressure (PEEP) helps keep the alveoli open and greatly aids the treatment, although excessive PEEP may paradoxically decrease cardiovascular function. The incidence of posttraumatic fat embolism is reduced but not eliminated by early stabilization of long bone fractures. Once you get the great-grandmother stabilized, you go back to see the motorcycle passenger with the external fixator on her pelvis. Now she too is restless, has tachypnea, and is disoriented, but has no evidence of petechiae or fat in her urine. Her blood gases show low Po_2 and low Pco_2. What's wrong with her?

    a. Adult respiratory distress syndrome
    b. Toxic shock syndrome
    c. Malignant hyperthermia
    d. Pulmonary embolus

You look around. You are alone for some strange reason, so you check your notebook. Adult respiratory distress syndrome (ARDS) is a disorder that can follow severe systemic or pulmonary injury. It is the end result of a complex cascade involving inflammatory mediators and the biochemical reactions they initiate. Direct lung damage occurs from smoke or water inhalation, gastric aspiration, lung contusion, or pneumonia. Indirect causes include trauma with severe shock, multiple blood transfusions, sepsis, pancreatitis, and diffuse intravascular coagulation, to name only a few. Trauma and shock can lead to ARDS if they are accompanied by massive blood transfusion or severe tissue damage. As treatment of ARDS is often prolonged and riddled with complications, prevention is far superior. In the trauma setting this means prompt and aggressive treatment of shock and blood loss while avoiding excessive hydration. Early rigid fracture fixation may likewise be preventive.

Just as you get this patient stabilized on a ventilator, the residents and attending physicians appear for the evening rounds. Later they congratulate you on your knowledge and skills. You try to whistle "A Night in Tunisia," but for some strange reason a ditty comes out. The notes happen to be the answers to the questions in this chapter: abcba abcebca.

ADVANCED READING

Collins DN, Temple SD. Open joint injuries. Classification and treatment. Clin Orthop Relat Res 243:48-56, 1989.

Olson SA. Pulmonary aspects of treatment of long bone fractures in the poly-trauma patient. Clin Orthop Relat Res 422:66-70, 2004.

Osler W. Aequanimitas. With Other Addresses to Medical Students, Nurses, and Practitioners of Medicine. New York: Blakiston, 1904.

Pryor JP, Reilly PM. Initial care of the patient with blunt polytrauma. Clin Orthop Relat Res 422:30-36, 2004.

Shafi S, Kauder DR. Fluid resuscitation and blood replacement in patients with polytrauma. Clin Orthop Relat Res 422:37-42, 2004.

Roberts CS, Pape HC, Jones AL, et al. Damage control orthopaedics. Evolving concepts in the treatment of patients who have sustained orthopaedic trauma. J Bone Joint Surg Am 87:434-449, 2005.

Robinson CM. Current concepts of respiratory insufficiency syndromes after fracture. J Bone Joint Surg Br 83:781-791, 2001.

ten Duis HJ. The fat embolism syndrome. Injury 28:77-85, 1997.

Ware LB, Matthay MA. Medical progress: The acute respiratory distress syndrome. N Engl J Med 342:1334-1349, 2000.

Wolinsky PR. Assessment and management of pelvic fracture in the hemodynamically unstable patient. Orthop Clin North Am 28:321-329, 1997.

61

Mission: Impossible

Michiyuki Kono ✦ *Roy A. Meals*

The airport is empty except for a janitor mopping up on his graveyard shift and two servicemen sleeping fitfully on benches as they await their red-eye flight. A well-groomed, middle-aged gentleman inconspicuously approaches the locker bay. Glancing furtively around, he removes a digital recorder and an envelope from one of the lockers and steals away to a phone booth. Once inside, he starts the recording and removes the contents of the envelope.

[TAPE]   Good evening, Quent. The middle eastern country of Onok has recently put a hold on peace talks while it investigates the reported attack on Prince Ihcim, 8-year-old son of the emir and first in line to the throne.

Last week the Onok News Agency reported that the prince suffered a fracture of the femur while being attacked by one of our government's operatives. Allegations have been made that this fracture represents an act of terrorism designed to coerce the country of Onok into signing an unbalanced treaty. Our undercover agents, however, were present when the injury occurred and report that the prince was merely running around playing soccer when he suddenly fell to the ground complaining of a painful hip. They were able to smuggle out copies of the x-rays taken at the time of the injury.

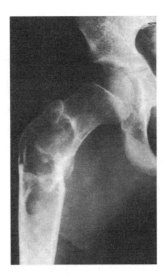

[RADIOGRAPH]   There is an expansive, multilocular, radiolucent lesion of the proximal femur involving the femoral neck and the intertrochanteric region at a distance of 3 cm from the physeal plate. The cortex is thinned and there is a minimally displaced distal neck fracture. There is no periosteal new bone formation or cortical breakthrough to suggest a malignant neoplasm.

[TAPE]   Our experts have examined the film and are certain that this is a unicameral, or simple, bone cyst with a pathologic fracture of the femoral neck—not a fracture from trauma alone. Although the differential diagnosis includes histiocytosis X, fibrous dysplasia, aneurysmal bone cyst, and cystic degeneration from a neoplasm such as chondroblastoma, osteoblastoma, or osteosarcoma, our experts are certain of the characteristic appearance on this x-ray and believe that further evaluation is not necessary. Unicameral bone cysts are benign, fluid-filled lesions found almost exclusively in children. Ninety percent occur in either the proximal humerus or the proximal femur. The prince is an 8-year-old boy with no previous medical problems, thus giving him the typical profile of a patient with a unicameral cyst.

PRINCIPLE: Preliminary diagnosis of a bone tumor is based on location, radiographic appearance, and age of patient. The final diagnosis requires histologic assessment.

In the absence of a pathologic fracture, these cysts are asymptomatic, discovered at times as incidental findings on x-rays obtained for other reasons. In the absence of structural compromise of the involved bone (most notably the high stress regions of the proximal femur), no treatment other than observation is warranted. Bone cysts are thought to resolve gradually with skeletal maturity, which is supported by their distinct rarity in adults. Unfortunately, however, the cortical thinning caused by unicameral cysts may lead to fractures from minor trauma, as appears to be the case with Prince Ichim, and further treatment is necessary.

Unfortunately, our operatives inform us that the Onok government is planning to use this injury, along with the false allegation of terrorism, to withdraw completely from the peace talks. They also plan to withhold proper treatment from the prince so that his eventual crippling from varus malunion or avascular necrosis of the femoral head will serve to further foster hatred against our nation.

Proper treatment in this case would involve a long course of orthopedic care. First, the prince needs an operation to internally fix the fracture and place bone graft in the cavity. Treatment of the fracture will prevent the complications of varus deformity or collapse of the femoral head from avascular necrosis. There is, however, approximately a 50% chance that the cyst will recur within the next year. The likelihood in the prince is diminished somewhat by the fact that his cyst is not an "active" lesion (within 1 cm of the growth plate). If the cyst should recur, or if one is fortunate enough to identify a cyst before fracture occurs, currently accepted treatments include percutaneous injection of the cyst with corticosteroid. Although multiple injections a few months apart are usually needed for complete resolution of the cyst, there is low morbidity from this operating-room procedure. Other options include injection of the cyst with either bone marrow aspirate or various bone graft substitutes such as a demineralized bone matrix. Reports suggest that recurrence rates following injection of these substances are low compared with corticosteroids.

[FILE PICTURE] Intraoperative photograph of an Onok surgeon preparing to inject a unicameral cyst.

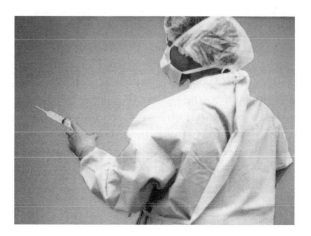

[TAPE]   If this is not successful, the other major treatment is curettage and bone grafting, but this is usually not done unless the cyst has diminished to a "latent" state, more than 1 cm from the physis, where damage to the growth plate from curettage is less likely.

[RADIOGRAPH]   Here is a series of x-rays from a similar case in Onok several years ago. The cyst was injected shortly after its discovery when the child was 7. By 11 years of age, the humeral head had grown away from the involved cyst, and at age 17 the cyst had nearly disappeared.

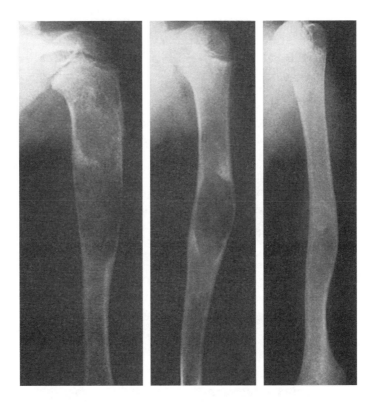

[TAPE]   Your mission, should you choose to accept it, is to infiltrate the medical staff treating Prince Ichim and ensure that he receives the proper orthopedic care. In addition, you must make it widely known to the country that the prince was not attacked but suffered a pathologic fracture from a developmental condition. As before, if you are caught the government will deny any knowledge of your existence. Good luck. This tape will self-destruct in 10 seconds.

ADVANCED READING

Aboulafia AJ, Temple HT, Scully SP. Surgical treatment of benign bone tumors. Instr Course Lect 51:441-450, 2002.

Biermann JS. Common benign lesions of bone in children and adolescents. J Pediatr Orthop 22:268-273, 2002.

Capanna R, DalMonte A, Gitelis S, et al. The natural history of unicameral bone cyst after steroid injection. Clin Orthop Relat Res 166:204-211, 1982.

Docquier PL, Delloye C. Treatment of simple bone cysts with aspiration and a single bone marrow injection. J Pediatr Orthop 23:766-773, 2003.

Dormans JP, Pill SG. Fractures through bone cysts: Unicameral bone cysts, aneurismal bone cysts, fibrous cortical defects, and nonossifying fibromas. Instr Course Lect 51:457-467, 2002.

Temple HT, Scully SP, Aboulafia AJ. Benign bone tumors. Instr Course Lect 51:429-439, 2002.

Wilkins RM. Unicameral bone cysts. J Am Acad Orthop Surg 8:217-224, 2000.

◆ *What happens when you try to walk after your foot has gone to sleep from sitting with your legs crossed too long? Which nerve and which muscles are affected?*

62

Donut's Great Adventure

Kevin Mikaelian ✦ *Roy A. Meals*

Donut, a 62-day-old red cell, was having a major midlife crisis. He had traveled extensively throughout the body and felt that he had pretty much seen all there was to see. Sure he had lots of friends and related cell lines, but there was just nothing left to accomplish. He had done his job, always the same thing, day in and day out. He knew exactly where to go and when, and how long each oxygen run took. "Could this be all there is?" he wondered, "Where did I miss out?" For the last few days, he had been vegging out in his favorite splenic sinusoid. "Why couldn't I be a helper T cell and mastermind an entire immune response?" he thought. "Heck, I don't even have any DNA."

Suddenly a rumble and a loud crash swept through the spleen, and Donut was thrown nearly 80 microns. "Yikes! What was that? I'd better find out what's happening." Donut traveled directly to the brain to find Sparky, the neuron.

"Donut, it was wild!" Sparky shouted above the buzzing. "This guy lost control of his motorcycle. The rest is quite hazy, but damage reports are indicating that the left leg is painful, very unstable. And get this—early reports from the visual center say that something is sticking out of the skin; some even say it's bone!" Donut was concerned and intrigued, but he also was getting blue, so he had to make a quick oxygen run.

"I'll see the damage for myself," asserted Donut. He took his favorite route: a straight shot through the aorta down to the anterior tibial artery. "Wow, traffic is bad. Either I'm in LA or there's thrombus ahead." Just above him bright light glinted in through jagged openings—the ripped skin Sparky had heard about. Donut dodged sideways into an arteriole and traversed a network of small vessels to get a good look at the injury.

"I'm below the knee, probably about mid-leg. The tibia and fibula are both broken."

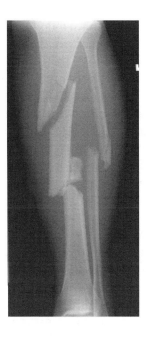

Comminuted segmental fracture of the tibial shaft with associated fibula fracture. The degree of associated soft tissue damage from high-energy mechanisms of injury can only be ascertained by a physical examination.

"The broken surfaces are slanted slightly, and a few little pieces are broken off and floating free. The main arteries though, despite a couple of sharp kinks, are still running straight to the foot."

PRINCIPLE: To describe a fracture, note its location, orientation, the presence of multiple fragments, and any angulation or translation of the distal fragment.

Donut was shocked by the damage. He hoped Rocky, the osteocyte, could console him. "I'm really sorry about the leg, Rocky."

Rocky nodded his head and smiled. "You know, the tibia is the most commonly fractured long bone in the body, and about a sixth of them are open—you know, bone exposed to outer space. It's a big injury. The associated fibular fracture allows increased displacement and instability, which are important prognostic factors. But with proper treatment this leg could be as good as new. Initially the leg needs to be stabilized with a splint to prevent further damage. For closed tibia fractures that are not displaced or only minimally displaced, placement in a long leg cast for 6 to 8 weeks followed by a brace and rehabilitation therapy is adequate."

Donut groaned, "I'll never live long enough to see. . . ."

"But this fracture is severe, and proper alignment with adequate soft tissue support will not be achieved by casting. Depending on the severity of the soft tissue injury, a large nail can be placed inside the medullary canal to support the fracture. This is especially useful when displacement is significant or if slow healing is anticipated because of missing bone fragments or severe comminution. But if the soft tissues are in bad enough shape, an external fixator is helpful to stabilize the fracture fragments while the wound site remains accessible for the multiple debridements that are often necessary."

"So is that all one has to do to make everything right?"

"Not exactly," Rocky continued. "Because the tibia is so close under the skin and has a relatively poor blood supply, severe complications can occur, especially with open fractures. Infection of the soft tissues or the bone itself is always a risk, so antibiotics and timely irrigation and debridement of devitalized tissue are a must. Bone healing can also be very slow, and if healing isn't secure by about 5 months, we call it a delayed union. Some further treatment, such as a bone graft, may be required to achieve good stability. Complete lack of healing is also a real possibility—nonunion." Both cells shuddered at the sound of this frightful word. "If a fractured tibia hasn't healed by 8 months, it's unlikely that it has the potential to do so without assistance. Nowadays they can use recombinant BMP—you know, bone morphogenetic proteins—those growth factors that I used to munch on back in my uncommitted, preosteoblast days. Oh, that was the life. . . . Anyhow, they can inject BMP directly into the fracture site to help recruit young mesenchymal cells to promote bony healing.

"At other times the bone will heal but at a funny angle—malunion. Angular deformity of up to 10 degrees is well-tolerated in the tibia. Greater side-to-side deformities—varus or valgus deformities—as well as flexion and extension deformities are unsightly and dysfunctional because of gait disturbances. Rotational malalignments are really kooky, such as when the knee points west and the foot points south. That's not as bad as infection, though."

Donut's eyes bulged out, and he looked carefully around to see whether any bacteria were sneaking up on his friend. In a lower tone Rocky continued: "The likelihood of infection increases with open fractures, severe displacement, and the presence of avascular bony fragments. During treatment it's very important not to deprive the bone of any more of its sparse and vital blood supply. Otherwise infection can lead to disastrous complications such as nonunion, chronic osteomyelitis, and amputation."

Donut was spooked, and by this time almost completely blue, so he decided to leave. "Thanks, Rocky. Take care of yourself."

"Come back again with more oxygen. Hey, by the way, I've got a riddle for you to think about: What's the only solid tissue in the body that heals without a scar?"

Donut pondered that along with the fright of infection as he fought his way upstream to find his friend Harry, a skin cell, who had narrowly missed getting tattooed some years previously and was an expert on infections. "Harry, what's the deal with open fractures and infection? Is this guy's leg going to be amputated?"

Harry soothed him. "Have a nip of plasma, Donut. There are three types of open fractures, and the likelihood of infection increases exponentially from one type to the next. The first type has only a small opening in the skin, usually from the sharp bone end punching out from the inside, accompanied by only minimal soft tissue damage. Infections are uncommon in these wounds unless severe contamination is present, such as with farm injuries. In the second kind the skin opening is larger, and moderate soft tissue damage is present, but there is still adequate healthy soft tissue available to keep the bone covered after the surgeon cleans things up. The third type is a massive injury with extensive soft tissue tearing and major bone displacement, comminution, and possible segmental loss. These factors mean less blood supply to the bone ends. Serious nerve and artery damage can further complicate this type. But you know, Donut, with proper debridement, irrigation, and prophylactic antibiotics, the complications Rocky mentioned can frequently be avoided. So it's very important to quickly take the patient to the operating room for a thorough removal of any foreign material, hematoma, devitalized bone, and soft tissue fragments. This procedure may have to be repeated several times in the first week. 'Never give the bacteria a handout,' we like to say."

Donut still did not understand the concept of soft tissue injury very well, so he visited his old friend Arnold, the muscle cell. Arnold explained: "The most important factor in soft tissue injury is the extent of vessel and nerve damage. Without you guys to supply oxygen and nutrients, a muscle cell dies within 6 to 12 hours, depending on its temperature. Furthermore, muscle cells are useless without functioning nerves, and various parts of the limb would also be nonfunctional. This is why it's so important to check sensory and motor functions in detail as well as tissue perfusion in the injured limb. But be careful; pulses can be deceptive. For example, a palpable dorsalis pedis pulse does not mean the anterior tibial artery is intact, because blood could be coming backward into the dorsum of the foot through the posterior tibial system. Therefore complete vascular assessment includes color, temperature, and capillary refill. When the nerves and arteries are disrupted, many, many months can be wasted trying to salvage a limb that eventually requires amputation."

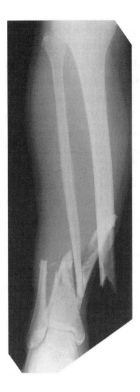

Severe open tibia fracture. Significant bone and soft tissue loss from both the injury and operative debridement may dramatically impair fracture healing.

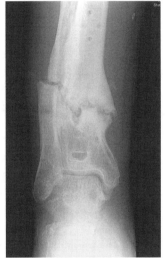

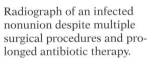

Radiograph of an infected nonunion despite multiple surgical procedures and prolonged antibiotic therapy.

"So primary amputation is probably best when the posterior tibial nerve is transected or when warm ischemia time is more than 6 hours. Other relative indications for early amputation include polytrauma to the same limb and the triad of severe skin loss, bone loss, and muscle damage."

"OK, enough about amputation. That word gives me the creeps," Donut interrupted. "Imagine if I was downstream when. . . ."

As he floated away, Donut began feeling better about himself; he had so many good friends, and they really depended on him for oxygen. Cruising through the anterior tibial vein, he noted that the vessel was smaller than usual and the walls were collapsing on him.

He felt sluggish as he pulled up to Spindle, a fibroblast, to talk about this weird sensation.

"Hi, Donut. Looks like you're under some pressure. Easily explained. We're in the anterior compartment of the leg, rather rigidly bound by the tibia, the fibula, the intervening interosseous membrane, and a tight fascial sheath under the skin. With any hemorrhage or edema, the pressure in here goes up because the compartment can't expand. As you already know, this pressure compromises blood flow and can produce ischemia with eventual occlusion of the blood vessels. Because early detection is critical and treatment is simple, one must always be concerned about compartmental pressure. This must be monitored closely, not only after any injury to the leg, but also with injuries in the forearm, hand, and foot where the fascial restraints over the muscle are equally unyielding."

Donut winced. "The thought of being crushed and suffocated is frightening."

Spindle nodded. "The first sign of compartment syndrome is muscle pain from ischemia. The compartment becomes tense, and passive movement of joints distal to the compartment causes excruciating pain. Hypoxia causes nerves to become irritable at first—paresthesia, pain, and the sort. Then comes numbness and weakness, but that's a bit later in the game. All the while, though, the distal pulses may remain strong; but if the compartment pressure is unrelieved, the muscle dies. Then if it isn't scraped out, all that dead muscle contracts, permanently rendering the limb rigid and dysfunctional."

Donut shivered at the thought. "Can't something be done to relieve this pressure before the damage is irreversible?"

"Once the diagnosis is made during physical examination, sometimes aided by intracompartmental pressure measurements, the treatment is relatively easy. One must split open the fascia enclosing the compartment to let the tissues expand and thereby reduce the tissue pressure so capillary perfusion can resume. Skin grafting may be necessary later to cover the exposed muscle. Now get out of here before all your floating friends panic in this pressure pot. I'll be OK because I don't need much oxygen."

Donut floated back to the spleen. He had learned a great deal about fractures and himself that day. Prompt and thorough treatment can frequently preclude the complications that often accompany tibial shaft fractures; and red cells play an indispensable part in bringing extra nourishment that the injured tissues need to heal and defend themselves against invaders. With his sense of self-importance rediscovered, Donut was last seen in his usual sinusoid sipping a warm potassium and telling stories about the day of his great adventure.

ADVANCED READING

DeCoster TA, Gehlert RJ, Mikola EA, et al. Management of post-traumatic segmental bone defects. J Am Acad Orthop Surg 12:28-38, 2004.

Einhorn TA. Clinical applications of recombinant human BMPs: Early experience and future development. J Bone Joint Surg Am 85(Suppl 3):S82-S88, 2003.

French B, Tornetta P. High-energy tibial shaft fractures. Orthop Clin North Am 33:211-230, 2002.

Goulet JA, Templeman D. Delayed union and nonunion of tibial shaft fractures. Instr Course Lect 46:281-291, 1997.

Olson SA, Schemitsch EH. Open fractures of the tibial shaft: An update. Instr Course Lect 52:623-631, 2003.

Rosenberg GA, Patterson BM. Limb salvage versus amputation for severe open fractures of the tibia. Orthopedics 21:343-349, 1998.

Sanders R, Swiotkowski MF, Nunley JA II, et al. The management of fractures with soft-tissue disruptions. Instr Course Lect 43:559-570, 1994.

Sarmiento A, Latta LL. Functional fracture bracing. J Am Acad Orthop Surg 7:66-75, 1999.

Schmidt AH, Finkemeier CG, Tornetta P. Treatment of closed tibial shaft fractures. Instr Course Lect 52:607-622, 2003.

Tornetta P. Compartment syndrome associated with tibial fracture. Instr Course Lect 46:303-308, 1997.

◆ *Flex your right elbow 85 degrees, fully supinate your forearm, and internally rotate your shoulder 45 degrees. Now flex your left elbow 95 degrees, fully pronate your forearm, and internally rotate your left shoulder 45 degrees. Extend and adduct your digits on both hands, and keep your wrists in neutral. Through 5-degree arcs, rapidly and repeatedly extend your left elbow and flex your right elbow. You deserve congratulations.*

Index